VISION

Its Development in Infant & Child

Arnold Gesell, M.D.
Frances L. Ilg, M.D.
Glenna E. Bullis

Assisted by Vivienne Ilg, O.D.
and G.N. Getman, O.D.
with
Foreword by
John W. Streff, O.D.

Optometric Extension Program Foundation

Reprinted and Published by arrangement with Lippincott-Raven Publishers
Originally published in 1949
Reprinted in 1967, 1970

Optometric Extension Program Foundation, Inc.
1921 East Carnegie Ave., 3-L
Santa Ana, CA 92705-5510

Printed in the United States of America

Library of Congress Cataloging in Publication
Gesell, Arnold, 1880-1961.
Vision : its development in infant & child / Arnold Gesell, Frances L. Ilg, Glenna E. Bullis.
p. cm.
Originally published: Darien, Conn. : Harper and Row, 1949.
Includes bibliographical references and index.
ISBN 0-943599-92-X
1. Vision. 2. Child development. 3. Infants—Development. I. Ilg, Frances Lillian, 1902- . II. Bullis, Glenna E. III. Title.
BF723.V5G4 1998
155.4'1214—dc21 98-15403
CIP

Optometry is the health care profession specifically licensed by state law to prescribe lenses, optical devices and procedures to improve human vision. Optometry has advanced vision therapy as a unique treatment modality for the development and remediation of the visual process. Effective vision therapy requires extensive understanding of:

- the effects of lenses (including prisms, filters and occluders)
- the variety of responses to the changes produced by lenses
- the various physiological aspects of the visual process
- the pervasive nature of the visual process in human behavior

As a consequence, effective vision therapy requires the supervision, direction and active involvement of the optometrist.

CONTENTS

PART TWO— DEVELOPMENTAL OPTICS

PART THREE—DEVELOPMENTAL APPRAISAL

APPENDICES

List of Illustrations

PHOTOGRAPHIC SOURCES

Figures 1, 2, 6, 7, 8, 10, 39, 41, 46 are reproduced from Gesell et al., An Atlas of Infant Behavior, New Haven, Yale University Press, 1934.

Figures 23-35 (Chapter V) are derived from Gesell, Arnold (in collaboration with C. S. Amatruda), Embryology of Behavior, New York: Harper & Brothers, 1945.

Figure 40 is reproduced from the Encyclopaedia Britannica Film, Life Begins.

FOREWORD

When approaching the request to write a forward for the reprinting of what I consider my most prized book, I spied an inscription on the fly cover of my original copy. In 1956, Dr. Ilg penned: "To John Streff—our spaceman. One last copy just for you! See that you read it and prepare yourself for its future revision."

I have agreed to write this forward and to abstract some of the basic concepts stated by Gesell. Because I have been writing a review of the Gesell Years, I have recently re-read this book several times. I am amazed that the concepts and central ideas continue to be contemporary and pertinent. While *Vision Its Development in Infant and Child* is not a clinical text, it contains critical information for vision care practioners. It is a tome with many momentous concepts and pearls of wisdom, a book that should be read over and over again.

My copy is copiously highlighted, from the last paragraph on the first page of the preface to the last chapter, The Conservation of Child Vision. As I again became engrossed with this book, I often took pause. How could such insight have been elucidated in 1949 and be so ignored in 1998? What has prevented the understanding of the implications related to vision development, especially in our daily clinical lives and clinical services?

Gesell's comment to me, when I last met with him in 1956, succinctly summarizes his efforts in vision development. He observed, *"The goal of evolution and development is not to make a more perfect end organ (the eye), but rather to develop a system to serve the needs of the organism."* This statement should be kept in mind when one reads this valuable book.

Often members of the vision care professions continue to be caught up in an effort to make *more perfect eyes*. The major concern is health, ocular health, and optical neutralization. While these are laudable goals, they are limited in scope and fall short of Gesell's stated mission....to assist in developing vision to better serve a patient's needs. This can only be accomplished by providing care programs to facilitate visual functions, guide development, and enhance vision performance.

Gesell recognized a fresh view of vision. He saw a developing system which had a basic species pattern, overlaid with individualized heredity patterns. He also was acutely aware of a system which grew, developed, and interacted in response to the organism's environment. What allowed Gesell to look at and see vision so differently? He approached development from a point of view that it was a lawful constitutional process. There was logic and order to development, and he viewed the evolutionary process as significant. Gesell was usually considered to side with heredity in the heredity-environment controversy. But in vision development, he is faulted for being too environmental. The position I came to know from him was that there was a strong evolutionary-heredity base which developed and grew through interaction with the environment in an effort to meet one's needs.

Throughout his research and writing, Gesell's model was neuro-motor. It would probably be more accurate to label it as a motor-neural model because his observations were motor responses; his explanations were neurological. When Gesell's model is understood, one can easily recognize how he was instrumental in discovering an increased role of visual-motor function. He saw that visual-motor aspects were far more significant than they had previously been credited. He noted in *Infant Development* that muscle function precedes neural; motor nerves are functional before sensory. The role of vision-motor function as afferent continues to lack appreciation.

Gesell's emphasis of visual-motor was often misinterpreted within the optometric profession. Many clinicians understood the meaning to be general body motor with visual controls. While Gesell did not ignore this aspect of motor function, his meaning was more specific. From my interactions with Gesell, he was focusing upon the motor functions of eyes and the visual system. He recognized that the visual-motor functions formed the foundation for discernment and perception of visual sensory information.

Because of his recognition of the importance of vision motor processes, he was able to look at vision from a different prospective. He noted, "...vision is an act which is mediated by eye and brain, but which emanates from a growing action system. Specific acts of vision always occur within the total unitary pattern of the organism. Mentally, they have a motor basis."

Gesell noted that a child was born with a pair of eyes, but not with a visual world. Ocular movement and control were mechanisms to help define an experienced environment. Likewise one can propose that the meaning of accommodative movements are to serve as the mechanism for reaching out and grasping the experienced world. But accommodative movements are also the mechanism of give and take, to bring in as well as to project out. They allow our eyes to "finger" the object of regard. Together, the ocular motor control functions serve to plot and map the experienced environment as well as interact, associate, and grasp to develop a level of trust. The level of trust is a level of confidence in the ability to predict a coincidence in one's vision, action and experienced environment. And thus the visual system serves the needs of the organism.

Further Gesell notes, "We have called vision an act, but this should not blind us to the fact that vision is also a process". As a process, we might think of vision as a complex process, a growing "corpus". He noted in this sense we could gain different views in terms of speed in the visual domain, developmental patterning of visual behavior, visual acts, zones of regard, visual manipulation of space, and the localization of projection. Gesell held that the visual process was the leader from birth in taking hold of the world; the eyes take hold of the world long before the hands.

Gesell's pronouncement is clear and distinct. When we accept the responsibility and take charge of providing care for the visual needs of children, we should look beyond eyes and ocular measures. At the same time, the eye is the mediator, so ocular measures are important and critical. Programs of care should not be based upon any one finding; they should be based upon an understanding of a changing, dynamic, visual activating system. Vision is an active creative dynamic process. Prescribing lenses is not limited, or even directed, to neutralizing eyes . Our goal should be to stimulate change, not to stymie function and development.

The optometric department of the Gesell Institute of Child Development, under the able and steady guidance of Richard Apell, was instrumental in developing clinical regimens to meet the goal of serving the needs of the organism. This required an increased level of observation, an ability to view optometric findings as dynamics. Emphasis was placed upon measuring and understanding flexibility, especially in visual-motor areas. Use of lenses, prisms, and vision therapy was expanded to increase quality of life. This lead to the recognition of the value of small lens amounts, differences between +0.75 spheres and a Plano/+0.75 bifocal as well as prisms oriented in the same direction (yoked prisms) all because of how these lenses changed visual motor demands. Lenses and regimens of care were not constrained by optical neutralization and maximum acuity, but evaluated in terms of positive changes in the quality of a patient's life.

John W. Streff, O.D.
Lancaster, Ohio
February, 1998

PREFACE

The background, scope, and genesis of the present volume are outlined in an introductory chapter which follows. There is not much more which needs to be said by way of preface.

The investigations of the Yale Clinic of Child Development since its founding in 1911 have been mainly concerned with the growth aspects of early human behavior. All told, the behavior characteristics of 34 age levels have been charted, encompassing the first 10 years of life. An intensive longitudinal study of a group of five infants in 1927 established methods for a systematic normative survey. These methods included developmental examinations and inventories at lunar month intervals during the first year of life. Concurrent cinema records were analyzed to define significant behavior patterns and growth trends. Special attention was given to the ontogenetic patterning of posture, locomotion, prehension and manipulation.

Cinemanalysis, both of normative and experimental data, demonstrated that the eyes play an important role in the ontogenesis of the total action system of the total child. The nature and the dynamics of the role constitute the subject matter of the present study.

The adult human eye has been likened to a camera. This analogy has had some truth and much tradition in its favor. But it has tended to obscure the developmental factors which determine the structure and the organization of the visual functions during infancy and childhood. The development of vision in the individual child is an extremely complex and protracted process for the very good reason that it took countless ages of evolution to bring human vision to its present preeminence.

Our culture is becoming increasingly eye minded with the advancing perfection and implementation of the organ of sight. What is that organ? It is more than a dioptric lens and a retinal film. It embraces enormous areas of the cerebrum; it is deeply involved in the autonomic nervous system; it is identified reflexively and directively with the skeletal musculature from head and hand to foot. Vision is so pervasively bound up with the past and present performances of the organism that it must be interpreted in terms of a total, unitary, integrated action system. The nature of the integration, in turn, can be understood only through an appreciation of the orderly stages and relativities of development whereby the integration itself is progressively attained.

The authors have attempted to achieve a closer acquaintance with the interrelations of the visual system per se and the total action system of the child. This finally entailed the use of the retinoscope and of analytic optometry at early age levels where these technical procedures ordinarily are not applied. The examinations of the visual functions and of visual skills were really conducted as behavior tests, not only to determine the refractive status of the eyes, but also to determine the reactions of the child as an organism to specific and total test situations. The objective findings have been correlated with the cumulative evidence furnished by the developmental examinations, numerous interviews, and naturalistic observations of the children at home and in a guidance nursery. Although the conclusions of our study are preliminary in character we may hope that they will contribute to a better understanding of the child in terms of vision and a better understanding of vision in terms of the child. The two should not be sundered.

With increased knowledge it is possible that the visual behavior of the individual child will become an acute index for the appraisal of fundamental constitutional traits. Periodic examination of these traits in dynamic activity would throw diagnostic light on their developmental significance. The ocular fundus, being an integral component of the brain, offers a unique avenue for observation of subtle behavior events. In this broadest sense, visual symptoms, both normal and atypical, are closely allied to problems of personality and of mental hygiene. The observable and potentially recordable reactions of the retina may thus yield a more intimate glimpse into the basic individuality of the growing organism. These possibilities cannot be realized without long-range projections of developmental research.

Our own preliminary research has had generous support from the American Optical Company through its Bureau of Visual Science. We are deeply indebted to the officers of this company and to the Director of the Bureau, Dr. Paul Boeder, and to his former associate, Dr. Marion Stoll. At an earlier stage of our study (1942-43) we received small but significant grants from the Graduate Clinic Foundation, the Optometric Extension Program, and from the Fluid Research Fund of the School of Medicine, Yale University. In this connection we are especially indebted to Dr. A. M. Skeffington and to former Dean Francis G. Blake.

During the prosecution of the present study over a period of 10 years, we have had the benefit of innumerable instances of cooperation, both professional and lay. We have drawn freely upon various specialists in the fields of optometry, ophthalmology, orthoptics, and psychology. We are particularly indebted to Dr. George Crow, Dr. Frederick Brock, and Professor Samuel Renshaw. Mrs. Louise B. Ames, as Curator of the Yale Films of Child Development, rendered generous assistance in the preparation of the illustrations of this volume. Her own studies in the field of child development have proved of great value in our investigation. Miss Elisabeth Wetsel has given unstinted service in the details of preparing the manuscript and index for publication.

We have been in long-continuing indebtedness to the staff of the Yale Guidance Nursery, including Miss Janet Learned, Miss Anne Lockwood, and Mrs. Ludmila Glasscock. In a similar way we are indebted to Headmaster Henry Welles, to Supervisor Paulina Olsen, and to the teaching staff of the New Canaan Country School, who facilitated in every way our periodic contacts with the children under developmental investigation from year to year. Finally, and comprehensively, we should like to express our debt to the truth-seeking spirit and intelligence of the parents who cooperated so consistently throughout the long program of investigation. Equally impressive and essential was the spontaneous cooperation of the children at every age level—in infancy, the preschool period, and the school years. They responded to every reasonable demand. We owe them a return in improved understanding and more enlightened guidance.

ACKNOWLEDGMENT

American Optical Company, through its Bureau of Visual Science, has given generous support of the research program of the Yale Clinic of Child Development. This support has made possible the special investigations in the field of Developmental Optics published for the first time in the present volume.

The eye is the first circle; the horizon which it forms is the second; and throughout nature this primary figure is repeated without end.

—Ralph Waldo Emerson

CHAPTER 1
The Eyes of Today and Tomorrow

Among all living creatures, man is the most eye-minded. Nothing does he treasure more than the apple of his eye. Myth, language, folklore, proverbs, art, and poetry abound in allusions to the magic, the mystery, the power, the evil, and the charm of the eye. To Thoreau the human eye is "a noble feature." ... "It is the focus in which all rays are collected. It sees from within, or from the center, just as we scan the whole concave of the heavens at a glance, but can compass only one side of the pebble at our feet ... The eye revolves upon an independent pivot which we can no more control than our own will. Its axle is the axle of the soul, as the axis of the earth is coincident with the axis of the heavens."

Less poetic, but still superlative, is Aristotle's realistic comment: "All men by nature desire to know. An indication of this is the delight we take in our senses; for even apart from their usefulness they are loved for themselves; and above all others the sense of sight. For not only with a view of action, but when we are not going to do anything, we prefer seeing to everything else. The reason is that this, most of all senses, makes us know and brings to light many differences between things."

All the vast science and technology accumulated since Aristotle's day have strengthened the truth of his words. The science of biology has demonstrated that the human eye is virtually a vestibule to the brain, and that stereoscopic vision with its cortical elaborations is the crown jewel of organic evolution.

The preeminence of vision in the sensory-motor construction of the human action system is reflected in the input and output arrangements of retina and brain. The retina, with its multibillion sensitive points and polarities, is receptive to an enormous range of impressions. Retina and brain are sensitive enough to detect the light of a candle 14 miles distant. Speaking as a neurophysiologist, McCulloch points out that the eye alone has more than 100,000,000 photoreceptors, each of which is either signaling or not signaling at a given moment. This means that the eye can exist in $2^{100,000,000}$ states, each of which corresponds to a unique distribution of stimulation ... Each eye transmits as much information to the brain as does all the rest of the body. It can send in a million impulses per millisecond. For the whole organism, including eyes, the input has a maximum of three million signals per millisecond.

Modern technology reflects a significant emphasis on the function of vision. It has clothed the naked eye with light-gathering devices which penetrate deeper and deeper into microscopic and into sidereal space. The visual hunger of cultural man is insatiable. He can never see enough. Inaudible sound he translates into visible waves. Hearing alone does not sate him. If the pulsation of brain potentials is

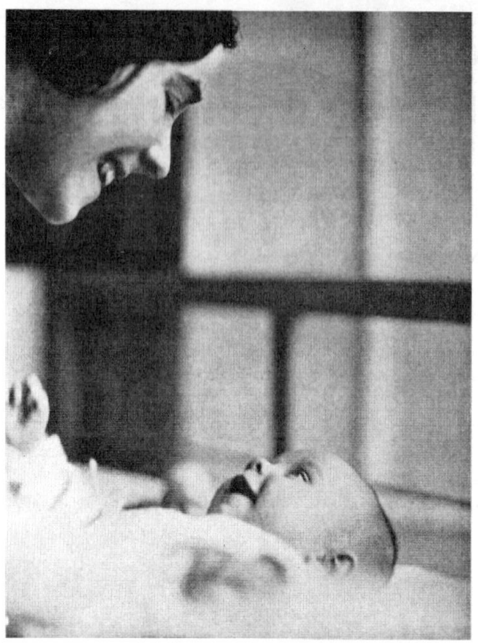

Figure 1. Eyes fixate eyes. The infant is 12 weeks of age.

communicated to him through sound magnification, that does not suffice. He must *see* the waves graphically recorded on a smoked drum for his closer scrutiny and for the sweeping glances impossible by ear. It is not enough to infer a gene; he must behold it through the agency of ultramicrophotography. The cathode ray oscillograph is used to expand time and to show visually on the end of a luminescent tube what happens in as small an instant as .000000001 of a second. Photographic records have recently been made of subatomic particles which survive for only a millionth of a second and which are only 50 to 60 times larger than a single electron.

Photography affords supercyclopean vision. It is a third eye. The camera collects the images; and the chemical emulsion of the film serves both as a receiving and as a recording retina. But even the most sensitive photographic plate has limitations. So the insatiable astronomer contrives lead-sulfide photoconductive cells which will lift the veil of interstellar clouds and enable him to see the invisible. He builds at Palomar a 200-inch camera which reaches to stars and universes a billion light-years away. With the aid of photography and this gigantic eye, he has moved his farpoint vision to a distance of 60 x 60 x 24 x 365 x 1,000,000,000 x 186,000 miles, for light travels at a speed of 186,000 miles per second. The human eye is attuned to this velocity which, according to the doctrine of relativity, is the top limiting velocity in the universe.

The function of vision, as Aristotle hinted, is to reveal. Technologic vision does not replace organic vision; it enhances and enriches it. The most remarkable technologic extension now developing in "the womb of time" is television—an instantaneous electronic method of transmitting visual images over the long reaches of earthly space. This miracle, at one paradoxical stroke, both penetrates and abolishes space. It brings the visual and the auditory world into simultaneous focus. It should in time bind distant peoples into closer psychologic unity and understanding.

Already we are promised transoceanic interviews, which will bring participants separated thousands of miles onto the speaking screen of a family living room.

Leaders of nations from opposite sides of the earth will appear face to face through two-way television.

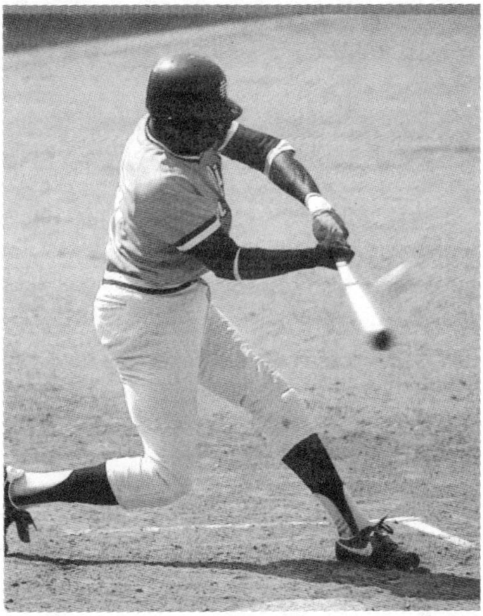

When millions, as individuals in their households, witness the same spectacle, they will not be so subject to mob psychology. On the basis of what they see, they may frame calmer judgments. One prophet reports that a push-button device for registering opinion is in an experimental stage of development. Millions of such video votes could be instantaneously totaled and classified by an electronic computer! Vision as language thus assumes a role in socialization, and in molding the social psychology of the individual.

Figure 2. Organized sport places a high premium on visual skills. In baseball, all eyes fixate, with postures poised for sudden unpredictable shifts. The ball speeds across the plate in 3/10 of a second. The batter has 1/50 of a second in which to connect. "It's all in your eyes and timing," says a champion batter.

Television will enormously diversify the channels of vision because telecasting is not under the restrictions of the beholder's own oculomotor fixations. Using multiple, mobile cameras, television can transmit a spectacle viewed from multiple, shifting angles. The optimal scenes are continuously selected in the control room. Through montage manipulation, modulated intensifications and coincident projection, reinforced by sound effects, the television screen will mirror what an Argus-eyed son of Zeus might witness.

Not only the eyes of scientists and technicians, but the eyes of common men, women, and children have been tremendously augmented through modern invention. And the end is not yet. Our civilization is becoming increasingly eye-minded. The tasks for the growing eyes of children are multiplying and intensifying. Radio, with its exclusive appeal to the ear, has somewhat lightened the environmental pressures, but radio is now uniting with video, and voice and vision merge. We are entering an electronic Look-See-Pic-Screen age, and education will place a relentless premium upon alert, accurate, and swift vision.

The culture sets its visual premiums in many different ways—in science, in the arts, in recreation and sports, in craftsmanship and industry. The challenges, rewards, and competitions are innumerable. For example, the American glorification of baseball has various psychological sources, but not the least is the extraordinary visual tension it creates in the players, the umpire, and the keenly watching crowd, which through television may embrace a nation.

The visual demands of school, factory and urban life are often excessive and distorting. Fortunately, vision is the most adaptable of all physiologic functions, and the chemical events of eye and brain are the least fatigable for they have amazing powers of rapid restitution. But statistics show that the eyes are not altogether ready to meet the strains of present cultural conditions. Visual maladaptations, not to say defects, are mounting alarmingly in the years from 5 to 10. The increase of myopia among children and adults has serious portent. The frequency and varieties of strabismus in the early years of life indicate numerous unsolved problems—optometric, ophthalmologic, and surgical. A deeper insight into the complicated development of the visual functions of infants and school children is essential to further scientific control.

The development of vision in the individual child is complex because it took countless ages of evolution in the race to bring vision to its present advanced state. Human visual perception ranks with speech in complexity and passes through comparable developmental phases. Moreover, seeing is not a separate, isolable function; it is profoundly integrated with the total action system of the child—his posture, his manual skills and coordination, his intelligence and even his personality make-up. Indeed, vision is so intimately identified with the whole child that we cannot understand its economy and its hygiene without investigating the whole child.

Vision, therefore, may become a key to a fuller understanding of the nature and the needs of the individual child. He sees with his whole being. Eye care involves child care. The conservation of vision, particularly in the young child, goes far beyond the detection and correction of refractive error. Acuity is only one aspect of the economy of vision. How does a child use his eyes in personal and in practical situations? How does he shift from far to near tasks and vice versa? Are central and peripheral vision in balance? Do his eyes team coordinately? If not, is his strabismus resolving? Does he show visual competence in his handling of toys, tools, eating utensils, crayon, pencil, primer? If he has any difficulties, are they due to his temporary immaturity or to a more permanent intrinsic visual deviation, or to faulty cultural arrangements? How does his visual behavior comport with his general behavior? Do we need a broader kind of visual hygiene to protect the growing eyes of today and the eyes of tomorrow?

To answer such questions we need a more ordered knowledge of the child as a growing organism. His visual history begins in the darkness of the uterus. His patterns of visual behavior transform in lawful sequence through the stages of infancy, of preschool childhood, and the school years.

CHAPTER 2
Orientation: The Background and Scope Of this Study

"The hearing ear and the seeing eye, the Lord hath made even both of them."

In the present volume we attempt to examine some of the natural laws and wonders which are inherent in the formation of man's supreme sense: vision.

Visual science has made brilliant contributions to our knowledge of the eye as an optical organ. There is a vast amount of basic information on the efficiency, the mechanism, and the neurophysiology of seeing derived from studies of the mature, adult eye. There is, however, a relative paucity of information on the genesis and growth of visual functions. Somewhat paradoxically, we know rather more about the evolution of vision in the race than we do about its development in the child. Perhaps this is because the eye and the connecting brain have had such a venerable history and the salient stages of their structural transformations are, therefore, writ large in the anatomies of living species, from fish to man.

In the gestation and growth of the individual child, this venerable history is condensed and revised within the narrow limits of years as contrasted with eons. The development of visual functions in infancy and childhood is so subtle, swift, and esoteric that it does not declare itself in conspicuous stages. Moreover, one tends to think of the eyes and the vision of the child as operating in the same manner as they operate in the adult.

This, of course, is a gratuitous assumption. Unfortunately, the human infant cannot tell us exactly how gratuitous. He cannot report to us the subjective essence of his visual experience; nor can microscopic sections of his retina and cortex tell us precisely how and what he sees. But evidence is not altogether wanting. By careful attention, the curious-minded observer can detect the outward signs of vision and can cautiously deduce some of its underlying processes. The baby uses his eyes to perform overt acts of vision; presently he uses his hands to perform yet more complicated acts in which the eyes lead or follow. Later he points with a gesturing hand. Still later he names what he points to, thus bringing hand, eyes and speech into union. Even during his preschool years he responds cooperatively to tests of visual experience adapted to his interests and capacity. At the age of 4 he begins to report visual introspections by word of mouth, and thus he becomes an articulate participant in a formalized examination. As he grows older, the reciprocity between child and examiner increases and it is possible to analyze the visual functions in considerable detail. But to interpret the nature and the import of these functions, it is always necessary to observe the *total child.* For the Lord hath made the seeing eye part and parcel of an indivisible, integrated, growing action system.

The intimate interdependence of the visual and action systems is nowhere more significantly displayed than in the sequences and trends of child development. Some 30 years ago, the Yale Clinic began a series of studies of the forms and the growth of the behavior patterns of the human infant. Our approach was inclusive rather than topical, for we were systematically interested in the total child and the total aspect of advancing stages of maturity. In due course, we charted the behavior characteristics of normal subjects at 34 progressive age levels from birth to 10 years. The original charting took into account four major fields of behavior as follows:

1. *Motor Behavior*: posture and locomotion; prehension and manipulation; gross and fine motor coordination
2. *Adaptive Behavior:* self-initiated, induced and imitative behavior; learning; resourcefulness and exploitiveness in new situations
3. *Language Behavior:* vocalizations; vocal signs; gestures; comprehension of words; speech and reading
4. *Personal-social Behavior:* reactions to persons; responses to overtures and commissions; adjustments to life situations in home and school.

Various methods of approach were used to secure systematic data in the foregoing behavior fields: periodic examinations of behavior, naturalistic observation, parent interviews, and analysis of cinema records. For a detailed description of these methods the reader must be referred to previous publications (a list of titles appears on page 11) which report the basic developmental surveys as follows:

a. A normative survey of infant behavior at lunar month intervals from 4 through 56 weeks
b. A naturalistic survey of a small group of infants at lunar month intervals
c. A period study of the feeding behavior of infants
d. A normative survey of the preschool period at tri-monthly and semi-annual intervals from 15 months to 5 years
e. A sequential study of the maturity traits of school children at annual and semi-annual intervals from 5 to 10 years of age.
f. A developmental study of a group of fetal infants, with post- conception ages of 28 to 40 weeks
g. Clinical studies of maldevelopment throughout infancy and childhood

The developmental investigations listed above built up a cumulative background for the special researches reported in the present volume. Indeed, a special study of visual behavior evolved as a natural culmination of the preceding studies of child development. Among the thousands of behavior items which are identified by the developmental protocols (and the cinema records), those which pertain to vision are numerous and outstandingly important. The biologic and cultural role of vision becomes apparent when the patterns of eye behavior are viewed in the context of associated behavior, and in the perspective of ontogenetic sequence. No one of the major fields of behavior—motor, adaptive, language, and personal-social—is normally devoid of visual content or visual controls. So interfused are vision and action systems that the two must be regarded as inseparable. To understand vision, we must know the child; to understand the child, we must know the nature of his vision.

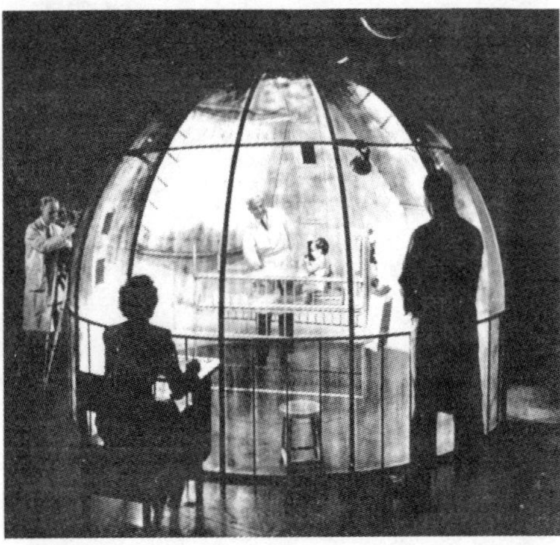

Figure 3. Photographic dome used to secure systematic cinema records of infant behavior patterns at lunar month intervals. (Courtesy of LIFE Magazine.)The delineative action photographs of An Atlas of Infant Behavior were selected from the cinema records. Two silent cameras ride on the quadrants of the dome. The infant is examined in the crib. The dome is encased in a one-way vision screen, which conceals the observers from the infant, but permits full view of his behavior.

The child and his eyes reveal themselves conjointly in outward patterns of behavior. Behavior is a convenient term for all the reactions of the organism which are mediated by the neuromotor system. All behavior tends to assume characteristic forms. A behavior pattern is simply a definable formed response to a specific situation. Our normative surveys were designed to elicit for inventory those patterns of behavior which would serve as useful criteria in the interpretation of the developmental status and potentialities of the growing child.

Scores of behavior tests were devised and repeated at successive age intervals under comparable controlled conditions. For example, at lunar month intervals from 4 to 28 weeks we examined the reactions of the supine infant to a ring dangled in the field of near vision. The physical arrangements and procedures were simple, but were carried out with careful regard for standardized technique. The infant lay on the platform of a clinical crib. The examiner slowly moved the ring (a four-inch red wooden ring) headward and into the line of the infant's vision. The ring was then moved through an arc of 180°, from left to right and right to left (see Figure 8).

We also wished to observe the reactions of older infants (age 28 to 56 weeks). These infants were seated at a test table and the same ring-and-string was placed upon the table top within easy reach and view. From 26 to 48 infants were examined at each lunar month interval. The stenographic reports of their responses were later analyzed and tabulated. The accompanying table (Table A) lists the percentage distribution of 49 behavior items and patterns in the Dangling-Ring Situation. Table B lists the percentage distribution for 37 behavior items and patterns in the Ring-and-String Situation.

TABLE A
DANGLING RING BEHAVIOR (4-28 weeks)
SITUATION: DANGLING RING (RD)

RD	Behavior Items	4	6	8	12	16	20	24	28
1	Regards after delay	77	54	64	65	27	13	14	5
2	Regards immediately	26	46	36	35	68	97	96	95
3	Regards momentarily	53	85	71	38	35	..	..	..
4	Regards prolongedly	47	43	29	62	87	47	38	5
5	Regards consistently	..	..	..	..	17	26	59	90
6	Disregards in midplane	77	39	46	46	14	..	..	..
7	Regards in midplane	29	61	54	54	86	..	..	..
8	Regards in midplane (long head)	22	25	12	50	83	..	..	..
9	Regards in midplane(round head)	32	75	70	56	88	..	..	..
10	Regards ring in hand	..	..	..	..	66	82	100	100
11	Regards string	..	..	..	..	7	13	46	53
12	Shifts regard	94	100	100	96	93	46	38	41
13	Shifts regard to surroundings	75	68	61	35	13	16	14	5
14	Shifts regard to examiner's hand	28	64	61	77	48	..	..	..
15	Shifts regard to examiner	41	54	57	65	64	27	24	27
16	Shifts regard to hand	0	4	7	8	19	5	3	..
17	Follows past midplane	44	62	50	58	84	..	..	..
18	Follows past midplane (lg.h.)	20	33	25	37	83	..	..	..
19	Follows past midplane (rd.h.)	55	75	60	67	77	..	..	..
20	Follows approximately 180°	16	43	46	50	68	..	..	..
21	Follows approximately 180° (lg. h.)	0	11	25	25	83	..	..	..
22	Follows approximately 180° (rd. h.)	36	55	55	61	62	..	..	..
23	Approaches	0	0	11	12	62	89	96	100
24	Approaches after delay	..	..	..	..	58	30	19	9
25	Approaches promptly	..	..	..	..	32	66	81	91
26	Arms increase activity	0	4	11	42	64	..	..	..
27	Arms separate	0	0	4	15	17	19	7	..
28	Approaches with one hand	0	0	4	12	20	24	39	55
29	Approaches with both hands	0	0	0	0	50	76	82	77
30	Approaches with arms flexed	0	0	0	12	44	60	54	14
31	Hands come together	0	0	0	8	20	38	11	5
32	Contacts ring	3	4.	4	15	43	81	100	100
33	Dislodges ring on contact	3	4	4	8	20	35	28	5
34	Grasps	0	0	0	8	22	73	96	100
35	Grasps after delay if grasps	..	..	..	..	..	75	46	14
36	Grasps interdigitally	..	..	..	..	..	61	45	7
37	Retains entire period	..	..	..	..	20	19	40	65
38	Holds with both hands	..	..	..	..	10	33	56	67
39	Hand opens and closes on ring	..	..	..	..	30	1	10	14
40	Brings ring to mouth	..	..	..	..	38	58	82	74
41	Free hand to midplane	..	..	..	..	25	51	56	84

42 Transfers	..	..	..	..	3	18	41	74
43 Drops	..	..	..	..	78	56	41	32
44 Drops immediately	..	..	..	..	42	32	7	0
45 Regards dropped ring if drops	..	..	..	..	10	37	43	100
46 (If drops) pursues dropped ring	..	..	..	..	7	16	29	100
47 (If drops) resecures dropped ring	..	..	..	..	7	5	29	60
48 Rolls to side	3	4	8	4	35	42	38	18
49 Frets	9	14	4	8	27	23	32	21

ATLAS DELINEATIONS

RD
1 Regards after delay: 8-12 weeks
2 Regards immediately: 16 weeks
3 Regards momentarily: 4 weeks
4 Regards prolongedly: 12 weeks
6 Disregards in midplane: 4 weeks
7 Regards in midplane: 8 weeks
10 Regards ring in hand: 16 weeks
11 Regards string: 28 weeks
14 Shifts regard to examiner's hand: 8 weeks
17 Follows past midplane: 8-12 weeks
20 Follows apporoximately 180°: 12 weeks
23 Approaches: 16 weeks
27 Arms separate: 20 weeks
28 Approaches with one hand: 24-28 weeks
29 Approaches with both hands: 16 weeks
30 Approaches with arms flexed: 20 weeks
31 Hands come together: 16-20 weeks
34 Grasps: 20 weeks
35 If grasps, grasps after delay: 20 weeks
38 Holds with both hands: 28 weeks
40 Brings ring to mouth: 24-28 weeks
41 Free hand to midplane: 20 weeks
43 Drops: 20 weeks

It will be noted that fully one-half of the items in the *Dangling-Ring Situation* refer explicitly to eye behavior. Similarly, 10 items in the Ring-and-String Situation refer specifically to visual regard. The participation of vision in other items is readily inferred: for example, items 28, 29,and 36 suggest that, owing to new postural propensities, the infant is beginning to pivot while in the seated position. By pivoting, he expands the area in which he deploys his eyes and his hands, bringing the objects of visual interest to the platform and the side panel. All this suggests that the action system and the eyes are very closely interrelated. The changing space structure of the child's visual domain is primarily determined by growth factors, which shape the basic postural orientations of the organism.

TABLE B
RING AND STRING BEHAVIOR (28-56 weeks)
SITUATION: RING AND STRING (R-S)

R-S	Behavior Items	28	32	36	40	44	48	52	56
1	Regards ring	100	94	85	97	94	94	100	95
2	Regards ring first	89	68	65	69	77	81	79	84
3	Regards string	71	90	88	83	74	61	76	74
4	Regards string first (regard before appr.)	11	32	35	28	23	19	17	21
5	Shifts re. from ring to str. or ring-str.-ring	54	58	53	64	55	52	55	58
6	Approaches ring	54	28	26	8	6	6	5	8
7	Approaches ring first	50	28	26	5	6	..	5	8
8	Approaches string	50	81	92	97	94	97	100	100
9	Approaches string first	43	69	83	95	94	97	100	92
10	Contacts string before ring	46	75	92	95	97	95	100	100
11	Grasps string	18	53	83	92	91	92	100	92
12	Hand closes on string ineffectively	21	41	32	27	24	..	8	8
13	(If hand closes on string)grasps ineffect	55	71	53	46	36	25	11	8
14	Grasps string immediately	0	16	32	65	67	89	90	83
15	Pulls or drags string in	29	53	83	95	94	95	97	96
16	Regards str. only as reaches and pulls str.	4	16	23	5	15	8	3	17
17	Regards ring as approaches and pulls string	18	34	60	87	82	78	74	50
18	Regards ring only as appr. and pulls string	4	3	34	46	52	44	42	25
19	Regards ring only as ring approaches	7	25	80	81	85	75	69	42
20	Manipulates string before securing ring	0	22	6	5	15	8	0	0
21	Pulls ring off table top before secural	0	9	9	11	15	25	5	8
22	Dangles or bounces ring before secural	0	9	6	8	3	25	16	17
23	Secures ring using string	29	47	86	95	97	92	97	92
24	Hits or bangs ring on table top	17	27	14	16	35	9	24	17
25	Brings ring to mouth	46	58	39	30	32	24	13	20
26	Transfers ring	46	42	43	43	16	18	16	17
27	Turns ring	17	23	18	35	23	6	11	0
28	Brings ring to platform	13	15	7	38	42	33	26	50
29	Brings ring to side panel	0	4	0	5	10	24	21	13
30	Manipulates string after contact with ring	33	58	79	73	84	73	66	71
31	Holds ring in one hand; string in other	0	12	36	19	29	12	29	29
32	Dangles ring by string	0	8	29	49	48	58	58	58
33	Dangles ring by string after con.with ring	0	0	25	43	45	36	50	58
34	Drops ring completely	33	31	36	33	39	55	45	50
35	Resecures ring	25	15	21	27	29	39	21	17
36	Turns or pivots	0	0	0	15	37	34	47	33
37	Postural activity	0	0	12	19	40	47	53	58

R-S 7 Approaches ring first: 36 weeks,
9 Approaches string first: 28 weeks,
22 Dangles or bounces ring before secural: 48 weeks
23 Secures ring using string: 36 weeks
24 Hits or bangs ring on table top: 44 weeks
28 Brings ring to platform: 44 weeks
30 Manipulates string after contact with ring: 32 weeks
33 Dangles ring by string after contact with ring: 52 weeks
36 Turns or pivots: 48 weeks

In addition to the systematic normative survey, special studies were undertaken which served to show the influence of growth factors on specific patterns of visual behavior. These studies include the following investigations, some of which will be referred to in more detail in subsequent chapters.

- Eye movements and optic nystagmus in early infancy (McGinnis)
- A genetic study of sustained visual fixation and associated behavior in the human infant from birth to 6 months (Bing Chung Ling)
- The development of handedness; directionality in drawing. The infant's reaction to his mirror image (Gesell and Ames)
- Early individual differences in visual and motor behavior patterns (Ames)
- Handedness and eyedness of children referred to a guidance clinic; predictive signs of potential reading disability (Castner)
- The tonic neck reflex (Gesell)
- The influence of congenital blindness on mental growth (Gesell)

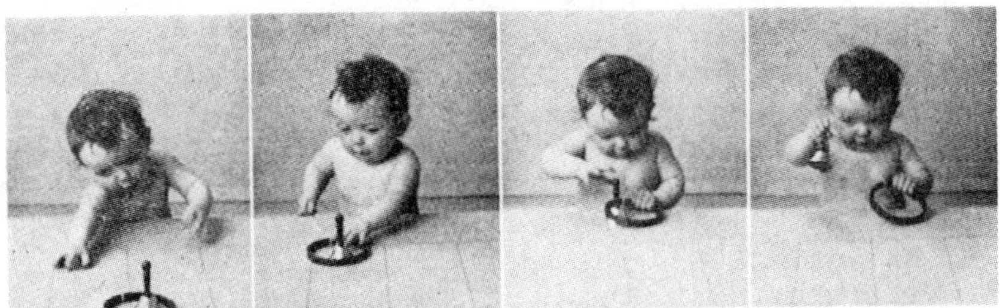

Figure 4. Action photographs of behavior patterns. The action photographs delineate the behavior patterns of a 44-week-old infant in the ring, string, and bell situation, in four consecutive phases, at 0.0, 2, 5, and 10 seconds.

- Correlations of behavior and neuropathology in a case of cerebral palsy from birth injury (Gesell and Zimmerman)
- Twinning and ocular pathology (Gesell and E. M. Blake)
- The mental growth of a blind infant: a four-year study of a case of congenital anophthalmia (Gesell)

From this sketchy outline of the earlier work of the Yale Clinic, it is apparent that the present study of child vision is a natural outgrowth of a systematic program of

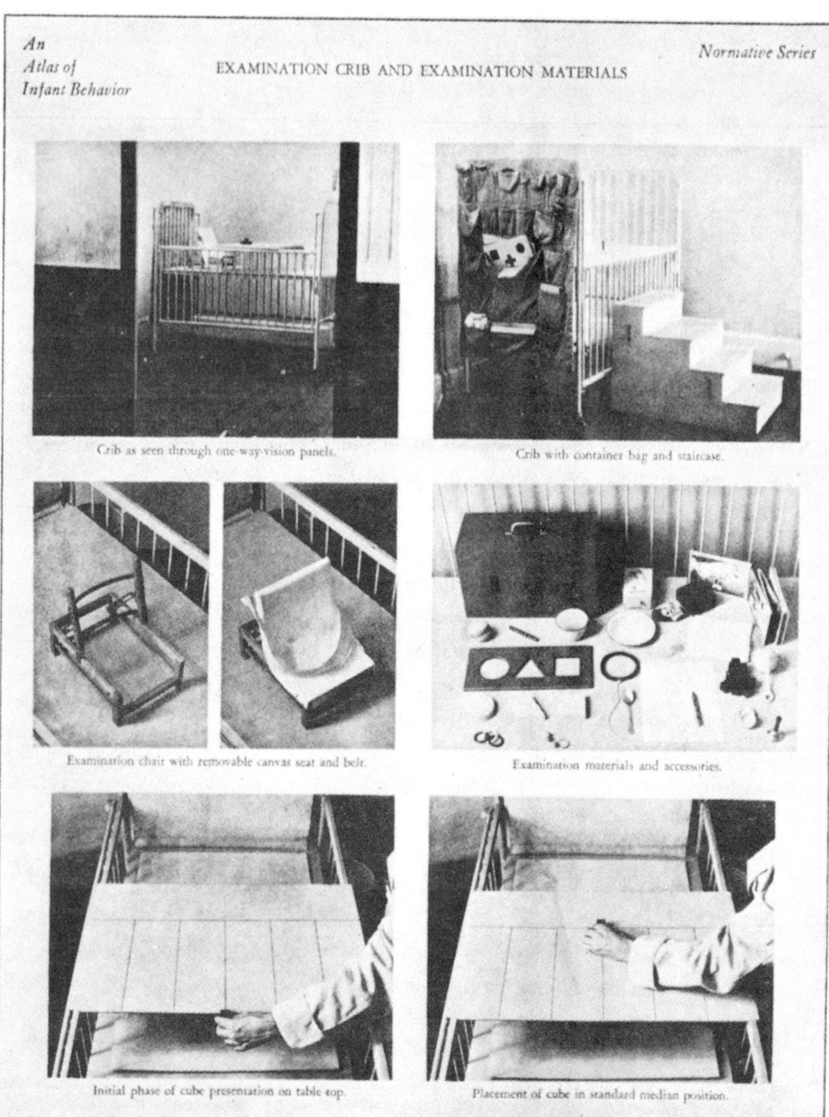

Figure 5.

developmental research. This program eventually included infants, preschool children and children of school age. It has been primarily concerned with the ontogenetic sequences of normal behavior, but defects and deviations of development were likewise investigated by similar methods—normative, naturalistic, experimental and clinical. Our approach, moreover combined both cross-sectional and longitudinal (biogenetic) data. Individual differences were analyzed in terms of maturity

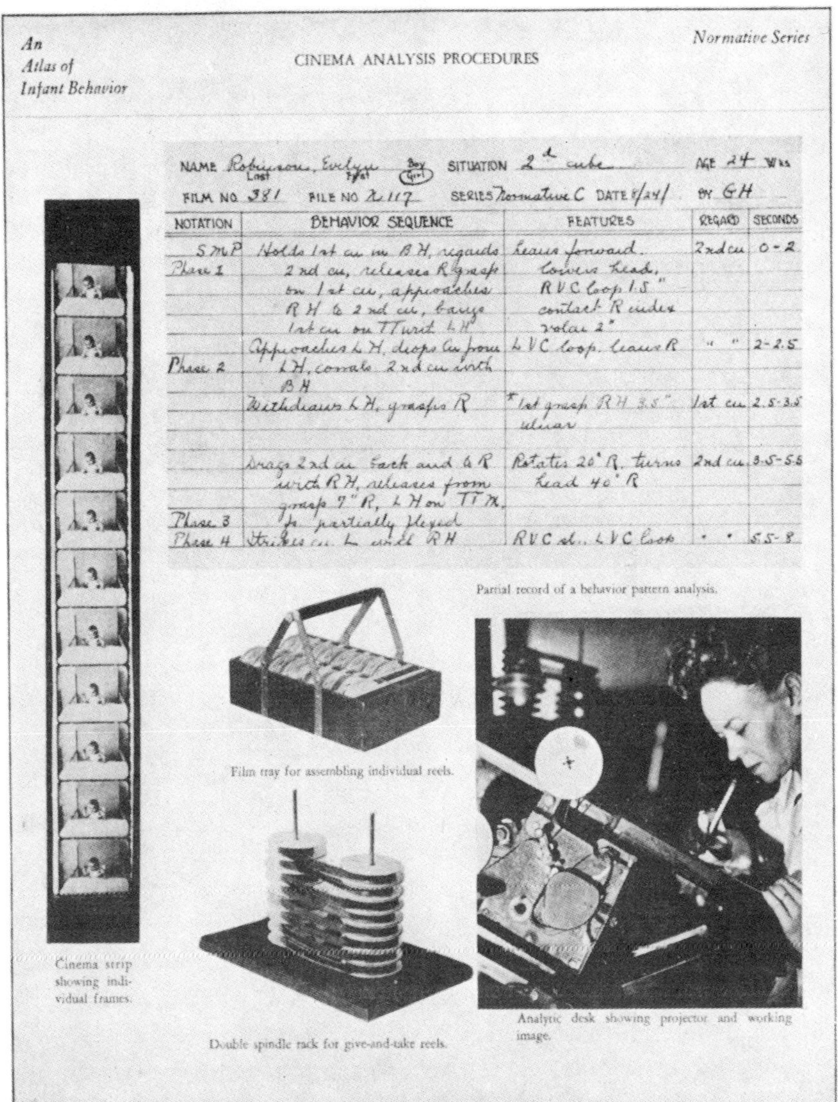

Figure 6.

traits, and for each of the older subjects we had development data for the period of infancy or the preschool period, or both periods.

The survey of the age period from 5 to 10 years brought into clearer focus the developmental aspects of visual behavior. Fifty or more children were examined at 5, 5 1/2, 6, 7, 8 and 9 years of age, and a smaller number at 10 years. Three-fourths

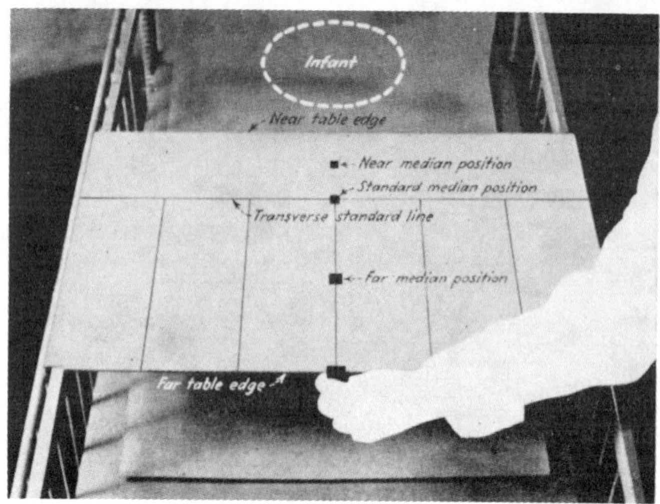

Figure 7. Photodiagram showing the standard location points of the examination table. The table top surmounts the two adjustable side panels of a crib. The infant confronts the near table edge. Test objects which elicit visual and manual responses are presented from the far table edge and are placed on the following location points in accordance with standardized procedure: near median position, standard median position, far median position: respectively, 9 cm., 17 cm., and 41 cm. from the near table edge.

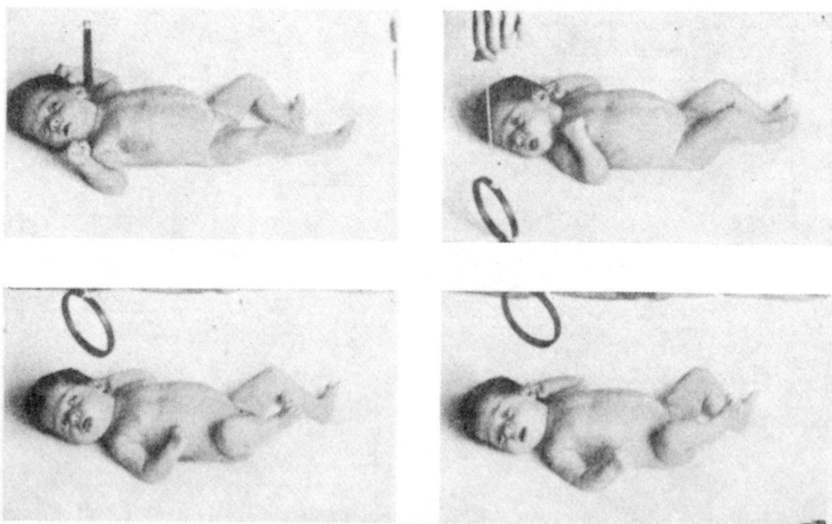

Figure 8. A 6-week-old infant reacts to the dangling-ring situation in an interval of 12.5 seconds, as follows: (a) The ring is dangled in the midplane. The infant stares vaguely into far distance (0.2.5 seconds). (b) His eyes fixate as the ring comes into the line of vision (6.75 seconds). (c) Turning his head slightly to the left, he pursues the ring with his eyes to within 15 degrees of midposition (11.25 seconds). (d) His eyes release, the head turns fully right, and he resumes the asymmetric tonic-neck reflex (TNR) attitude (12.5 seconds). Individual photographs in this and following figures are arranged from left to right in a, b, c, d order.

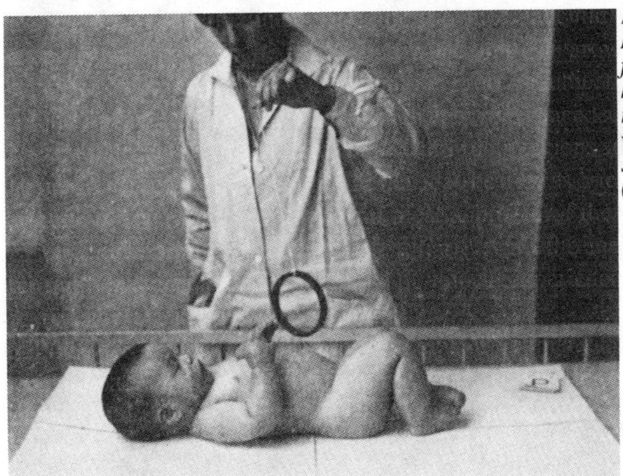

Figure 9. The Dangling-Ring Test for a supine infant (age 20 weeks). The head favors a midposition and hands move toward the midplane by a symmetrotonic reflex (STR).

of these children had attended the Guidance Nursery of the Yale Clinic and some had been examined as infants. Most of them are now attending a public elementary school. We are continuing our contacts with them. They are generally of high average intelligence and come from homes of comfortable socio-economic status. In 1942 we made a fortunate association with a private country school at New Canaan, Connecticut. A special group of 14 children from this school were examined at semi-annual intervals from 6 through 11 years. Throughout all these studies we have profited from the generous and well-informed cooperation of parents and teachers. Our knowledge of the children is based on personal clinical familiarity with their individual careers.

For the reader's orientation it should be stated that the survey of visual functions began with a study of visual skills at consecutive annual age levels from 5 to 10 years. This initial study suggested developmental trends, but did not give sufficiently precise information for developmental interpretation. Accordingly, analytic tests were made with spheres and prisms, and with a full refractive examination beginning with the age of 8 years, followed by extensions downward and upward from this age level. During this period of exploration, we made fixation and projection and other tests at preschool age levels in the hope of establishing some developmental continuity with the older age levels. This hope was not realized until the retinoscope came to the rescue. Retinoscopy of the 3-year-old child dramatically revealed a complex visual process which yielded to further analysis at the age levels below and beyond 3 years. These findings furnished the basis for a developmental interpretation which established a continuity from the period of infancy through the first 10 years of life, and which imparted a new developmental meaning to the analytic and skills tests with which the survey began. Further investigation will utilize the retinoscope in order to elucidate more dynamic correlates in especially devised behavior-test situations.

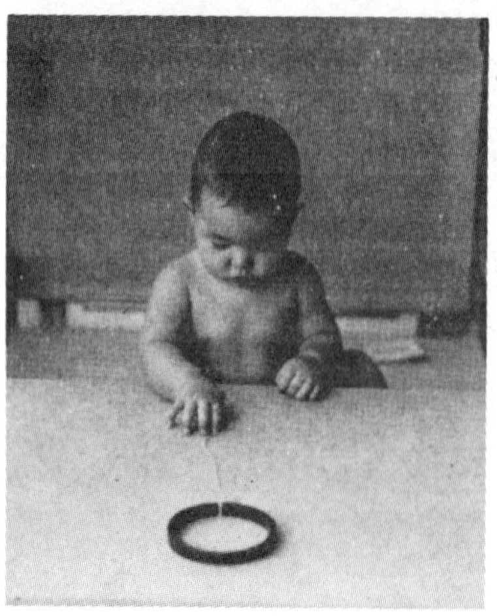
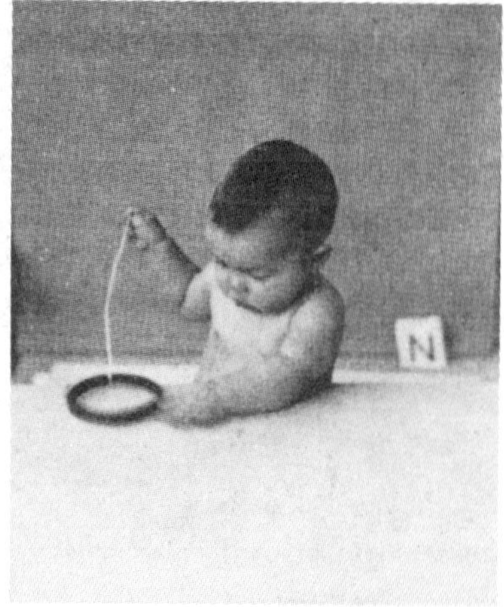

Figure 10. Ring-and-String situation for the free-sitting infant (age 36 weeks).

The typical case record for a given child included developmental and visual data as follows:

a. Consecutive examinations at advancing ages based on the Yale Developmental Schedules
b. Reading-readiness tests, including the Monroe battery
c. Performance tests, including the Arthur series
d. Visual skills tests—pursuit fixation, fusion, acuity, stereoscopic perception, etc.
e. Naturalistic observations of the child's school behavior, postural reactions and tensional behavior
f. Wide-ranging interview with a parent, detailing behavior at home and school.

In due course, over a period of four years, we secured the expert assistance of two research optometrists who made objective determinations of visual functions at both preschool and school ages. Retinoscope, phoropter, and other analytical procedures were brought into requisition. These procedures had to be especially adapted to the maturity of the children. Extremely favorable environmental conditions, combined with skilled management by the nursery staff, made it possible to secure reliable findings at the younger age levels, where such detailed observations have not previously been made. In the developmental examination of a preschool child the observer is concealed by a one-way vision screen.

The findings were reviewed and discussed in seminar sessions, and were brought into correlation with the previous developmental and visual examinations. It was not always possible to make a tenable distinction between individuality traits and developmental factors. Developmental interpretations were not made unless the total weight of the evidence of several examinations at different age levels denoted the presence of a growth process. When more knowledge is available, we shall have better criteria for making a differential appraisal of developmental versus individual-constitutional factors. The problems are complicated, but they will yield to the refinements of a developmental approach.

The present volume is based upon the concept of developmental morphology. In the study of human vision, and doubly so in the study of child vision, one cannot escape problems of pattern and form. Morphology is the science of form. It is equally applicable to physical and to functional phenomena. It applies to behavior as well as to skulls and bones. Behavior grows and as it grows it assumes characteristic forms.

These forms are structured; they can be investigated from the standpoint of a dynamic morphology. As a process, vision is so complex and inclusive that it needs all possible elucidation from the chemical, physical and physiological sciences. But vision also comes within the scope of embryological science—not only by way of somatic morphogenesis in utero, but also postnatally as a growing complex of reaction patterns.

If we set aside metaphysical distinctions between psyche and soma, we may think of this visual complex as a growing "corpus" which has patterned structure and calls for morphological description. It is in this sense that one may speak of the "visual domain," of "the density of space," of "the developmental patterning of visual behavior," of "visual acts," of the organization and reorganization of "zones of regard"; the "visual manipulation of space," "the direction of developmental drift," "the localization of projection," etc. Vision always remains a process, but the process is a manifestation of an action system which has structured form, and which is subject at all ages to maturational (embryologic) mechanisms of form regulation.

This outlook upon visual phenomena is reflected in the content and arrangement of the chapters which follow. The concept of the total action system is set forth in Chapter 3 in terms of phyletic history. The motor basis of vision (Chapter 4) has its origin in the phylogenetic processes which molded the racial action system. The ontogenesis of vision in the individual child is complex because it took countless ages of evolution in the race to bring vision to its present advanced state.

The progressions and the complexities of the ontogenesis of the action system are outlined in Chapters 5-8 of Part One. A score of growth stages from the embryonic period to the age of 10 years are considered in sequence. Here, with the aid of photographs, we should like to convey an impression of the child as an organism and as a person, living and having his being in a culture. We describe how he uses his eyes, his hands, and his postural abilities to come into contact and communication with both his physical and his personal-social environment. In these chapters, we do not discuss vision as a specific function. We portray the total child of whom vision is part and parcel, but only a part. This is a growing child. He grows and he reacts as an integer. Growth is, of course, a continuous process subject to many individual variations, but a separate delineation of each age level is needed to bring into view the growth trends of the total action system. These delineations are typical but they should not be regarded as rigid standards. They may be used as orientational norms and as a frame of reference. An accurate clinical appraisal of the maturity status of any given child presumes a technical familiarity with the methods of developmental diagnosis and an ample background of clinical experience.

The Chapters of Part Two deal more specifically with the developmental morphology of visual behavior patterns. The visual system is considered in terms of several functions which interact as an organic complex. The components of this complex are schematically shown in a chart, Chapter 10. The relationships of the components vary from age to age. Vision does not develop in a symmetric proportionate manner. The complex undergoes many transformations which are summarized in a separate chapter. This chapter (12) outlines the transformations in their ontogenetic sequence, with special reference to far and near fixation, the retinal reflex, projection, etc. Data which elaborate this chapter are tabulated in Appendix B. The ontogenetic patterning of visual behavior is distorted by visual impairments and defects. A special chapter deals with the developmental aspects of amentia, cerebral palsy and blindness. These brief case studies of abnormal and atypical development are presented to accentuate by contrast the role of vision in normal development.

Part Three briefly sets forth the implications of a developmental approach to techniques of appraisal and supervision. We undertake to show that developmental concepts and methods of procedure may be applied in the early examination of visual functions, both normal and deviant. A developmental approach broadens the scope and the goal of visual hygiene. It shifts the emphasis from acuity and refraction to the total visual economy and developmental welfare of the child. Such a shift of emphasis can be made only by taking into account the growth status and the growth trends of the total organism.

In this sense, we may venture to offer this volume as a preface to Developmental Optics. It is hoped that such an introduction will call attention to the conceptual and the practical values of a developmental philosophy in safeguarding the vision of the growing child.

Developmental Optics is concerned with the ontogenesis and the organization of visual functions in their dynamic relation to the total action system.

CHAPTER 3
The Evolution of the Human Action System

SENSATION AND MOVEMENT have been closely linked in evolution. Even in plants, even in a unicellular fungus, photosensitive structures serve the functions of movements. The phototropisms of the sea squirt have some of the basic elements of human vision. One need not speculate as to whether sensation or movement ever came first. They are now indissolubly associated. The eye may have originated as a photosensitive spot somewhere in the protoplasm of a very lowly creature, but even this primitive receptor was related to a motor system in such a way as to influence the creature's movements; and the movements of the creature, in turn, affected the time and mode of the next succeeding photic stimulation. To this day, a primary function of vision is to direct movements.

In this chapter we shall stress the interrelation of sensory and motor functions as they evolve in a total action system. The comparative anatomy of eye and brain supplies many clues to this long and tedious evolution. By reconstructing the types of behavior which were associated with advancing animal forms, we may gain a better appreciation of the mechanisms which determine the supremacy of human vision.

It takes a tortuous journey for the human child to reachieve what it took the race so long to attain. There will be much to say about the reciprocal relationships of eyes and hands in the racial ascent. The child is not like a chick, whose ocular-prehensory powers are almost perfect at the time of hatching. The chick, lacking hands, strikes with its bill, and from the first it strikes and seizes with a high degree of accuracy. Man strikes with his hands. The coordinations of his eyes and hands with the rest of the action system are enormously complicated and required ages of evolution.

This evolution brought about a refinement and a multiplication of both the sensory and the motor components of vision. The retina, phylogenetically, was derived from the brain. The visual cells originated from photosensory ependymal cells and trace back to a primitive tubular, chordate form of nervous system (Walls). The most ancient cells were probably filamentous, with simple dendrites as foot pieces. After many millions of years, they developed extremely rich and diversified connections with other nerve cells, for the retinal cells are essentially specialized neurones. The cones are more ancient than the rods. Chemical elaborations accompanied the refinements of microscopic architecture. The photochemical reactions involved in the translation of the stimulus of light into nervous response are now extremely sensitive. A single quantum of light which can activate one molecule of visual purple is sufficient to excite a single rod cell, and it is estimated that only six rods must be excited to elicit a threshold effect.

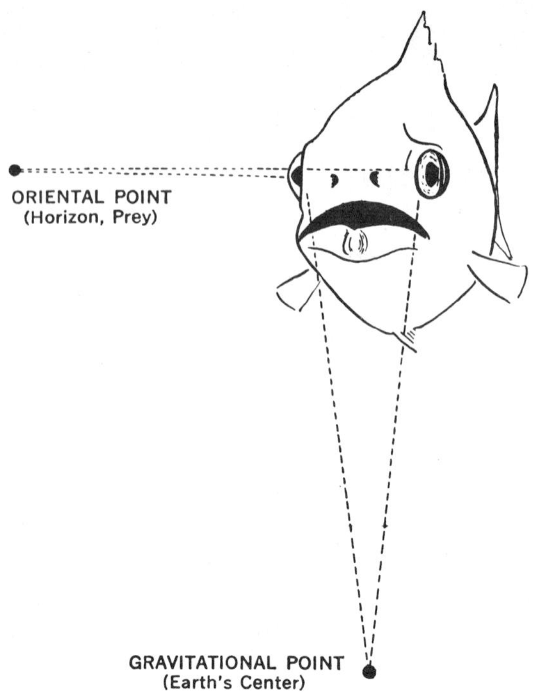

Figure 11. Formation of the conditioned retinal-oriental-fixation reflex, on the basis of the unconditioned labyrinthine-compensatory-fixation reflex. The oriental object effects the fixation of the two eyes, which previously had been effected by gravitational stimuli alone. (Adapted from Worth's Squint.)

The human eye has some 100,000,000 photoreceptors, each of which has two potential states. It may be that the evolution of the sensory apparatus has far outdistanced the motor apparatus, but sensory possibilities are always limited by the reactivity of the action system.

The complexity of muscular tissue, however, must not be underestimated. Muscles are made up of extremely numerous, delicate fibrils, and these, in turn, are composed of countless cables of giant protein molecules, as many as 150,000,000 in the cross-section of a single fibril.

The immense scope of the ocular apparatus is determined by the complexity of its neural connections. The optic nerve consists of about 1,000,000 fibers that connect with the cortex, which is composed of billions of neurones, and each of these neurones is directly or indirectly connected with the subcortex and every other part of the total neuro-motor system. The eyes are intricately interlocked with this enormous communication system. No organ focuses more concentrated energies. The function of human vision is in many respects near the acme of the evolutionary process.

It does not follow that the summit of visual powers has been reached. Evolution may continue indefinitely into a remote future, pressing our present modes of vision into the basal brain and freeing the cortex for higher functions. Such has been the evolutionary trend throughout eons. Nature's goal does not seem so much to be a more perfect eye, but rather a plastic seeing mechanism which will permit a higher type of action system. If the eye should become excessively specialized it might too soon spell doom for the species.

The comparative biology of the eye, brilliantly summarized by Walls, shows that the pattern of the vertebrate eye has been modified in different species to adapt itself to varying conditions of life. This process of "adaptive radiation" is very evident as early as the Devonian age, a few hundred million years ago. The vertebrate eye originated in water, and had to acquire many special adaptations to an aquatic medium; but the ground plan of the human eye was already foreshadowed in the eye of the fish. Indeed, the evolutionist blithely reminds us that man is but a modified fish.

A brief sketch of how these biological modifications have taken place in relation to the behavior characteristics of ascending species should give us some insight into the visual demands made upon the human infant. The race evolved; the child grows. During his period of growth the patterns of his functioning eyes are progressively adapted to the changing tasks of his changing action system. Although the infant does not repeat in precise sequence the stages of racial evolution, he is confronted with comparable problems of harmonizing equipment and environment in an ontogenetic kind of adaptive radiation.

Consider, therefore, a typical fish. It has no neck to speak of and is therefore below the phyletic threshold of the tonic-neck reflex. But the fish eye is equipped with a full set of oculomotor muscles, internal, external and oblique. The function of these muscles is to maintain a constant visual field, which is a prerequisite for detecting movement. The movement denotes food or danger and the eyes are gyroscopically stabilized to be constantly aware and alert. Not having a neck, the fish turns the whole body in order to keep the object of interest within its narrow binocular field. The field is narrow because the fish wears its eyes, as well as its ears, on the side.

In the course of evolution, the eyes have moved forward to a frontal position, and the binocular field of primates is thereby greatly widened. Our ears, however, have remained in a lateral position, which places limitations on the sense of hearing. It is interesting to speculate what would have happened to our action system if Nature had reversed her procedure and had placed the hearing receptors in our eye sockets, compelling us to wear our eyes in the ancient lateral position.

A fish in water scarcely needs a neck, but when a fish aspires to life on land, the lack of a neck is a disadvantage. Nature had a solution even for this problem, as represented by the mud skipper fish, *periophthalmus,* an amazing creature. In this organism the eyes are set in high turrets and they move on universal joints. The eyes are elevated in their conning tower by a cat-cradle arrangement of the inferior rectus and the inferior oblique muscles.

This outlandish fish has a pair of enlarged and somewhat specialized pectoral fins to assist it in its locomotion on the mud flats, but they are extremely crude structures without importance in visual economy. Nevertheless, they were the forerunners of

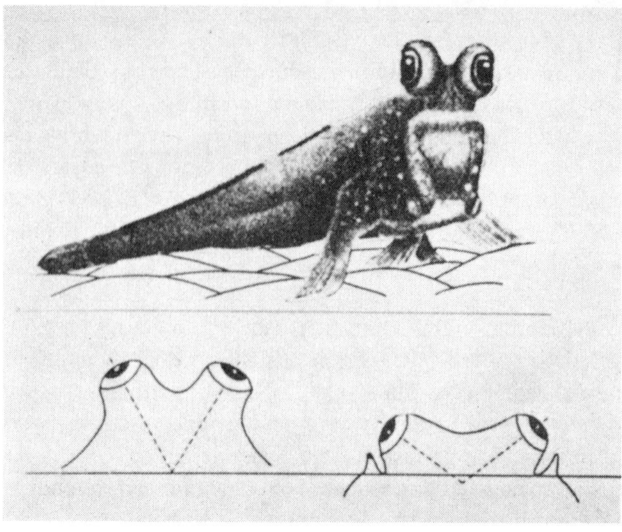

Figure 12. Periophthalmus. The eyes of this amazing creature are set in high turrets and move on universal joints. They are elevated by a cat-cradle arrangement of the inferior rectus and inferior oblique muscles. (About half natural size, after Hess, Hein, and Walls)

the forelimbs which, in arboreal vertebrates, were destined to play a significant role in the evolution of vision. In reptiles, both ancient and modern, the skeleton of the forepaw, with its five digits and wrist, radius and ulna, is amazingly like the human hand in ground plan. In the land turtle, this "hand" is connected with a brain cortex and is thus brought into simple association with vision. For the most part, however, in amphibia, reptiles and ground-going quadrupedal mammals, the "hand" serves mainly to support and to propel. It figures only to a limited degree in the sensory life of the animal.

Snout, tongue, and vibrissae are relatively more important in the daily lives of creatures who roam the solid earth. The snout functions as the organ of prehension: the animal sniffs, noses, grasps, and "handles" with its projecting muzzle. Under these circumstances, touch, smell and hearing are of more primary value than vision. The uses of the visual sense tend to be restricted, even though the animal may have a high degree of acuity for significant slight changes in the environment.

Vision cannot become versatile until the forelimbs are emancipated for prehension and manipulation, allowing the creature at the same time to sit up and take notice with frontally placed eyes. Although the universal joint of the turret eyes of the *periophthalmus* would seem to be an ingenious arrangement, Nature discarded this expedient in favor of a freely moving neck and a diminished snout.

All these revised specifications are embodied in the small furry animal whose intriguing face stares from the next page. This remarkable creature interests us greatly because in him the optical apparatus assumes a new, prophetic relation to the action system. If not a primate, *Tarsius Spectrum* is at least a preprimate, representative of the early Eocene primitive placental mammals, which lived about 50,000,000 years ago and were in some way ancestral to modern man.

Tarsius is scarcely as large as a small kitten but exceeds a kitten in agility, particularly at dusk and nighttime. He hops from bough to bough with supra-sonic speed, using the powerful leverage of his elongated ankle bones and the balance of a long, tufted tail. His hind limbs are much longer than his forelimbs and the latter are equipped with "beautiful little hands." He is free to use them because he habitually progresses and sits in an upright posture. His eyes are enormous, occupying two-thirds of a rather delicate face, in which the snout has been reduced to a slightly rounded hillock. Skull and eyeballs are spherical. Although supplied with a full set of oculomotor muscles, the eyeballs are almost locked into the cuplike orbits. The ears, in contrast, are mobile, unilaterally as well as bilaterally. One ear may be cocked forward, the other being cocked backward to sense danger from the rear.

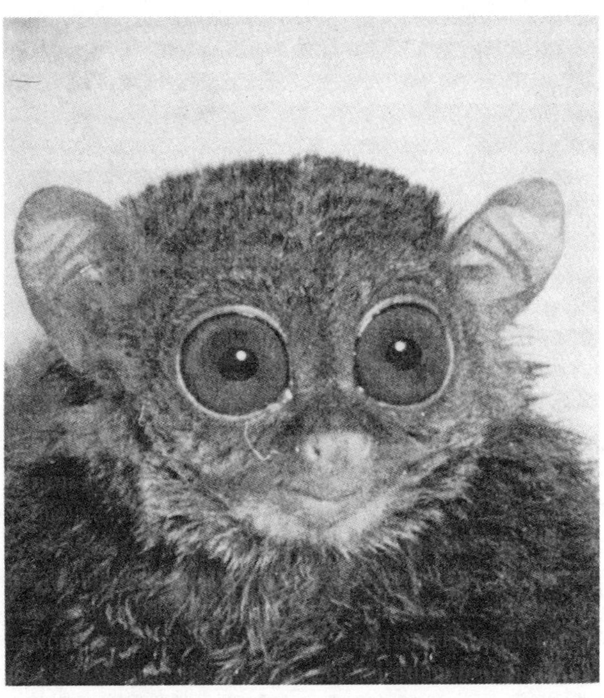

Figure 13. Tarsius Spectrum. The specimen pictured herewith was captured in the Philippines and, thanks to the skill of Dr. John R. Fulton, was safely transported to this country and kept in captivity in the physiologic laboratory at Yale University. It was remarked at the time that this Tarsius was certainly the most ancient mammal to arrive in the United States since Eocene times. I am much indebted to Dr. Fulton for the photographs and observations placed at my disposal.

The relative immotility of the eyes is more than compensated for by the extraordinary motility of the head, which *Tarsius* can swivel like a capstan through an arc of 180 degrees, so that the eyes look directly backward. Nature has not neglected his rear defenses.

His eyes face squarely front from their sentry boxes. They have almost completely migrated from the sideways position characteristic of the fish stage. The optic nerve carries about 400 nerve bundles and the fibers decussate completely. At a more advanced evolutionary stage, the fibers will semidecussate to insure combined transmission of impulses from each eye to one and the same cortical area. Vision, however, is acute if not stereoscopic. *Tarsius,* perched stock-still, spies a cockroach;

the arms, held in outspread poise, suddenly flex. With a pounce, he seizes and decapitates the prey. He may eat the meal at leisure, using his hands in a squirrel-like manner.

It is said that the eyes of *Tarsius* do not converge despite the fact that he is equipped with a full set of oculomotors. Being a two-handed feeder, after the manner of the squirrel, he needs only a limited degree of projection. The higher primates, in contrast, developed high powers of convergence along with unilateral postures and one-handed swinging from branch to branch. Diversified and precise projection was achieved through noncrossing of temporal optic fibers. *Tarsius,* however, fixates with superb intensity as he holds, manipulates, and eats his morsel.

Tarsius merits the space we have given him because his action system prefigures the trends of later evolution, which for many millions of years continues an interweaving course from hand-to-mouth-to-eye-to-hand-to-mouth. The elementary relationships of the human visual complex were established in a primitive primate. The fossil remains in Eocene deposits give mute testimony that a creature closely akin to *Tarsius* lived in that ancient era.

All that has happened since to the anthropoid-humanoid stocks which emerged after the *tarsiers* has tended to enhance and to enrich the visual functions. The brain nucleus for accommodation was remodeled in the primates and was split so that each eye can be focused independently upon any object. The sense of smell, once in the lead, has declined and the eyes have maintained a priority in the constellation of the sense organs. Yet, in the process, the eye has not become overspecialized. It has shown a remarkable adaptability by meeting environmental demands without exaggerated development of any one of its several components at the expense of others. Overspecialization would have led to isolation from other areas of sense and movement. This generalized biologic adaptability suggests that even under cultural stress the human eye will prove equal to new demands, maintaining a supremacy without weakening the unity of the action system. Its evolutionary potentialities have by no means been exhausted.

The human hand likewise remains in a primitive and very generalized condition and may well continue capable of many new refinements in the evolution of the action system. To this day the hand, and also wrist and arm, bear a striking resemblance to the ground plan of the forelimb which made its appearance in the age of reptiles.

Something, however, should be said about the foot of man. Although it is not directly concerned in the mechanisms of vision, the human foot is the most specialized and distinctive feature of his anatomy. In a very real sense, it is the foundation of his distinctive visual skills because his feet have become the "arch platforms" which enable him to maintain an erect posture and to bestride the earth as a master of destiny, eyes forward. This posture and this distinctive mode of locomotion have also favored reorientations and new conquests in the sphere of vision. The forces of evolution had to provide continuously for a harmonious interadjustment between eyes, hands and feet. In this sense, feet do figure in the economy of vision and we shall find that they cannot be left out of an account of the development of visual behavior in infant and child.

It is possible that the evolution of human stereopsis did not require a brachiating ancestor. Recent fossil finds in South Africa indicate that 7,000,000 years ago there lived a prehuman Plesianthropus who walked erect, with frontal eyes under an arching forehead and small brow ridges. Presumably, the forelimbs of this creature, even though they did not flex freely at the elbow, were sufficiently mobile to release hands and eyes for evolutionary advance in the direction of space manipulation.

Early man probably did not begin to contrive and use tools with his hands until he had command of his feet. His brain grew in size and complexity, assuming increasing control of his eyes and hands. Even in the tarsiers, the occipital lobes had expanded to give additional cortical representation to the retina. Vision, henceforth, became the guiding cue for the emancipated hands and they, in turn, directed the eyes into new pathways. With respect to the interaction of eyes, hands, brain and feet, it is idle to differentiate between cause and effect. We do know that, with increase of brain tissue, the human species greatly exceeded all others in ocular and manual skills. And the artifacts produced by these skills were destined to have a profound reflex effect upon the psychology of vision.

The origins of tool making are, of course, wrapped in obscurity because most of the works of man are perishable. Implements of stone, however, have been found which must have been made and used as early as the beginning of the Pleistocene era, a full million years ago. These implements—pointed fist axes, choppers, knives and hide scrapers—were fashioned from flint by strokes of a hammer stone. They were not accidents; they denoted a purposeful coordination of eye and hand. It took millions of years of evolution to bring remote man to this level of workmanship, his inventiveness and insight being restricted not only by the limitations of his brain, but by the absence of an accumulated culture. Throughout the long Pliocene epoch, which began some 7,000,000 years ago, he had to confront life with his bare hands.

What did he do with them? Did he not gradually apprehend that his arm and hand were a kind of crowbar with which he could move and impress objects? He pushed a stone, he grasped it, dropped it, hurled it. Under the stress of excitement, or in a mood of play, he beat one stone against another, noting the sound with his ears, noting the collision with his eyes. Perhaps he fractured a stone without, however, appreciating the implication of his creative act. In a more distant generation the implication was duly noted: the upper stone became a constructive hammer and the nether stone a preconceived implement, designed and even polished for a future purpose. All this represents a complicated chain of thought and action—a chain which was long in the making. But there was ample time at disposal! *Tarsius* lived 50,000,000 years ago and *Homo sapiens* (modern living man and his recent forebears) dates back to say 50,000 years B.C.

During all this vast reach of time, the action system with varying tempo was evolving from lower to higher levels of performance. It is not suggested that this advance was due to mere self-instruction, although experience served to channelize activity, and ultimately led to the organization of a culture, transmitted by material possessions, by language and tradition. In terms of geologic time, this culture has formed with remarkable swiftness. Just now, with the approach of an atomic age, it is in a phase of acceleration never exceeded in human history. But if we are to appreciate the nature and the complexity of the eye-hand-brain complex, which underlies a technologic culture, we must consider the slow, elementary stages through which the action system passed in the prolonged precultural era.

The bare, precultural hand harbored great potentialities. It was a flexible instrument, almost a kit of tools in itself, a system of levers which could be flexed, extended, more or less at will. At first, the finger movements were crude and hardly separated from shoulder and arm movements. The hand curled into a fist and the fingers moved conjointly. The flat nails, successors to claws, were diminutive tools, of a sort, and could be used to dig, to burrow, to scratch. The fist could pound, rub to and fro, and even swirl in circles through shoulder motion, although pestle and mortar were still far in the future.

In time, the wrist became more flexible and the fingers could be moved more independently. The thumb swept in with a sideways pincer movement which plucked small objects. The index finger participated in this thumb opposition and acquired a significant priority, both sensory and motor, among all the digits. It became a forefinger used with dim inquisitiveness to probe and pry.

Thus the hand, by progressive stages, became more sophisticated, not only because it grew more agile, but because the eyes took note of the doings of the hand. In due course, the eye indicated what the hand might do. In this manner, spontaneous hand behaviors developed into voluntary behaviors.

Volition and insight were long in the making. They grew by small increments in close association with the two prime necessities of life—food and shelter. Then, as now, wits were sharpened (though not produced) by the pressure of making a living. Whether the food was vegetable, fruit, insect, or beast, it had to be pursued, secured and macerated for consumption. All this required visual-manual skills, expedients and, in time, tools, to say nothing as yet of feeding utensils. It was serious business, but there were also long spells of idleness.

The leisure time was by no means empty. The hands indulged in playful, experimental activity. The intrusive forefinger traced a groove in the sand. The palm scooped up a handful and scattered the pebbles for the eye to see. A trailing vine was plucked, pulled—behold, the far-off leaves came within the hand's reach—an elementary experience in the mastery of space! The irrepressible forefinger extended again to probe a hole in the tender leaf—an elementary step toward apprehension of a third dimension. For the moment, the index finger was used as though it were a tool, an awl to bore with. In a yet more dramatic moment, the primitive hand seized a stick and probed the stick into the tender leaf and into the plastic stand—one more step toward cultural tool behavior.

In some such manner, through lawful evolutionary gradations, which could not be short-circuited, the race acquired its capacities for practical and also for esthetic workmanship. Eyes and hands became not only more expert in contriving useful things, but more eager to create beauty for enjoyment. It is as though the eyes demanded approval of what they helped to make; they desired to be delighted. The genesis and the nature of the visual functions in man cannot be fully understood without a recognition of this important esthetic component. The eye seeks beauty wherever it can be found.

And so the rough stones were in time made smooth. The stone implements of the Neolithic period have both geometric and functional beauty. Even in the Old Stone Age, some 15,000 years ago, graphic and plastic art reached a marvelous development in the dark recesses of cave life. These cave dwellers must have had a veritable visual hunger, for they decorated ceilings, as well as walls, with paintings and sculptures, working by the flare of torches and stone lamps.

These Cro-Magnon artists worked with sure strokes. Using a stylus upon limestone, they etched the silhouettes of mammoth, reindeer, and bear. Upon a great mass of clay they modeled the bulky figures of a male and a female bison. The sculpture, preserved to this day by the moisture of the cave, is still soft to the touch and the clay bears the imprints of the ancient modeling hand.* Polychrome murals on walls and ceilings were made with crayons whittled from ochre, and with paints kept in skulls and big bone tubes. Yellow, brown, red and black pigments were used with vivid effect. But most remarkable was the lifelike accuracy of the silhouettes of animals, delineated both at rest and in motion.

**Roy Chapman Andrews has given a lively account of the art of the Aurignacian caves in his readable volume, Meet Your Ancestors, Viking Press, New York, 1945: p. 259.*

There were no models in the caves from which to draw. This circumstance suggests an interesting possibility in the evolution of human vision. Did Cro-Magnon man have a primitive kind of eidetic imagery which could dispense with models? An eidetic image is not a mere memory image, nor yet an afterimage such as one experiences after looking at a strong light. It is a reinstated image which is reperceived with hallucinatory clearness. It tends to reproduce the original stimulus with photographic fidelity. We may ask whether in the flush of early creative expression the primitive artist did not entertain such imagery. If so, this enabled him to bring realistic, as well as mystic, portrayals into the darkness of the caverns. In the abstractionism of contemporary art the pendulum is swinging to an opposite extreme, as though present day man were searching for the conceptual essence, rather than the perceived contours, of visual experience. The reduction of eidetic recall may indeed represent a forward evolutionary step.

At the close of the last glacial age, some 150 centuries ago, did *Homo sapiens* have the same visual-behavior equipment that he boasts today? Probably not. The question is unanswerable, for the mind leaves not even a fossil to support a speculation. But in view of the tremendous acceleration of cultural progress, it is likely that there have been associated organic changes in both the receptor and the cortical mechanisms of seeing: In contrast with caveman, the vision of the city dweller is probably more agile, more ubiquitous, less naive, less fatiguable. Even in prehistoric times, however, alert vision was an aid to success and survival.

CHAPTER 4
The Motor Basis of Vision

THE RACE EVOLVES. The child grows. The capacities and, to no small extent, the directions of growth are the end products of ages of evolution. This profound fact requires us to think of vision as an act which is mediated by eye and brain, but which emanates from a growing action system. Specific acts of vision always occur within the total unitary pattern of the organism. Mentally, they have a motor basis.

From the standpoint of developmental optics, we may think of the unitary action system as a labile postural mechanism. By posture we mean the position assumed by the body as a whole, or by its members, in order to execute a movement or to maintain an attitude. No sharp line can be drawn between attitude and action. Action presupposes a postural set and any moment of an action may be regarded as a postural attitude. Postural attitude issues into postural action. Fixation of posture is sustained inhibition of a potential or completed action. Posture may thus be either static or dynamic. Static posture produces station, steadiness and stance. Dynamic posture translates attitude into adaptive reactions such as locomotion, prehension and inspection. Both static and dynamic postures entail tonal discharge and expenditure of energy.

The first and foremost function of this postural apparatus is to adjust to the ceaseless pull of gravity, and to changes of position registered by otoliths and semicircular canals. With the development of distance receptors, the motor system must adjust to a complex of interacting sensory stimuli. A sharp line cannot be drawn between receptor and effector mechanisms, but the motor component is basic. The development of vision is influenced at every turn by current and antecedent motor factors. Whether the eyes are immobilized for visual fixation, or whether they move in pursuit or in exploratory regard, the postural set of the organism is of primary importance. The sensitiveness of the retina and the complexity of the cortical associations, of course, play a prominent role in the refinements of visual perception, but even these refinements are derived from correlated refinements of postural set. It will therefore not be misleading to interpret the development of visual functions in relation to a basic motor system.

The muscular system of adult man and, for that matter, of fetal man, consists of some 400 paired or bilaterally symmetrical muscles. Only 47 pairs are visceral; all the rest, including the oculo-rotators, are skeletal and their function is the organization of postural tensions, attitudes and movements. (Another classification lists a total of over 600 distinguishable muscles.)

Embryologically, these muscles are for the most part formed from a series of mesoblastic segments or myotomes. A series of muscle plates extends throughout the entire trunk and neck and even into the head. From these are derived the axial muscles of the trunk and the appendicular muscles of arms and legs. It is well to note that the six oculomotor muscles of each eye also are derived from axial somites. Despite their very small size, these ocular muscles ultimately play an important role in postural orientation. They are phyletically extremely ancient muscles and are found in the lowest vertebrates, like the lamprey and the hagfish. In the embryology of the human infant they undergo early organization and ultimately they have an elaborate representation in the cerebrum.

Phylogenetically the deep muscles of the trunk may be regarded as among the oldest. They are arranged in long columns over considerable stretches of the back. The superficial broad, flat muscles which overlie the deeper masses are attached to the skeletons of the fore and hind limbs. This close union between axial and appendicular musculature is reflected in the patterning of postural behavior. The early movements of the limbs are part and parcel of dorsal, pectoral and pelvic girdle movements.

Since the axial and girdle muscles are phyletically so ancient, it is natural that they should be the first to become active in the ontogenesis of behavior. The earliest recorded movement (reported by Hooker) was elicited by stroking a fine hair across the right cheek of a surgical fetus with a crown-rump length of 25 mm (fetal age, circa 8 weeks). The long muscles of neck and trunk on the left side contracted, causing a contralateral body flexion. The shoulder muscles also contracted, causing arms and hands to move backward in a manner faintly suggestive of a swimming movement. This primitive behavior pattern represents a very first stage in the process of neuromotor organization which proceeds with great speed throughout the next 20 weeks of gestation. By the post-conception age of 28 weeks, the whole motor system is already so advanced that under favorable conditions a fetal-infant prematurely born at this time has a good chance of survival.

The foundations of visual behavior also are laid during this period of gestation. The neuromotor organization proceeds from the spinal axis to the distal segments, ultimately reaching forearm, hands, fingertips and likewise the toes. In the longitudinal direction, the course of organization proceeds in general from head to foot. The network of neurone fibers and muscle fibers, however, is so intricate that it cannot be built up piece by piece, but must be woven and interwoven like a complex fabric. Flexor and extensor muscles must be brought into counterbalance. Unilateral and cross-lateral and bilateral muscle groups must be harmonized. Forthcoming patterns of behavior are anticipated by threads of connection which block out and establish a basic design. This involves a complicated process of cross-stitching and interlacing, a process of reciprocal interweaving which knits together distant as well as adjacent muscle groups. Thus, the remote eyes are eventually brought into the sphere of the axial system. The shuttle of the morphogenetic loom flies well into the future after it picks up the past.

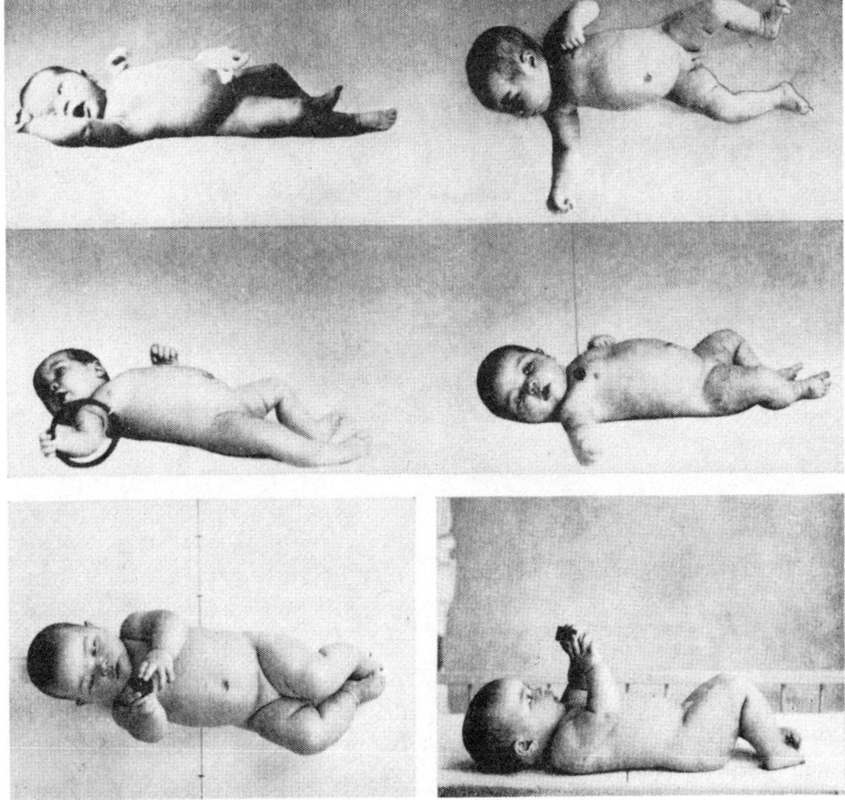

Figure 14. A developmental sequence in the patterning of eye-hand behavior in Infant B, at ages 1, 6, 8, 12 and 20 weeks. The infant spontaneously assumes a right TNR posture and keeps the head predominantly averted to the right. At 20-24 weeks of age, the TNR pattern gives way to an STR pattern (symmetrotonic reflex). The head now prefers the midplane, and hands and eyes converge upon an object of interest in the midplane, as shown in the two simultaneous pictures of the 20-week-old infant.

Histologically, it is impossible to see the multiform designs within the prodigious fabric of the neuromotor system. The designs are nevertheless evidenced in orderly modes of behavior which are usually called reflexes, but which also function in voluntary acts.

Three major kinds of postural reflexes may be distinguished:

a. *Attitudinal reflexes,* which orient the organism in space
b. *Righting reflexes,* which return the organism to a normal orientation
c. *Statokinetic reflexes,* which keep the organism moving in the right direction.

Attitudinal reflexes are of special interest to us because they determine orientations, and it is the peculiar function of vision to assist the organism in its adjustments to the plane and solid geometry of space. The most rudimentary attitudinal reflexes, however, are not dependent upon visual stimuli. They are mediated by propriocep-

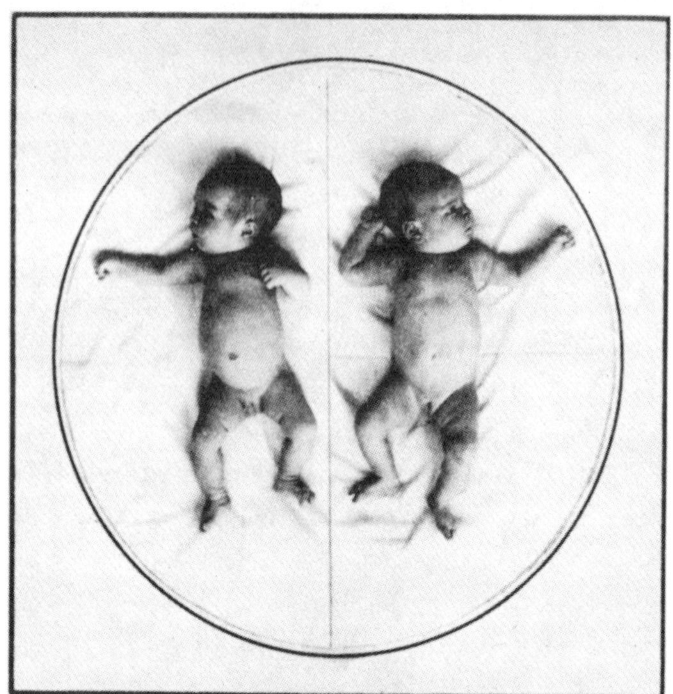

Figure 15. A contrast in laterality trends. The tonic-neck reflex pattern in two full-term infants, age 6 weeks. One infant was addicted to right TNR, the other infant to left TNR. Eyes tend to fixate in the direction of the extended arm.

tive impulses and by the more archaic labyrinthine mechanisms. The head and neck very early exert a controlling influence upon the postural attitudes assumed by limbs and trunk in the growing organism.

As early as the 12th week after conception, the eyeballs of the fetus begin to move, but these movements apparently have no effect upon the postural behavior. The habitus of the fetus at this age is symmetrical. The head maintains a midline position, and when the cheek is slightly stimulated, the head extends slightly, the arms and hands move bilaterally backward, and the hands approximate toward the midline. This symmetric behavior pattern foretokens a symmetrotonic reflex (STR).

At the postconception age of 20 weeks, torsion of the head of the fetus brings about an asymmetric attitudinal response. On the side toward which the head turns, the arm extends. This marks the genesis of a tonic-neck reflex (TNR), which figures so prominently in the patterning of ocular behavior of the human infant.

Although the eye movements at the fetal age of 20 weeks are already more complex, they do not as yet exert an influence. The early TNR may be ascribed chiefly to proprioceptive impulses arising in the neck. The TNR is not a stereotyped response, but undergoes progressive elaborations during the period of gestation and throughout infancy. It assumes a classic conformation in the fetal-infant* at a fetal age of 28 weeks, whether the eyes are open or closed. At a yet later age, when the oculomotor centers are riper, the eyes gaze in the direction of the extended arm.

The TNR thus serves as a morphogenetic matrix which promotes and channelizes visual fixation; it leads to perception of movement when the infant activates his arm; it leads also to hand inspection, to eye-hand coordination, top prehensory approach, and ultimately to unidextrous manipulation.

During the first 12 weeks of life, the full-term infant spends a considerable proportion of his waking time in exercising the TNR pattern, both in tonic immobilization and in windmill activity.

**A fetal-infant is an offspring born and living in what normally is the fetal period of existence. In the development of ocular controls, fixation of movements is quite as important as execution of movements. Innumerable patterns of visual behavior are functionally and genetically related to this most important attitudinal and also kinetic reflex, the TNR.*

Righting reflexes are occasioned by a wide variety of stimuli which stream toward nerve centers in midbrain and pons. The stimuli arrive in the otoliths (which react to change of position); in the semicircular canals (which react to accelerations of movement); also in head, neck, and body posturings and in the teleceptors, especially those of vision. The role of the eyes increases with advance in the animal scale, and it increases with the maturity of the child. Magnus locates the optical righting reflexes in the cerebral cortex.

Statokinetic reflexes are serial reflexes which are produced by movement, and which are designed to keep the movement going in the right direction toward a goal or conclusion. Such kinetic sequences consist virtually of a succession of attitudinal or righting reflexes, which set up tensions that lead to movements, which in turn lead to further adaptive movements. These reflexes figure in the execution of voluntary activities, as well as in the semi-automatic phases of locomotion, leaping, dodging, pursuing, and prehension.

Some statokinetic reflexes are mainly governed by proprioceptive, labyrinthine, and exteroceptive (pressure-contact) affectors; but most of them involve visual affectors and oculomotor effectors. In waking life, the eyes are rarely idle. They are constantly responding to shifts of body posture, or they initiate the shifts. Thus conceived, the action system is a labile complex of interacting statokinetic reflexes; and all acts of vision are influenced by the sensitive equilibriums of this total complex.

The basic equilibriums are motor rather than sensory. The retina as receptor originates cues and signals, but even "pure" perceptual responses have a nuclear motor component; and this motor component subtly or otherwise influences the total reaction of the unitary organism.

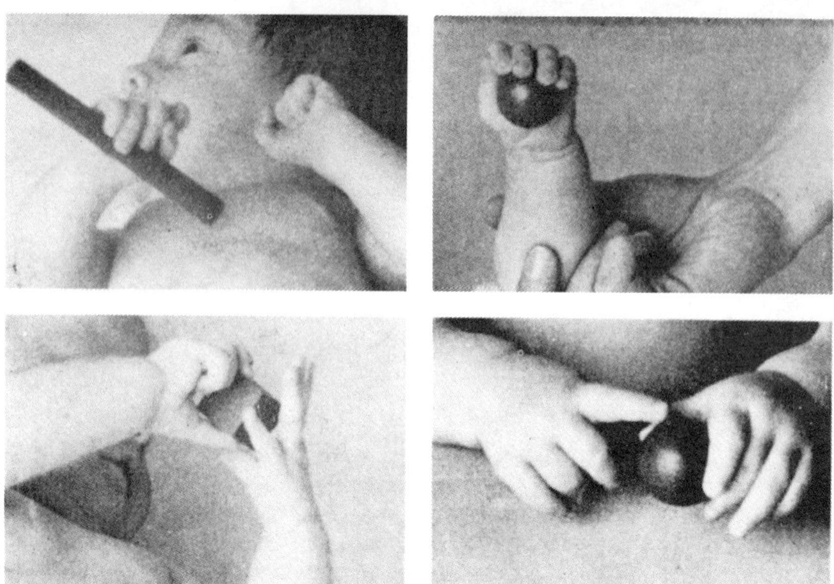

Figure 16. Eye-hand relationships: (a) The neonate clasps an object by an ulnar-heel grasp, without visual regard. (b) At 16 weeks, the thumb pivots to an adducted position to grasp an object. (c) At 28 weeks, the thumb opposes with its mesial surface. The child transfers the object from hand to hand. (d) At the end of the first year, full thumb opposition is achieved. The volar pad is applied to the presenting surface of the seized object.

The embryology of behavior points to the primacy of the motor components. Muscle cells exhibit function prior to nerve cells. Muscles acquire reflex tone when supplied by motor nerve fibers, and this primitive tonal reaction is a condition for overt movement. Motor innervation precedes sensory, and the requisite motor equipment for a behavior is established well in advance of the behavior itself.

The primacy of the motor aspects of vision has far-reaching implications for developmental optics. The growth of the visual functions must be interpreted in terms of a basic motor maturation. Indeed, life and growth are so constituted that the "sensitiveness" of the eye is always limited by the "sensitiveness" of the motor components of the reacting organism. The patterns of visual behavior are configured by pervasive muscular determiners—not only by the oculomotor activators, but by the total postural mechanisms and orientations.

Accordingly, as the child grows, his visual world transforms. It does not simply expand in scope or detail, it undergoes distinctive changes in topography and in its dynamic architecture. The metaphor of the camera has tended to obscure these significant developmental changes. Although his actual visual experiences are concealed, we can infer the developmental transformations from a study of his total action system.

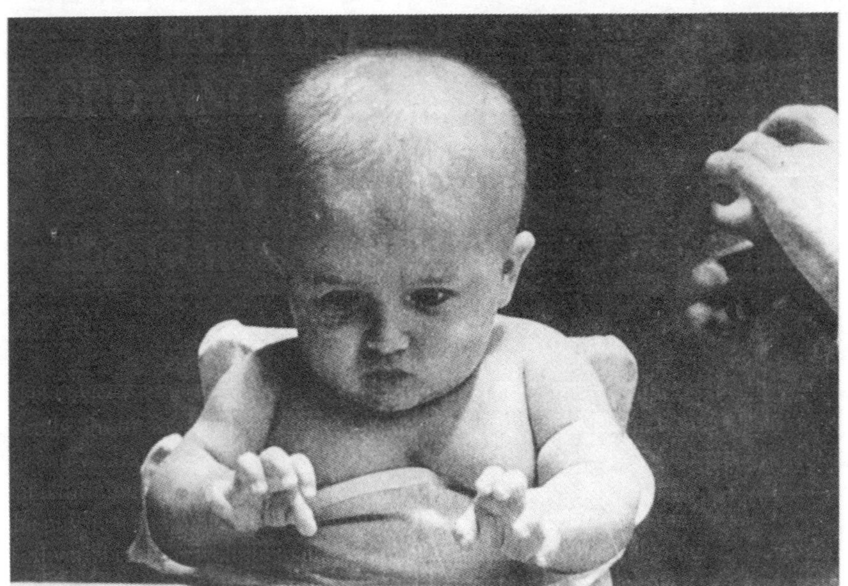

Figure 17. Reaction at 28 weeks to presentation of a 7mm. pellet. (Courtesy of March of Time.) Note the convergence of the total action system, including: (1) head leaning; (2) localizing eye fixation; (3) convergence of eyes; and (4) poised fingers.

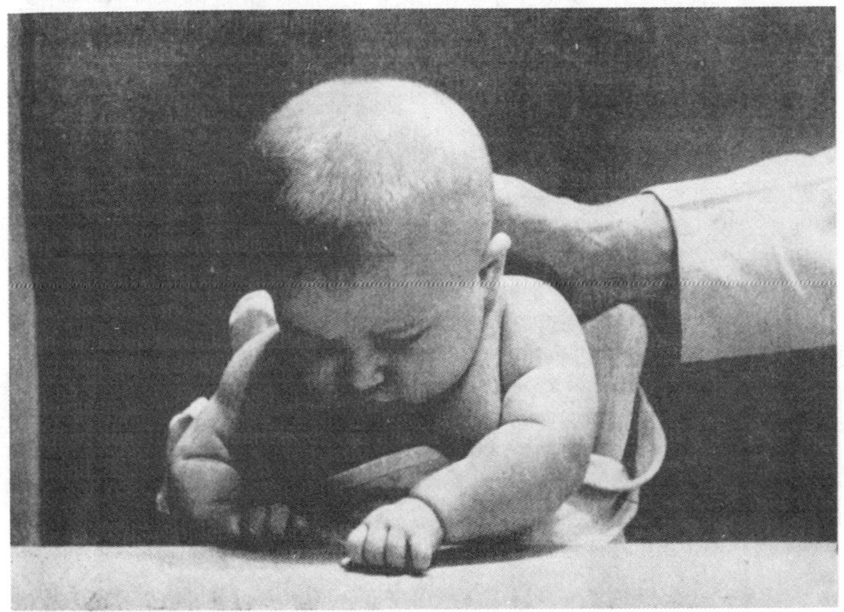

Figure 18. The prehensory approach. This results in intensified fixation, and placement of the hand near the pellet. The child rakes in a paw-like manner near the pellet, without grasping it.

Anatomically, the action system of the growing infant may be envisaged as a vast network of delicate neurone and muscle fibrils. This prodigious network is sustained and integrated through the body fluids and through electrotonic currents generated in one overall electrodynamic field which preserves the unity of the organism. The unity is maintained even during periods of rapid growth.

But this does not mean that the action system grows at a uniform and simultaneous rate in all its parts, expanding symmetrically like a balloon. On the contrary, the process of developmental organization is more like an intricate melody of rhythms, accents, crescendos, pauses, and diminuendos. These shifts in emphasis are reflected in patterns of adaptive movement, and in the spontaneous activities of the child. The eyes are always in the total behavior picture. At any given moment, either they are directing the postural set of the entire organism or they are registering the effect of local and general postural sets.

Classical theories of vision have emphasized its sensory aspects, to the neglect of motor factors. Newer theories recognize that even such refined "attributes" as fusion, projection, and stereopsis have a motor element, indeed a motor origin. They may be traced to eye-limb-body functions slowly evolved and subtilized but never divorced from the kinetic core of a unified action system.

Motorwise the action system is an exquisitely balanced machine. Not a movement can take place without affecting, more or less subtly, the equilibrium of the total machinery. The physiological interrelations of those movement patterns are so intricate that to mature them requires not only some 10 months of prenatal gestation, but a period of postnatal ontogenesis prolonged to over 20 years.

During the first decade of life, in particular, the components of the entire visual-motor system undergo ceaseless organization and reorganization, adapting not only to cultural demands, but even more to the structural changes within the organism itself. Infant, preschool, and school child are constantly confronted with problems of general body posture—supine, prone, upright; sitting, creeping, standing, walking, running, dodging, squatting, squirming, jumping. These movements involve the fundamental axial and appendicular musculature. But very early these fundamental postural patterns must be combined with increasingly refined eye-hand coordinations, mediated by the accessory musculature. Even the pupillary reflexes and the accommodation-convergence response of the intrinsic muscles must be brought into adaptive relation with the reflex and voluntary reactions of the extrinsic muscles which result in fixation, convergence and divergence, and pursuit and compensatory eye movements.

The oculomotor controls, with the still more primitive labyrinth controls, have from earliest times yoked the two eyes into virtually a single organ—"a physiological binoculas," as described by Worth. The eyes accordingly move conjugately, held in unison by three paired reflexes: (a) the *compensatory reflex,* which keeps the eyes fixed in relation to a gravitational point; (b) the *oriental reflex,* which keeps them fixed upon a motionless object of interest; and (c) the *vergence fixation and refixation reflexes,* which keep them on an object in motion. These three dynamic postural reflexes serve to maintain a panorama, and to continue a focus of regard within the panorama.

The component movements of vergence are horizontal, vertical and circular. During development, they are brought into functional relationship with a vast variety of movements of the body as a whole and of its members. The head rotates horizontally, it flexes and extends vertically, and it can also circumduct in a spiral or circular manner. The trunk, shoulders, and legs are capable of similar movements. But the arms, hands and fingers have the widest range of flexibility, combining flexions, extensions, ab-, ad-, and circum-ductions of great diversity.

Now all these movements, ocular and non-ocular, are correlated, partly through experience but chiefly through growth. Experience and training modulate the movements and improve their timing; but they do not engender the basic motor patterns. The basic patterns and the ontogenetic sequences are the product of organic maturation. They are beyond the ingenuity of man to contrive or to create. They are gene effects which it took Nature eons to evolve. An ontogenetic interpretation of child vision, therefore, must take into systematic account the growth of the motor patterns of a total action system.

PART ONE—
THE GROWING ACTION SYSTEM

CHAPTER 5
The Genesis Of Vision

Embryo and Fetus

THE GROWTH CAREER of the embryo begins when the zygote cleaves into 2, 4, 8, 16, 32 ... cells. Prodigious developments take place in the first month. Very early, the dorsal and ventral aspects of the organism differentiate. This is one of the most fundamental differentiations in the animal kingdom. It represents the impress of gravity on the physical and functional morphology of creatures more lowly than the worm, and all vertebrates as well. In man, this differentiation is complicated by the upright posture. Accordingly, visual problems of orientation are foreshadowed, even in the early history of the embryo.

The differentiation of the head also is precocious. This, likewise, is significant because the head plays an extremely important role in the mechanics of vision development. Nature has placed a certain premium on the head; hence, its priority and precocity. In the fetus, the head is one-half of the total height; in the newborn infant it is one-fourth; in the adult, one-tenth.

The human embryo pictured herewith is only 18 days old. The photograph of this famous specimen gives a dorsal view, as revealed through the transparent amnion. The embryo at this stage is a pear-shaped disc which measures 1.53 mm. in length and 0.75 mm. in its greatest breadth. The ground plan of the prospective child is already discernible in this tiny patch of protoplasm. The longitudinal aspect has been laid down; the embryo has a left and a right side, a dorsal and a ventral aspect. The primitive node, clearly visible in the photograph, marks the junction of the head and neck. The neck, as we have noted on a previous page, figures importantly in the evolution of vision. Three-quarters of the disc is already set aside for the formation of the head.

In a specimen only a few days older, the rudiments of the eyes would also be visible as optic pits, outpouchings of the open neural plate. At 4 weeks, when the embryo is approximately 7 mm in length, the optic vesicle has fully invaginated and the cerebral hemispheres are already present. The retina begins to differentiate about two weeks later.

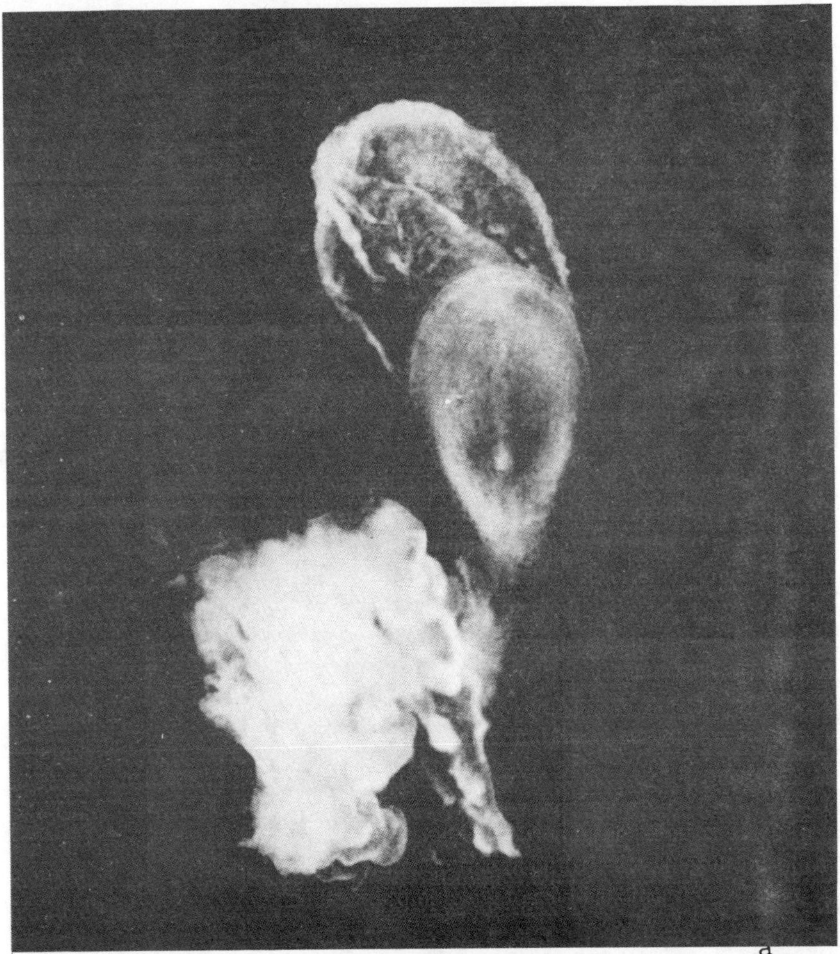

Figure 19. Human embryo, age 18 days. Dorsal view through the transparent amnion (a). The actual size of the embryo proper (the pear-shaped disk) is 0.75 mm x 1.53 mm, indicated in the small key outline. The primituive node (c) marks the junction of the head and neck structures. The head is derived from the region between b and c. d represents the thoracic region, e the lumbar region. (After Heuser, from Gesell, Embryology of Behavior.)

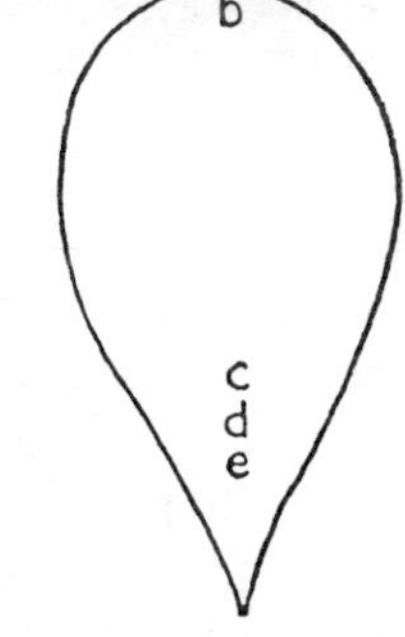

At 8 weeks, the embryo attains a length of 25 mm (one inch). At this stage, the eyes are moving in from their lateral position. (About a week later they are almost frontal, although the orbits diverge some 50 degrees). Eye muscles and eyelids are forming. Nerve fibers have already filled the inner layer of the optic stalk.

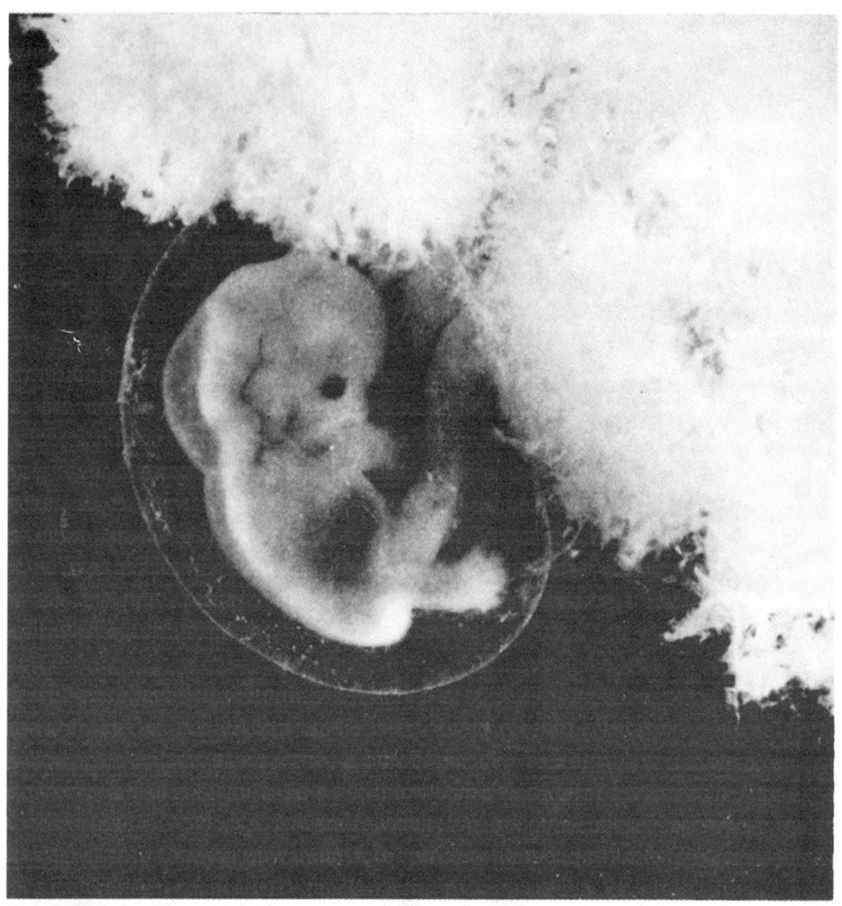

Figure 20. Human embryo, P.G., age 8 weeks. Cerebrum, cranial, and spinal nerves and fingers have formed. Secondary lens fibers are forming; the optic stalk is replaced by the optic nerve. The optic axes make an angle of 72 degrees. The embryo is approaching the fetal stage when the first overt movements make their appearance. (From Gesell, Embryology of Behavior.)

All these tissue changes are on a microscopic scale, but they would display a dramatic quality if the esoteric movements of growth could be witnessed. By fast-motion cinemicrophotographic technique, Speidel has demonstrated how the growing tips of single nerve fibers grope their way with ameboid movements into the intercellular spaces of living tissue. A neuroblast sends out a fine strand of naked protoplasm tipped with a growth cone. The growth cone advances, spinning the nerve fiber behind it. With certitude it moves toward its destination. Neighboring neuroblasts, myoblasts, and fibroblasts are also growing actively, setting up minute waves and pulsations in the intercellular fluids. All these events take place in an

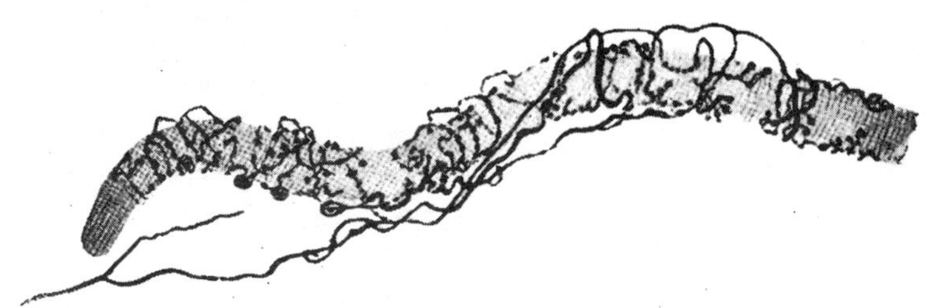

Figure 21. A sensory nerve ending enveloping a fiber of an ocular muscle. The nerve fibers end on the surface of the sarcolemma. The axis cylinders, after shedding their myelin sheath, envelop it with continuous circular and spiral twists. Their varicose twigs terminate with nodular swellings. (After Dogiel and Maximow and Bloom.)

electro-dynamic field, within which muscle cells and nerve cells are brought into functional relationship.

The very first movements of the skeletal musculature—and this includes the oculomotor muscles—are probably microscopic in extent and largely myogenic in origin. It is unlikely that the maturing muscle cells are completely quiescent during the interval which precedes their innervation. Their movements, however minute, may well have a directive influence on the growing nerve fibers, which seem to "seek" them. In this way, a physical union is finally created between a motor end-plate and the sarcoplasm of a muscle fiber. This leads to neurogenic, effector control. But sensory controls also are needed, and these are supplied through sensory fibers. Figure 21 pictures a sensory nerve-ending enveloping a fiber of an ocular muscle. The nerve fibers end on the surface of the sarcolemma. The axis cylinders, after shedding their myelin sheath, envelop it by continuous circular and spiral twists. Their varicose twigs terminate with nodular swellings. Such are the primary embryological arrangements for the oculomotor reactions which are so essential for vision.

Similar arrangements, both through the cerebrospinal and the autonomic nervous systems impart tonus to the developing skeletal musculature. Muscle tonus is a condition of tension which exists independently of voluntary effort, but which is a prerequisite for both reflex and voluntary movements. It is more than a condition, it is an active function—a mode of behavior. There may be tonus without overt movement, but there cannot be movement without tonus. Tonus is essential for both static and dynamic posture. The early embryology of behavior consists, to a large extent in the progressive organization of the tonus of the skeletal muscular system.

Primitive tonal responses to changes of position may occur as early as the 7th week after conception. The semicircular canals of the labyrinth of the ear are perhaps functional at this extremely early period, when the embryo floats in a fluid sphere contained by the amniotic membrane. Under these conditions, it is conceivable that very simple righting reactions are accomplished to keep the organism on an even keel.

Such reactions, however, can only be conjectured. They have never been directly observed. At about the age of 8 weeks, the tonal capacities and musculature of the embryo are sufficiently advanced to produce overt movements. The embryo now enters the fetal stage of development—a stage of development when labyrinthine mechanisms may play a role in orientation. The morphogenesis of behavior is under way. The pattern of the earliest overt movements of the fetus suggests the primacy of the axial musculature in the molding of the action system. This follows naturally from a basic dorsal-ventral differentiation, and from the ubiquitousness of the forces of gravity. These forces operate in utero as well as postnatally. The amniotic fluid and the buoyancy of the head of the fetus facilitate both passive and active adjustments to the pull of gravity, as registered by otoliths and the endolymph in the semicircular canals. The movements of the fetus while in its fluid habitat can be visualized as reactions to that environment, as well as preparations for the postnatal life.

The organization of its postural behavior proceeds with great rapidity, as indicated by observation of fetuses surgically removed for therapeutic reasons (Minkowski and Hooker). By the fetal age of 12 weeks, a wide variety of reactions appears; most of them involve the fetus as a whole. Rhythmic contractions of the body, alternating from one side to the other, are apparently spontaneous. On mild stimulus at a corner of the mouth, long muscles of the neck and trunk contract contralaterally. Stimulation of the palm elicits extension of the wrist and fanning of the fingers. At a later stage the fingers flex. By 12 weeks, the arms and hands have so rotated from their early paddle position that the palms now face each other. In reaction to a facial stimulus, they both move toward the median plane—an early version of the symmetrotonic reflex, which, in the full-term infant, at the postnatal age of 20 weeks, comes under visual and voluntary control.

At the fetal age of 12 weeks, the eyelids are still fused. Nevertheless, prerequisites for eye-hand coordination are already in the making. The oculomotor muscles are undergoing innervation and, under a high light, the eyeballs have been observed to move beneath their sealed lids. These eye movements gather in strength and pattern as the fetus matures. It is impressive to realize that the eyes are active, in a motor sense, throughout a period of 7 lunar months prior to full-term birth.

The fourth gestation month is, in many respects, the most variegated in the embryology of prenatal behavior, because the fetus now exhibits (even though it cannot command) an extremely diverse repertoire of elementary movement patterns. Almost its entire skin is sensitive to stimulation. Restricted specific reactions supplement the generalized responses. Within the confines of the amniotic sac,

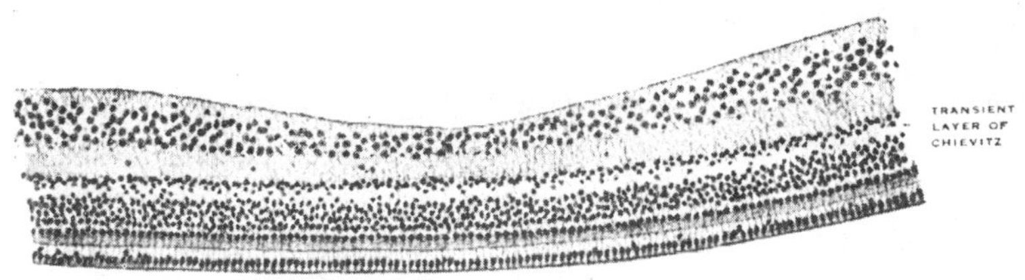

Figure 22. Microscopic cross-section of the fovea centralis of the human fetus at a fetal age of 24 weeks. (After Wolff and Seefelder.)

these movements are probably mild and vary from episodic twitches to protracted tonic contractions which wax and then wane into nothingness.

Of special interest to us are the head movements because the head is rightly considered one of the most important dynamic agents in the morphogenesis of behavior. Head movements which a short time ago were closely incorporated with trunk movements now show a certain degree of differentiation. Slight movements occur somewhat independently of total responses. The head nods, or tilts, or retracts and, even to a slight degree, it rotates. If these movements could actually be observed in utero, they might seem superficially to be isolated and somewhat disordered. But in the process of normal growth, such discrete movements are ultimately integrated into the unitary action pattern out of which they stem in the first instance.

The fetal period is a period of preparation. Every organ system is being prepared for the ultimate crisis of birth. During the 5th and 6th months (16-24 weeks), Nature adds one completing touch to another.

By the end of the 5th month, the fetus (approximately a pound in weight and a foot in length) is well advanced in its somatic organization. The countenance has taken on a not unpleasing appearance and is already somewhat stamped with individuality. Although the nervous system is far from finished, there is already the full quota of neuroblasts and neurones, 12 billion or more in number.

Even the mechanisms of vision are far advanced. Although the fetus does not have light to see, the anatomical arrangements for seeing have already been established. The optic nerve is equipped with a million fibers, 90% of them reaching the cortex via the lateral geniculate bodies which serve as a mediating mechanism for the macula. Up to the 4th month of development, there has been a close analogy between the layers of the cortex and those of the retina. By 7 months, the retina has assumed practically an adult arrangement. The macula began to differentiate as early as the 3rd month, and at about the age of 24 weeks (5 1/2 months) the development of the *fovea centralis* (the central pit of the macula) begins by a thinning of the ganglion cells, which recede to form a shallow depression, as pictured in the accompanying figure.

At this early age, the fovea is already as far distant from the optic nerve head at the time of its formation as it will be in the adult eye. This is a remarkable fact when one considers the tremendous anatomical changes which are yet to follow during the latter half of the gestation period and throughout the postnatal period of growth. The eye itself will more than double in weight prior to birth. It and the brain will increase 3 1/2 times from birth to maturity and the body will increase 21 times. Nevertheless, the distance between fovea and nerve head, established at the fetal age of 24 weeks, remains an absolute.

The Fetal Infant

By definition, the fetal infant is a child born prematurely and living in the fetal period which normally terminates approximately 40 weeks after conception. His status is rather paradoxical, for he is an extra-uterine fetus and yet also a neonate. Under favorable conditions, he may survive birth at a fetal (postconception) age of 28 weeks, or 12 weeks prior to full term. He thus serves as a touchstone for reconstructing the stages of behavior patterning, which are associated with the last 12 weeks of gestation. The characteristics of his visual behavior should be instructive because the precocious exposure to light will inevitably reveal the latent maturity of his ocular reactions.

Elsewhere we have reported in detail the spontaneous and responsive behavior of 22 fetal infants examined at periodic intervals.[1] A total of 80 systematic observations, supplemented by cinema records, were made. The following functions were observed by means of naturalistic and of controlled methods, adapted to the varying stages of maturity: (1) spontaneous supine behavior, (2) visual awareness, (3) manual grasp, (4) auditory awareness, (5) proprioceptive awareness, (6) functional laterality, (7) regard for face, (8) head station, (9) prone behavior, (10) muscle tone, (11) sleep-wake status. It will be noted that several of the foregoing categories have special significance for the ontogenesis of visual behavior.

The investigation embraced three stages of maturity as follows: (a) Early stage of fetal infancy (fetal age: 28-32 weeks); (b) Midstage of fetal infancy (fetal age: 32-36 weeks); (c) Late stage of fetal infancy (fetal age: 36-40 weeks)—all the infants included in this late age group had been born two or three months earlier.

Spontaneous postural attitudes and activities were noted as the infant lay in supine position. Laterality preferences and head movements were tested by gently and slowly rolling the trunk from right to left and left to right. The degree of alertness or somnolence of the infant was noted before and during the course of the examination. During a quiescent interval, soft light from a flashlight was gradually

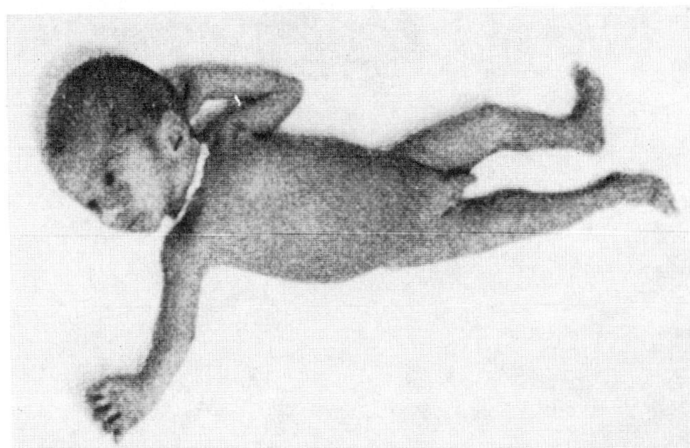

Figure 23. Tonic-neck-reflex pattern of a fetal infant (fetal age, 32 weeks). Note the head aversion: the extension of the faceward arm; and the flexion of the opposite arm, simulating a fencing attitude. This has an analogue in the shield and spear attitude, in which the extensor arm uses an aggressive weapon, and the flexed arm a defensive shield. (From Gesell, Embryology of Behavior.)

brought into the line of potential vision and was slowly moved from the side to the midline through an arc of 90 degrees.

This investigation demonstrated that there is considerable organization of visual behavior during the period of fetal infancy. Although the eyes of the infants were open only a very small fraction of the time, they showed a surprising degree of responsiveness. It cannot be said that the circumstance of premature birth fundamentally accelerates visual development, but it does bring into earlier evidence the otherwise dormant status of the visual structures.

The general aspect of behavior undergoes a striking change from the early to the late stage of prematurity, particularly with respect to the basic function of muscle tonus. This is a condition of muscle tension mediated by both the autonomic and cerebrospinal nervous systems. It is not, however, a generalized quality or quantity which simply increases in magnitude. *Tonus* is behavior and it is patterned through growth processes.

In the youngest fetal infants, tone is minimal, flaccid, and uneven, patchy and precarious. It rises, falls, and shifts above its low level. It may be comparatively high in one region, and low in another. As tonus tires, it seems to "wander" to fresher areas. This meandering characteristic is probably related both to morphogenetic factors and to the physiologic mechanism of recruitment. Muscle fibers are recruited and activated in squads, rather than in their entirety.

Even in the midstage fetal infant, the tonal responses are more integrated. The infant's gross postural activity comes in configured waves, rather than in small localized ripples. His general tonus increases on manipulation and rises to meet limited emergencies. He is not as fragile as he seems; but his tone does peter out readily.

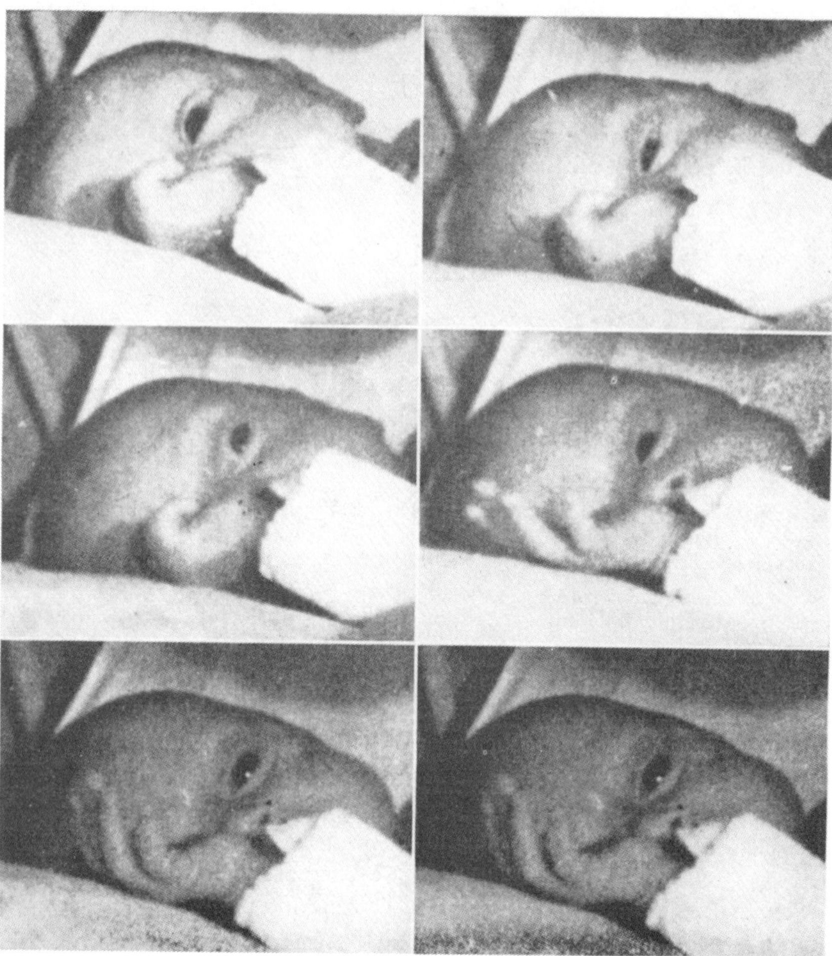

Figure 24. Ocular close-up of mature-stage fetal infant in incubator (fetal age, 38 weeks). The infant lies quiescent, with head averted. visual awareness is probably meager, but the eyes spontaneously make small, well-defined excursions. Only the left (occipital) eye is visible. It moves inward and slightly downward, holds this position for a second, moves laterally, and then returns to a yet more inward pose. Later, the eye directs forward and immobilizes, as though for sustained fixation. Meanwhile, the hand has opened and partly closed again. These eye-hand movements are intrinsically determined, and do not arise from retinal stimulation. Similar movements presumably occur in utero.

The late stage, near-term fetal infant has more tone on tap. He does not need to husband his tone as formerly because he has reserves of it to draw on. The whole substratum of tonus is more consolidated; he seems more firmly knit into a single, sturdy piece. He is more nearly ready to meet the buffetings of fate.

Early Stage. At the beginning of this stage, the fetal infant weighs only about two pounds and is so diminutive that he can be held in the palm of the adult hand.

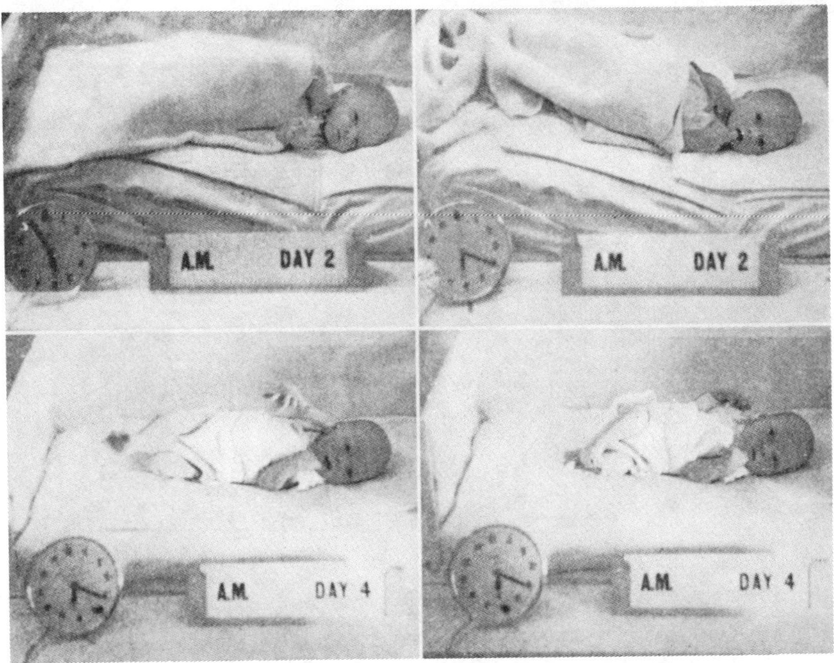

Figure 25. Eye and body postures of neonate at age 2 days and 4 days (Boy D.D.).

Occasionally he stirs but, even when he is a few weeks old, the distinction between activity and rest is not clear-cut. His ever-recurring torpor is, in fact, his most conspicuous and consistent behavior. His eyes are usually closed; sometimes one eye only is open, or semi-open. He winks with a sluggish blink.

Bodily movements are sporadic and meager. In the supine position, he lies with head turned to one side, with the arm on that side extended and his opposite (occipital) arm flexed. This is the classic tonic-neck-reflex pattern, which is of far-reaching significance in the patterning of visual behavior. At times, he may activate his extended arm and hold it in a transient catatonic pose, or he slowly elevates a flexed arm in a floating TNR attitude. Although general bodily activity is meager, he is seldom completely quiescent for any length of time. His complex facial musculature is busy; the forehead corrugates (sometimes only half of the brow, for bilateral integration is not yet firmly achieved); the oculomotors roll the eyeballs or weave them back and forth and up and down. The eyeballs usually move conjointly, but positive visual responses are scanty or quite absent. The early stage fetal infant will, however, make mild avoidance responses to a bright light even when eyes are closed, frowning and flinching slightly.

Midstage. In physical appearance, as well as in behavior capacities, the midstage fetal infant is definitely more mature. His anatomy is more compact, less mol-

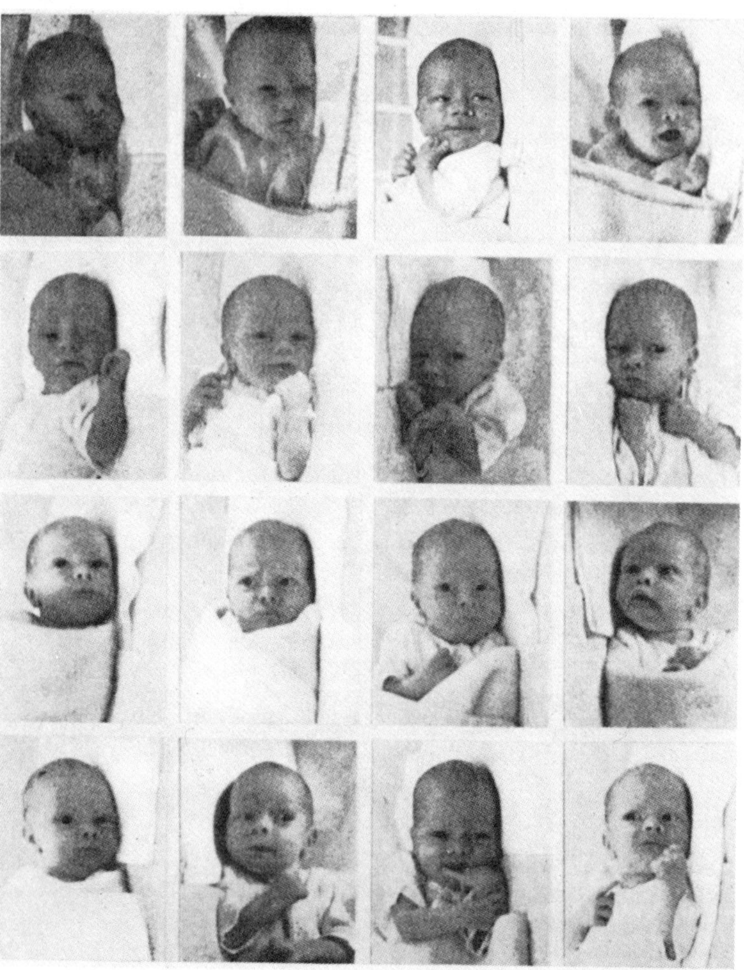

Figure 26. Head and eye posture: 2-13 days (Boy D.D.). The ocular attitudes of D.D. are progressively pictured for advancing ages, from 2 days to 13 days. A trend toward increasing alertness will be noted. In all but four instances, he lies in his preferred left TNR attitude. The pictures are vertically oriented in order to afford a better view of the eye posturings. The occipital eye (the right eye in the left TNR, the left eye in the right TNR) takes the lead. The opposite (resting) eye may be closed, or diverge to the nasal corner (a, c, e, n). The occipital eye is the active fixating eye. This is the stage of monocular fixation. Binocular fixation and true convergence become established after the second month. (Ages in days 2, 3, 3, 3—3, 4, 4, 5—7, 8, 9, 10—11, 11, 12, 13).

luscous. From the standpoint of vision, the most important developmental advance is reflected in his capacity for brief periods of wakeful alertness. He is still an indisputably drowsy individual, but again and again, during the day and the night, he pricks the surface of mere being with small acts of awareness which probably are not without at least dim visual content. Sometimes he keeps his eyes wide open, and he opens them oftener. He shows more vivid distaste of a bright light.

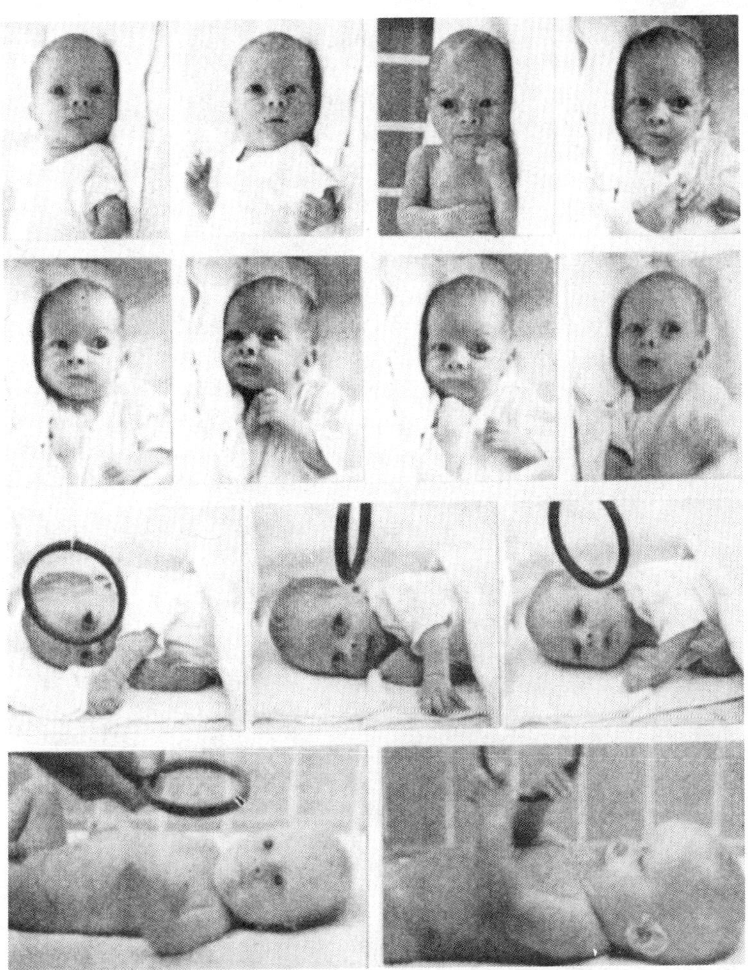

Figure 27. Head and eye postures: 13 days—24 weeks (Boy D.D.). Head and eye postures influence each other reciprocally. The right eye appears to be fixating in (a) and (b); the left in (d), (e), (f), and (g). The eyes move independently of the head, back and forth, up and down, and rotarywise (c-g). Associated head movements are absent or minimal, even when the eyes move laterally in pursuit of the dangling ring (i), (j), and (k). Eyes and head gain command of the midplane at about 20 weeks of age, with the ascendancy of the STR. Binocular fixation and convergence are organizing at 8 weeks (l). At 24 weeks, the infant grasps an object with hand, as well as with his two eyes (m). Eyes, head and hands are now in versatile coordination. But the eyes lead in taking hold of the physical world. (Ages in days: 13, 13, 14, 14—14, 14, 14, 15—15, 15, 15—8 wks., 24 wks.)

All his reactions, indeed, are more positive and sustained. His gross postural activity now comes in definite waves rather than in small localized ripples. Changes in trunk position tend to induce active rather than passive changes in the averted head position, for the head is now both anatomically and functionally more firmly united to the trunk. He may resist changes in head position because of an apparent unilateral preference. Functional laterality is already manifesting itself in postural

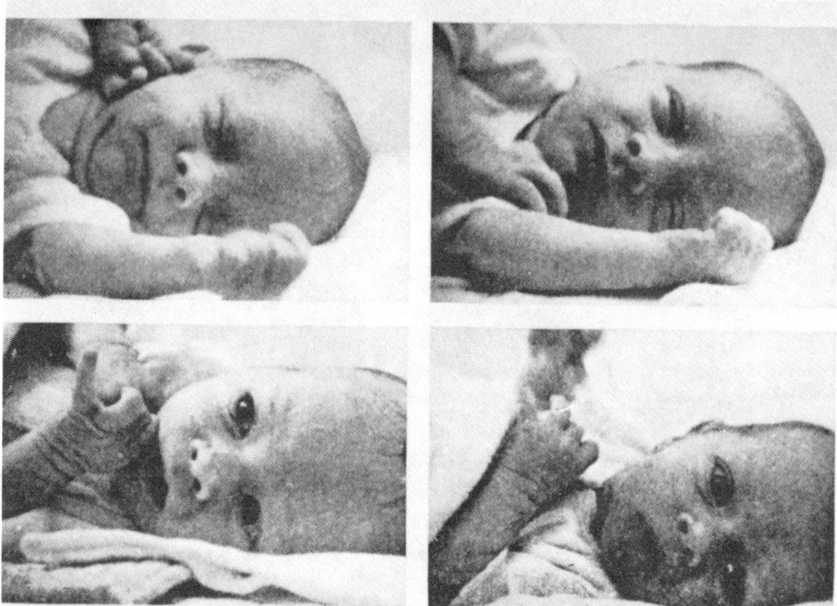

Figure 28. A drowsing neonate, age 9 days. The occipital hand churns the cheek in a TNR stretch; the heavy lids part unequally. By the age of 10 days, waking behavior is more clearly defined and the ocular postures and brightness suggest increased alertness.

sets, including ocular postural sets. He makes a definite, though primitive, ocular response in the dangling ring situation. He does not give the ring true regard as it is slowly moved across the field of potential vision. He does not even fixate upon it, but the eyes move saccadically in momentary afterpursuit. This is one of the very earliest components of visual function and it comes to unmistakable manifestation in the midstage of fetal infancy (fetal age: 32-36 weeks).

Late Stage. The late stage fetal infant presents a somewhat more finished appearance. Increased adipose has rounded his contours. He is physiologically more robust and his behavior patterns are more distinctly configured. He functions more smoothly, not only because of increased maturity, but because he has had prior experience in an atmospheric world. Accordingly, his behavior day has more character. Rhythms of activity and rest are assuming more distinct form. The mature fetal infant has caught the knack of sleeping. He falls off to sleep more decisively, sleeps more deeply, clings to sleep more tenaciously. He wakens spontaneously at intervals and stays awake with or without fussing.

Doubtless, the periods of wakeness result in lengthening periods of visual awareness. This awareness is beginning to show a faint aspect of interest and attention. The face assumes passing shades of expression which suggest inner springs of reactivity. The organism is beginning to take notice, and to stay awake long enough to take visual notice. This ability to wake up, like all complex behaviors, is based upon maturational changes in the central nervous system. The waking propensity

needs special neurological arrangements which, at the present stage, are pr
organized chiefly in the thalamic region, the equivalent, according to Kle
of the primitive waking center. This center is destined to undergo further
tions and by reverberating circuits will some day be joined to higher centers
cerebral cortex. But already the function of waking is intimately correlated with the function of vision.

The head has acquired increased mobility. It may move through an arc of 90 degrees, but the arc is confined to a preferred side, most infants showing a definite addiction to a rightward TNR attitude. If the antecedent period of fetal infancy has been a long one, the head may become so lopsided as to make aversion to the nonpreferred side all but impossible. A few such infants may even show a shortening and spasm of the sterno-cleido-mastoid muscle on the preferred side. This, however, is not a true torticollis but a transient developmental condition which usually undergoes self-correction when the head becomes more mobile and freely commands an arc of 180 degrees.

The mature fetal infant actively resists passive head rotation. His general postural set and his oculomotor postural set are delimited by a dominating tonic-neck reflex. At optimal moments, his ocular behavior suggests visual interest and, faintly, even a seeking kind of inspection. He definitely follows the movements of a dangling ring through an arc of 45 degrees in the preferred sector of his field of regard. At times, for brief moments, he immobilizes his eyes in pseudofixation as though drinking in visual impressions in a diffuse and passive manner. He blinks to a flash of light, but tolerates it far better than at an earlier age. He tends to open his eyes wide when he hears the sound of a bell.

When the late stage fetal infant reaches a postconception age of 40 weeks, he is chronologically equivalent to a newborn infant of full term. Premature birth lengthened his experience in a world of light and hastened some of his ocular adaptations. But has it conferred upon him any permanent visual advantage?

The Neonate

The neonatal period, by convention, comprises the first postnatal month. Normally, it follows 40 weeks of gestation. The mature fetal infant whom we have just described was born from 8 to 12 weeks prematurely. A full-term neonate spends these 8 to 12 weeks *in utero.* To what extent does this difference in the biological time of birth influence the patterning of visual behavior? That is an interesting question with both philosophical and clinical implications.

The mature (late-stage) fetal infant, having escaped some of the acute hardships of parturition, has also had some weeks in which to refine his adaptations to an extra-uterine environment. Consequently, for a week or more he may function more smoothly than the full-term neonate of equivalent postconception age. For a brief period the more experienced fetal infant appears better organized and physiologically more expert. He is less irritable, less given to trigger and tremor response. His homeostatic equilibrium is more stable, his ocular movements and postures are better defined.

These differences are readily explainable in terms of trauma and of habituation. The differences are transient and do not confer any fundamental advantage (or disadvantage) upon the prematurely born infants. By the time the full-term infant is 4 weeks old he has usually weathered the birth transition; he is physiologically more stabilized, and his visual behavior patterns are comparable to those of the premature infant (the former fetal infant) who has attained a corrected chronological age of 4 weeks. Having drawn these comparisons, we may now consider the behavior characteristics of the full-term neonate during the first month of his postnatal existence.

When does this newborn baby begin to use his eyes? He is visually sensitive to light from the moment of birth. Although his eyes are prevailingly close, they are far from inactive. The eyeballs frequently make short lateral excursions, even under closed lids. The lids themselves recurrently quiver, or they contract, participating in the grimacing which especially involves the ocular and oral regions. Repeatedly the eyes open, more or less completely, in unison or singly. The head extends or rotates slightly from time to time. Occasionally the eyes open and immobilize as though to stare. We cannot, of course, describe the subjective aspect of these moments, but one gains the impression that the function of vision is organizing at an extremely rapid rate through swiftly advancing stages of maturation. The overt ocular movements seem sporadic, but they are ordered by an underlying patterning process.

To gain a clearer picture of this patterning process, we arranged for continuous night and day observations of a healthy full-term neonate, as described elsewhere. Infant D.D. was placed on a self-demand feeding schedule and was permitted to sleep on his own terms. Beginning 20 minutes after birth, serial photographic records were made at half-minute intervals over a period of two weeks. Waking, sleeping and drowsing were recorded on continuous protocols. Drowsing was classified as either *sleep* or *wakeness* on the basis of predominant trend, and the distribution of periods of sleeping and waking was accordingly plotted for each 24-hour day in the fortnight of observation. Inasmuch as there is a very close correlation between wakefulness and "use of the eyes," the changing diurnal cycle of sleep gives important indications of the developmental status and nature of the visual functions in the first weeks of life.

There is no evidence that the neonatal infant is, *sui generis,* an expert sleeper. At a vegetative level he may sleep soundly enough, but the very fact that he is developing cortical mechanisms for a wakefulness of choice makes him somewhat awkward

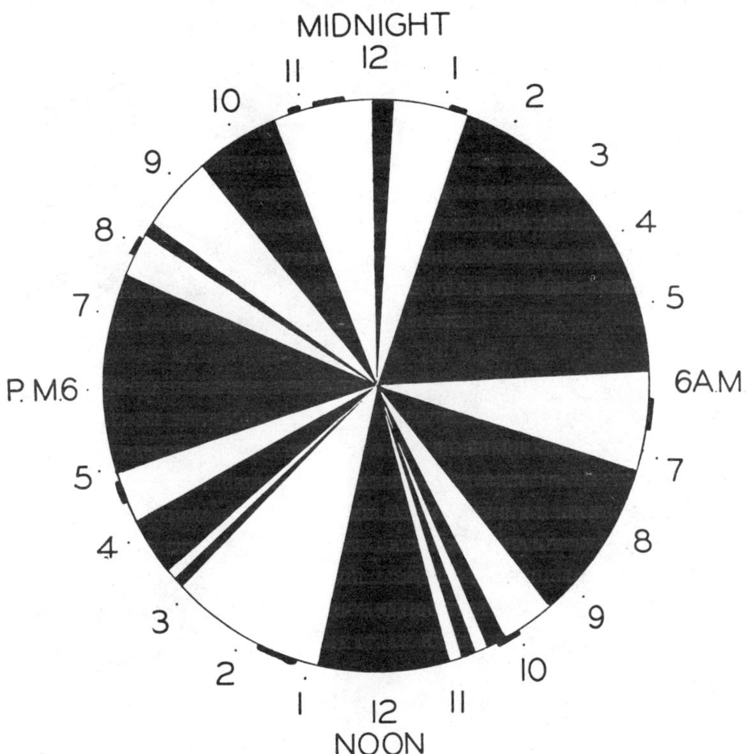

Figure 29. Diurnal cycle of Infant D.D., age 6 days. March 31: sunrise, 5:46 a.m.; sunset 6.23 p.m. Sleep, awakeness, and feeding shown on 24-hour clock dial. Solid segments indicate sleep. Feedings are shown at margin.

	6 p.m. to 6 a.m.	*6 a.m. to 6 p.m.*
No. of sleep periods	5	7
No. of awake periods	4	7
Total No. minutes asleep	472	381
Total No. minutes awake	248	339
Number of feedings	4	4
% of 12 hours asleep	65%	52%
% of 12 hours awake	35%	48%

(From Gesell: Embryology of Behavior)

in his transitions from one state to another. He opens his eyes in order to receive, to entertain and, in due time, to initiate visual impressions.

If quiescence (with closed eyes) is a criterion of deep sleep, then much of his sleep is poorly integrated, and he is ready for only a limited amount of visual experience. It was amazing to find that on Days 5, 6, 7, and again on Day 10, Infant D.D. was never completely quiet, whether asleep or awake, for a period as long as 15 minutes. The longest span of complete quiescence was a 30-minute period on Day 12.

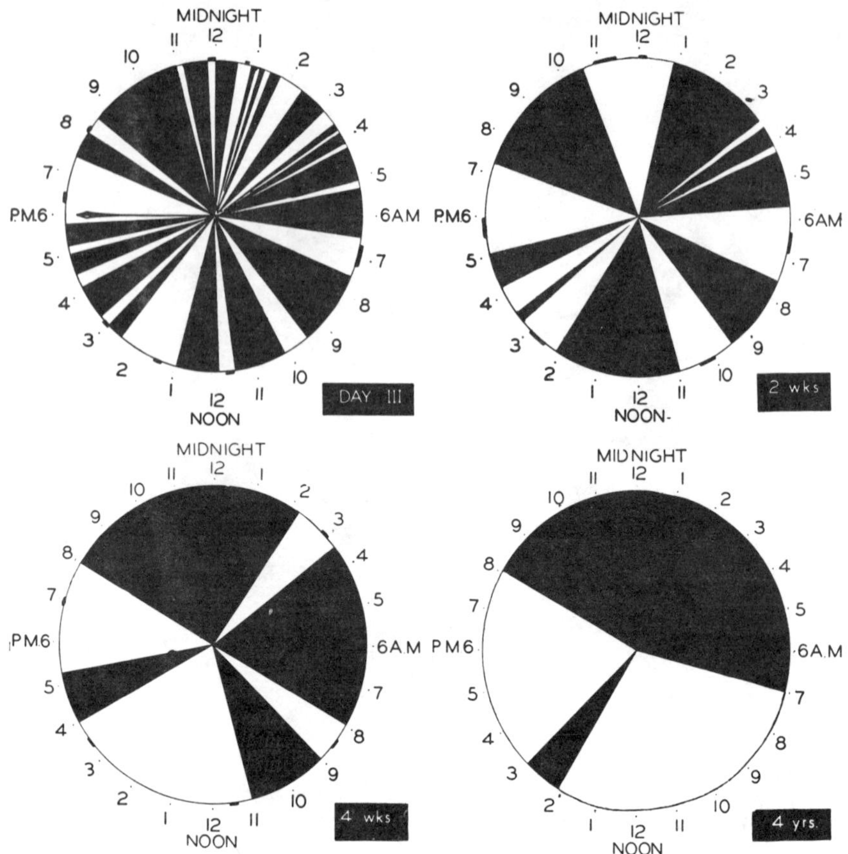

Figure 30. Diurnal cycle of behavior of Infant D.D. Day 3, week 2, month 1, year 4.

The accompanying 24-hour dials plot the distribution of periods of sleep and wakeness for the 3rd day, the 2nd week, the 1st month, and the 4th year.

The trend toward consolidation and toward a monophasic sleep rhythm is clearly demonstrated. Already, at the age of one year, the eyes are active, virtually throughout the livelong day. Of all the sense, vision is the most perpetually avid.

Photographs of the eye postures of Infant D.D. show a steady developmental trend toward increasing visual alertness during the first two weeks (see accompanying Figure 31). During sleep, the early body posture is reminiscent of the fetal habitus. On waking, one or both eyes open drowsily; occasionally they open decisively and widely as though drinking in vague but truly visual impressions. For brief periods the oculomotors heighten in tone. This infant preferred a somewhat poorly defined leftward TNR posture, which favored use of the right eye for monocular fixation.

The left eye closed, or diverged to the nasal corner, while the more active right eye immobilized.

Such monocular fixation is characteristic of the neonatal period, although there are great individual differences which already point to underlying constitutional factors. These differences relate to the action system, as well as to visual behavior, and they are so distinctive that they cannot be ascribed to environmental factors. Even the amount of visual experience and the degree of excitement and interest in the experience vary from child to child.

Vision has a preeminent place in neonatal development. Visual behavior patterns are among the first and most complex to assume form and function. In comparison, body and limb activities seem amorphous and unpredictable. On close examination, however, the ocular patterns prove to be closely correlated with total action-system responses. When the neonate fixates an object of interest, his sporadic bodily activities tend to subside; he stops fretting; he assumes a postural set. He may open his mouth and tense his lips. There are changes in rate and depth of respiration.

The fixational response, therefore, involves the entire action system to some degree. With the suppression of body-limb activity, there is a general reduction or a heightening of muscle tonus according to the maturity and the individuality of the infant. On the basis of outward tokens, we may infer that the early visual experiences of the infant soon become vivid and consuming. Similarly, he enjoys the sensory and organic satisfactions which come with warmth, snugness and feeding; but vision ranks as his supreme psychological achievement. The scope and complexity of his vision are delimited by the postural attitudes of his eyes, head, body and limbs. But as his eyes become more individuated and independent within the total complex, they also assume a directive role in determining body and limb attitudes. Even the tonic-neck reflex responds to changes of head posture, self-induced by the lead of the eyes.

Reference

1. Gesell A, CS. The Embryology of Behavior. New York: Harper & Brothers, 1945:107-122.

CHAPTER 6
Infancy

It is now our task to describe the changing action system and, incidentally, the visual world of the growing infant. This is no simple task because the human infant develops at a headlong pace and does not pause to report the many subtle elaborations by which he ceaselessly organizes his private visual experiences. These experiences, however, are not altogether private. Some are outwardly registered in the movements and the demeanor of his eyes, in his bodily attitudes, and in his active adjustments to physical and social environment. To determine the role of vision in the life of the infant, it is necessary to observe his patterns of ocular and postural behavior in their manifold interaction.

To trace the development of these patterns, it will be convenient to subdivide the period of infancy into six age zones, from 4 weeks through 15 months. There are many advantages in using lunar month intervals for the first year of life. The neonatal period comprises the first month. The remaining 12 lunar months divide themselves conveniently into quarters as follows: the First Quarter (4-16 weeks); the Second Quarter (16-28 weeks); the Third Quarter (28-40 weeks); the Fourth Quarter (40-52 weeks). The 15-month age level presents many interesting maturity traits transitional to the preschool period, which is reckoned as beginning at 18 months. The developmental sequences here described are fairly typical of normal infancy and may with caution be used as normative standards. The order of the sequence is similar from child to child, but the ages at which specific patterns make their appearance are subject to wide individual variations. Extreme variations occurring during infancy may have diagnostic import, and furnish a clue to visual difficulties which the child will show at later ages.

4-16 WEEKS

The characteristic visual acts of the *4-week-old* infant have already been suggested. He wakes not only to feed but to exercise his visual functions. He stares, albeit rather vaguely, at his surroundings. His countenance is impassive, but he quiets his activity when he regards a large area of light or when the face of his mother or attendant comes into his line of vision. He gives active, sustained attention to an object of interest brought within several inches of his eyes. He musters only feeble and sporadic glances when the object is farther away.

During the next two months, the scope of the infant's ocular fixations and movements increases. His eyes become more mobile; he fixates definitely on small objects of interest at distances ranging from one to three feet or more. As he lies supine in his crib, he can follow a dangling ring through an arc of 90 degrees. Eyes and head tend to move together, but his field of vision is restricted by the

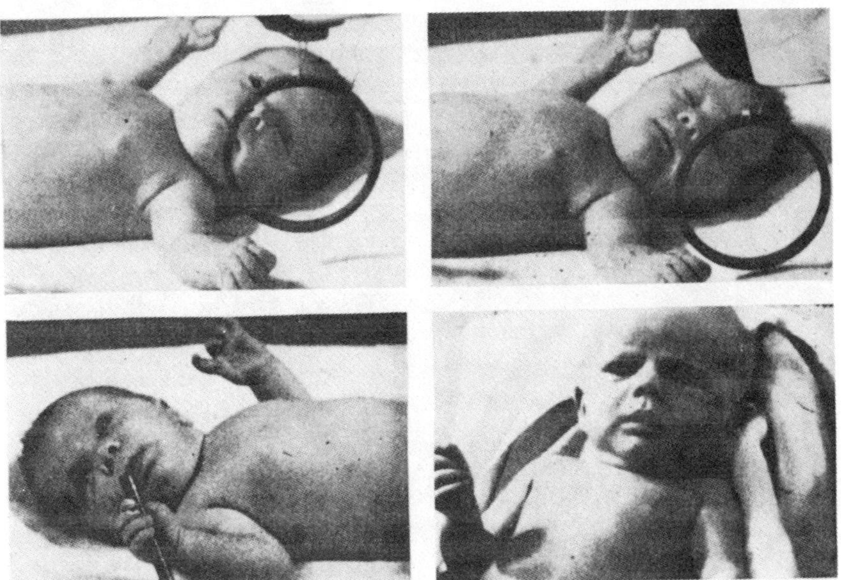

Figure 31. Visual behavior patterns at 4 weeks of age: (a) Diffusely fixates on ring, (b) Releases regard with blink, (c) Eyes brighten as he clenches rod, (d) Stares frowningly at person.

tonic-neck-reflex attitude, which is his preferred posture. His head may be habitually averted, right or left, his eyes directed forward. He seems to seek and enjoy stationary light; his regard intensifies when an object of interest moves or nods at a suitable tempo and rhythm. As he lies supine, he looks downward, but not upward, to pursue a moving person. His numerous, though limited, shifts of gaze indicate that the structure of his visual world is elaborating at a swift rate.

At *8 weeks* he is visually intrigued by bright objects—the shining surface of a mirror, a bottle of oil on a bath tray, a bit of gaily figured cretonne, a twirling, colored yarn ball, silhouettes and shadows on the wall. At *12 weeks* he enjoys the glisten of a brightly colored picture book as the pages turn; he likes the wavering light of a candle. Indeed, he may cry when a light is turned off, and he may fuss in the morning until the curtain is pulled up. Then, as the light streams in, he quiets with sheer visual satisfaction. He likes light.

In the ensuing month (12-16 weeks) these elaborations lead to a veritable visual heyday. Vision assumes an engrossing and exciting role in the mental life of the infant. He attains a new awareness of surroundings; he manifests both searching and absorbed regard for luminosities, shadows, and persons. When supine, he tilts his head backward and rolls his eyes upward to pursue the figure of his mother as she retreats around the corner of his crib. He can also look down his nose with increased facility. He pursues with improved smoothness the transit of the dangling ring (from right to left) through an arc of 180 degrees; he reverses this pursuit (from

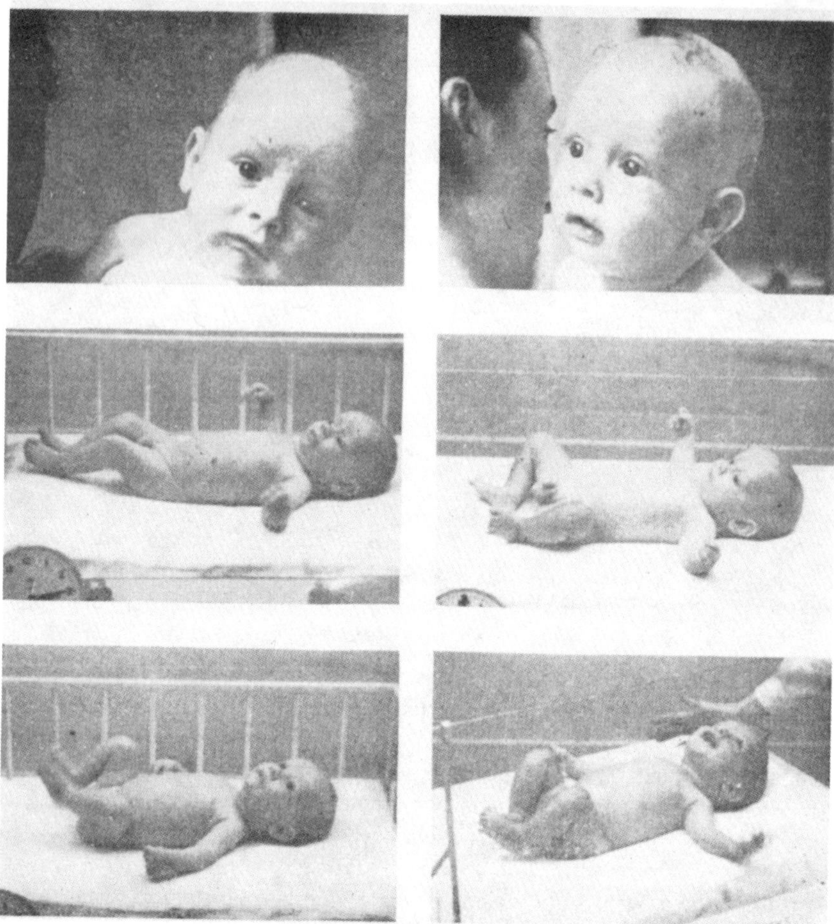

Figure 32. Comparative-action photograph of Infant D.D. at 8 weeks and at 12 weeks, showing differences in patterns, as follows: Forward regard (a) 8 weeks, Less diffuse, more direct, (b) 12 weeks, Sustained and absorbed; Footward regard (c) 8 weeks, Downward regard, (d) 12 weeks, More direct downward regard, with freer head and eye movements; Headward regard (e) 8 weeks, Limitation of head and eyes, on attempting to look upward (f) 12 weeks, Increased facility of eye and head movements.

left to right) with a pause for reposturing and refixation. Still more noteworthy, he can shift his regard from the ring to the string, and to the hand which suspends the string. He has a genuine visual predilection for hands. As he lies in his crib, he spends much time fixating more or less intently on his own hand, which he holds extended or near his chin. When he is supported in a sitting position, confronting a table top, he gives delayed regard to an object of interest placed on the table, and selective regard to the movement of the incoming and outgoing hand of the examiner.

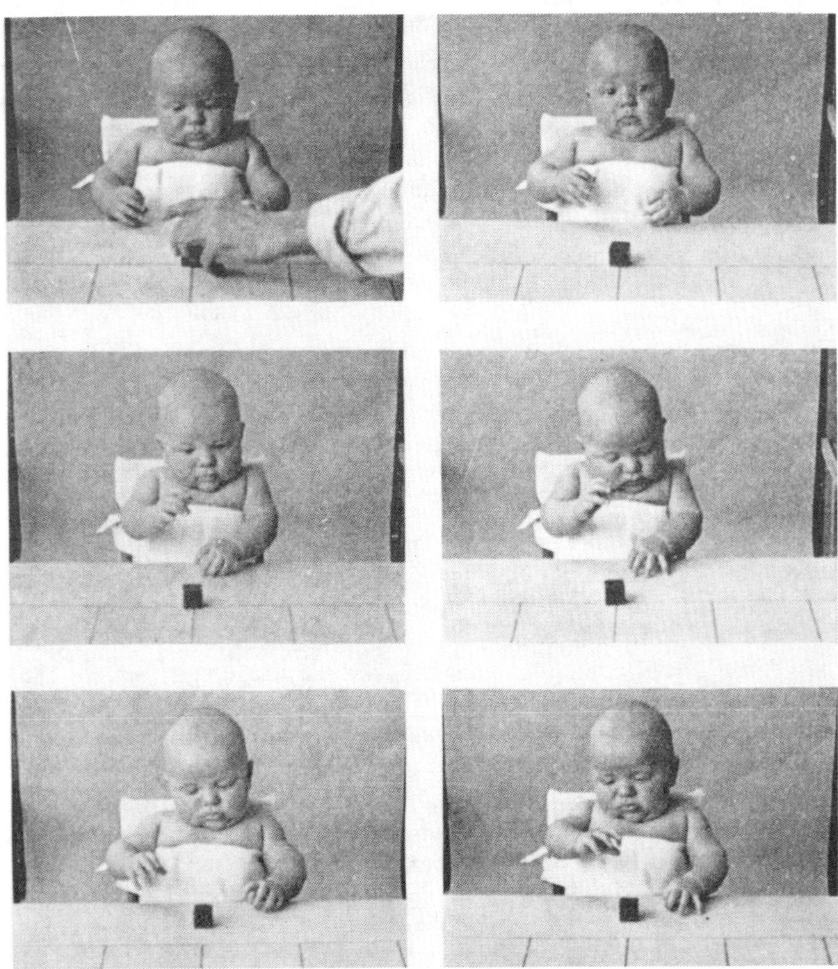

Figure 33. Visual-behavior patterns at 16 weeks. (a) Regards examiner's incoming hand, (b) Stares forward with minimal head lift, (c) Momentarily regards cube, (d) Regard shifts to own left hand, (e) Regard shifts back to cube, (f) Regard shifts to own right hand.

As he looks at the object of interest on the table top, he immobilizes his eyes; presently he activates his arms and legs, but especially his arms, thus indicating that some day he will appropriate the object with hands, as well as with eyes. But the heyday of prehension has not yet arrived. For the present he is content to pick up the physical environment with eyes alone.

16-28 WEEKS

During the second quarter, new patterns of prehension take shape—reaching and grasping both with mouth and with hands. Even at 16 weeks, we see anticipations of this era of prehension. The hands are opening—no longer are they predominantly fisted; and the arms activate on the sight of an approaching object. Although still given to protracted moments of starey fixation and of passive regard, the infant at 16 weeks responds vividly to visual challenges. He shifts his gaze more freely in the supine than in the seated position. He rotates his head to shift regard from one locus to another. He follows the transit of the dangling ring with greater facility and much less naively. He is likely to terminate his ocular pursuit while the ring is still in transit, directing his visual attention elsewhere. In an earlier, immature stage he tended to follow the transit through and to overshoot in his ocular pursuit. Now he is able to let his visual fixation shift with a facile release.

This ability to release regard smoothly is a prerequisite for exploratory inspection. Accordingly, when the infant is seated at a test table and an object of interest is placed on the table top, he shifts his regard from the object to his own hand, back to the object, back to his own hand, and sometimes to the nearby examiner. These more or less automatic shifts of regard do not denote confusion; instead they denote the emergence of a growing capacity for differential perception and finer visual discrimination. Even at the age of 16 weeks the infant is able to regard recurrently a tiny sugar pellet 7 mm. in diameter on the table top. Almost literally, he picks up the object with his eyes, drops it and picks it up again. This is truly a form of ocular prehension, a forerunner of manual prehension. The oculomotor organization which occurs in the first 16 weeks of life is prodigious. Never again will the infant advance at the same swift pace in the patterning of his visual functions.

He takes delight in his growing powers. Seeing has a certain priority in his daily life. Even when hungry, he will interrupt his feeding to regard a person in the room. Mere motor play does not suffice. He likes new horizons, likes to be translated in late afternoon to the wide expanse of a big bed. He is now happy with himself; he talks "to himself," but he can shift his regard to his mother as she moves about the room, and, as he releases with a laugh or chuckle, his eyes brighten as they never brightened before.

The 20-week-old infant, as he lies supine, gives sober regard to the dangling ring; he immobilizes his general postural activity, flings out his arms and closes in on the ring. He may grasp it with a short reach as it nears one of his hands.

Before a mirror, he gives regard to the image of his face and he activates his hands. Seated at a test table, he intently regards a cube, possibly corrals it with adduction or sweeps it aside with an abrupt abduction, or grasps it on favorable contact.

He appropriates with his eyes more successfully than with his hands. He fixates with great intensity and focalizes his whole action system when an object is in a near space sector above his chest, or in the near median position on the test table. If the object is moved only a slight distance away from him, the intense, closely bound fixation breaks. There is an optimal near area in space which evokes a maximum of focalized central regard. Bodily posture, prehensory approach, and oculomotor set are compactly knit together. Intent fixation dissolves with a flash release, often accompanied by blinking and eye-rolling.

Should he seize an object of interest, it goes avidly to his mouth and he tried to regard it even while he mouths it. The whole eye-hand-mouth episode is surcharged with optical implications. This mouthing may be interpreted as a form of tactual-spatial exploitation, which contributes a nucleus to the visual perception of form and substance. The infant seems to be impelled by a sensory-motor appetite. He definitely exploits the objects in a manner which indicates that he is seriously engaged in the developmental organization of visual-tactual behavior. When a toy drops out of hand, he pursues it with his eyes. In another month, he pursues it with his hands as well and retrieves it.

Even at 20 weeks, the infant shows signs of increasing visual sophistication based on remembered experience. He is becoming perceptually aware, and a little shy, of strangers. He cries when he is too suddenly left alone by his mother. He is aware of strange surroundings; he senses a reorientation when his crib is shifted to a new position.

At the 24-week maturity level, the infant's regard is obviously more relaxed and more versatile. He is ocularly less bound by a restricted focal area; his hands also have more independence; mouthing and head-reaching are less prominent. He regards an object as he brings it toward his mouth, but when the object touches his lips he releases his regard out into space and perhaps glances at the examiner. Before a mirror he regards his own face and also his hand as he pats the mirror surface. Again he shifts his regard from his image to that of the examiner.

Seated at the test table, he can similarly shift his regard from one cube to another, and he can manually pick up a cube on sight. Yet he is likely to drop it when a second cube is presented. His regard now is more inspectional, both in near and in far sectors. In near inspection he may give selective regard to details, looking, for example, at the dark handle of the bell which contrasts with the shining bowl. At the test table, he shows prompt and consistent awareness of all sizable objects, including a pellet. His shifts of head and hands, although more numerous and versatile, are slightly atactic and restricted because of immaturity. His discrimination of strangers, however, has become more definite. He is an intentful watcher. Sometimes watching and inspection even delay an outgoing hand response.

28-40 WEEKS

During the third quarter, the interests of the infant undergo a remarkable expansion and some significant projection. Note with what concentrated attention he exercises his growing powers of touch and vision. A spirited 28-week-old infant bounces,

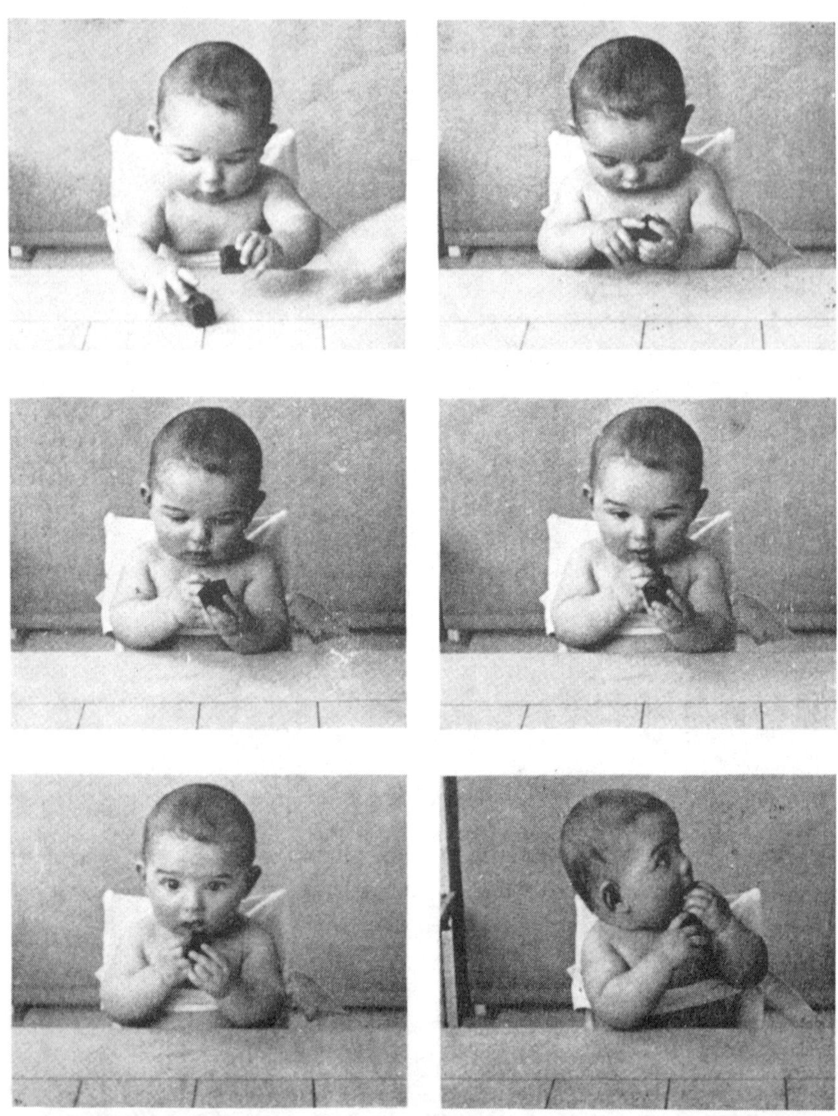

Figure 34. Visual-behavior patterns at 28 weeks (Boy D.). (a) Regards and grasps cube immediately, (b) Lowers head for close inspection, (c) Head lifts and eyes converge, (d) Eye slits widen with intensified convergence, (e) Eyes release with frontal stare, (f) Turns and tilts head to regard surroundings.

crows, vocalizes, bangs and brandishes with abandon. Present a cube on the test table and he seizes it almost before it is placed; after a swift glance he brings the cube to his mouth, senses its surfaces orally, while he looks into distance; speedily he withdraws the cube, rotates it with a twist of the wrist, noting the motion visually;

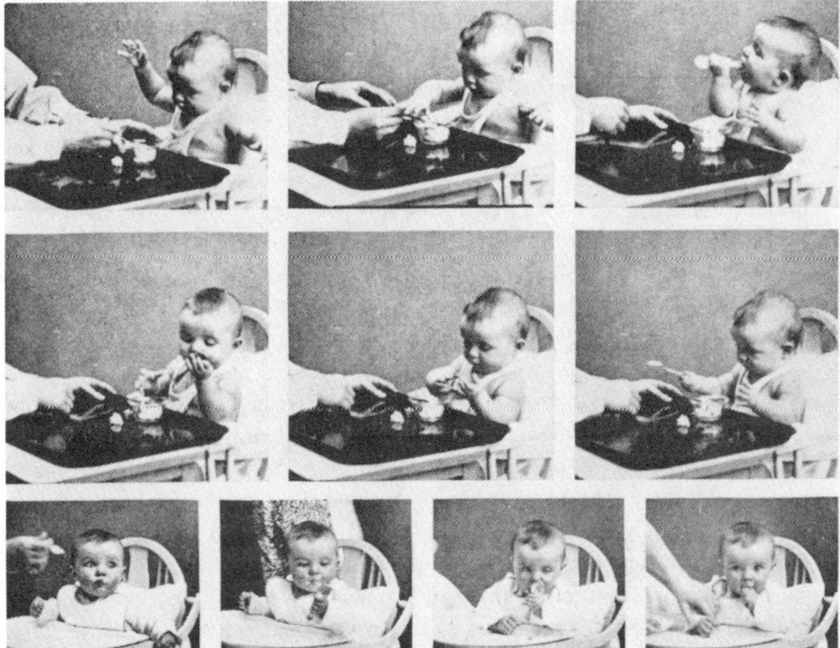

Figure 35. Eye-hand patterns at 32 weeks (Girl A.). At 32 weeks, alternate use of hands and repeated transfer are common. Although this child showed consistent leftward dominance, she uses her right hand during a bilateral stage, such as 32 weeks. (a,b,c) Grasps spoon with right hand and mouths handle, with rotation of forearm, (d,e,f) Transfers spoon to left hand; regards in transit and retransfers to right hand, (g,h,i,j) Manipulates spoon with left hand; eye incoordination tends to increase with attempts to insert spoon into mouth.

soon the cube goes back to the mouth or onto the table for further exploitation. The cycle of eye-hand behavior repeats itself with endless variations throughout the day, and throughout a series of days. The variations reflect the ceaseless morphogenesis which is transforming the total action system. A minutely organized structure is being laid down for more subtle and skillful visual performance.

Even now his eyes seize upon some identifying cue, as they show, for example, a preference based perhaps upon a visitor's hair color. He often discriminates strangers but usually adapts well to them. He has himself well in hand. He seems to take in a total situation and alternates with ease between self-directed and socially referred activity. He rather enjoys being passed from one lap to another in the family circle, but, left alone lying in his crib, he finds almost equal pleasure in bringing his feet into the field of vision for grasping and manipulation. Or his eyes may seize upon a piece of dangling string, which he will exploit with avidity.

Speed, dispatch, and abandon characterize his eye-hand behavior and his postural behavior. But he is in good equilibrium and typically presents an amiable union of self-containedness and sociality.

At 32 weeks of age he is not so self-contained. His reactions are less forthright and his face often wears a questioning, half-confused expression. He shows a greater sensitiveness in new situations and he needs more time to adjust to them. (This is not a favorable age for a visit to the doctor's office.) Even a familiar environment fatigues the child more readily because he has a deepening awareness of himself in relation to the environment. Such sensitiveness combined with assimilativeness is part of the process of growth and it involves his visual functions which are developing in close correlation with his social attitudes.

He watches with new penetration the actions and movements of people around him. He is more conscious of sounds in the next room, and betrays a dawning awareness of distance and of location. We cannot, of course, describe the subjective aspect of this awareness, but there is evidence of a heightened, even if diffuse, appreciation of the spatial intervals which separate him from an object of regard, or which separate two such objects. This appreciation is not a sophisticated judgment but a spontaneous interest. The infant senses in a new way his own personal status in a world of space. His motor reactions are less driven, more restrained, more tentative. He adjusts slowly to new surroundings because he apparently feels the spatial and the geographic novelty which comes with a change to an unaccustomed scene. Accordingly, he seems more sensitive than a month ago. He is quiet and watchful, often withdrawn.

Some of his timidities doubtless have their origin in the strangeness of his new visual experiences. Coincidentally, his auditory awareness takes on a projective character. He localizes sights and sounds well beyond the reach of his arms. He listens and looks expectantly when he hears approaching footsteps. Audition, now and later, serves to reinforce visual "projections" within the precincts of his familiar experiences. Language and social relationships play a part in the building up of his visualized space world. Folkways also help. It is almost a nursery game at this age to ask the baby: "Where is the kitty"? Where is Jimmy"? "Where is Granny"? His response is more than a mere conditioned reflex. Visual memory causes him to look in an accustomed place. This is an identification in space, a realization of a locus. Significantly enough, this interest in locality is, for the time being, more powerful and more conspicuous than the interest in motion. By the age of 36 weeks, he has a similar interest in motion as well. He likes to watch a ball as it moves toward him. He notices movements like the stirrings and gestures of persons nearby. He notes, in a mirror, the imaged movements of his own hands. His eyes follow a ball as it rolls across the field of his near vision. His auditory localization, likewise, is more formed and specific and goes further afield. He recognizes familiar sounds, such as the telephone bell. All this indicates a new projectiveness.

At 32 weeks, he used to cry for his meal as soon as he saw it. Now, at 36 weeks, he knows that it will move toward him and he can wait. He is less anxious; he has more mastery both of location and of movement. He is better oriented in space. He looks into distant space in a more penetrating manner. He peers into people's faces. He peers between the palings of his crib to see where an object has fallen. He peers into the cavity of an empty cup. We are not sure that he sees the bottom of that cup as bottom, but he is entering the domain of a third dimension. He even thrusts his hand part way into the cup. But his insight (this is almost a pun!) is very rudimentary. Optically speaking, his depth perception is still so meager that he has only a dim apprehension of container and contained.

Nevertheless, he is making new discriminations and exploitations of two side-by-side objects. This itself is a step toward tri-dimensional perception. At 32 weeks, he held a cube in each hand and looked from one cube to the other, and back again, without bringing them into decisive exploitive relationship—a visual forerunner of more definite combining manipulation. At 36 weeks, he takes a cube and pushes another cube with the one in hand; or he brings one cube against the side of another cube. He differentiates the string attached to the ring and manipulates it exploitively. By such tokens he shows a recognition of the posture and the relationship of two objects in space. He is just beginning to see them as solids and envelopes.

40-52 WEEKS

The motor equipment of the 40-week-old infant increases the radius, as well as the precision, of his occupations of space. He rotates his head and trunk with greater facility, sweeping his eyes freely across arcs of 180 degrees. His postural and arm movements are not as restricted as they were at 32 weeks, when he preferred the forward sectors of his environment. At 40 weeks, he tips his head well back to gaze upward. Vertical surfaces have a new appeal so he pulls himself to his feet. Oculomotor muscles, as well as legs and arms, share in that pull, which takes him into a new stratum of vision. He is also beginning to creep, and this further expands the scope of his ocular initiatives and of his visual experience.

During the last quarter of the first year, the infant identifies places by going to them. Given the freedom of the floor, he creeps to the threshold of the door and peers into the adjoining spaces. He is not likely to go too far out of bounds because his explorations are limited by his motor and emotional capacities. Freedom of movement, however, gives a new reality to distances, to locations, and to the grosser aspects of perspective. He is becoming sketchily oriented to major meridians of a radiating tridimensional space.

But the tridimensional world consists of minute distances, as well as of far reaches. And it is the minutiae of this world of intimate near vision with which the infant is preeminently concerned during the closing months of the first year. With his inquisitive index finger he punctures and penetrates the third dimension. He begins

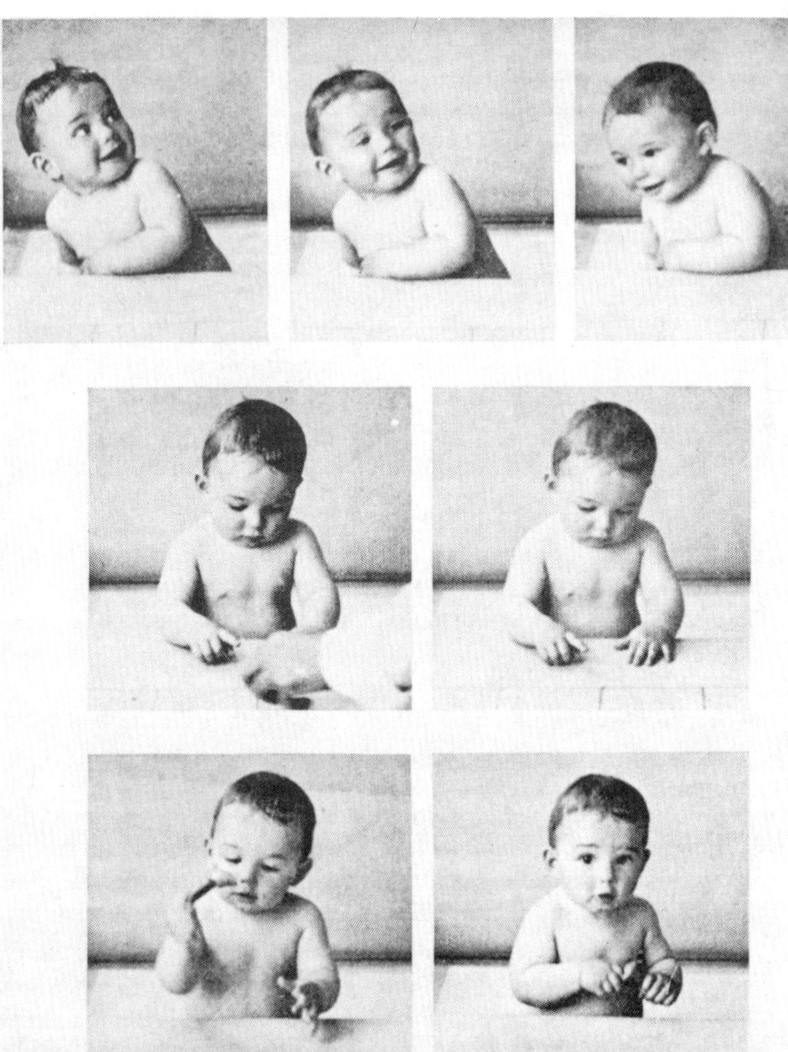

Figure 36. Visual Behavior patterns at 40 weeks (Boy D.). (a) Everts eyes leftward, (b) Everts eyes rightward, (c) Head everts rightward, following lead by eyes, (d) Regards incoming pellet and anticipates prehension with extended index, (e) Maintains regard on pellet, (f) Regards bell while manipulating, (g) Manipulates at times without maintaining regard on object.

to be analytic, both tactile-wise and ocular-wise. He segregates a single detail for attention, and he reacts in a successive and combining way to two details or to two objects. In the presence of more than one object, he manifests an awareness of more than one: a dim sense of two-ness, of container and contained, of solid and hollow, of top and bottom, of one side and the other side.

The 40-week-old infant also tends to respond to situations as a whole. He spreads his regard widely. Somewhat comprehensively he takes in a whole room, the whole mirror into which he looks, a whole mass of assembled cubes, and the whole person.

The 44-week-old infant is more given to focalized regard. In contrast to the 40-week age, he is apt to fixate a special object in a room and then spread his gaze to the rest of the room. Beginning with the face, he surveys a person from head to foot. An object does not have to be in motion to enlist his interest. He can sit and play with a single toy for a solid hour. During this play, he is likely to lift the toy obliquely and to regard it while he holds it aloft. This is another method of organizing the spatial domain.

By 48 weeks, this organizing takes on interesting refinements. For example, he pushes a ball a short distance then creeps for it, pushes it again for a distance and creeps toward it. He places an object with a decisive interest in the exact spot where it should go. During feeding, he exhibits a visually noteworthy pattern. Having placed a morsel of food in his mouth, he takes it out, looks at it intently and then puts it back again. (He is still organizing the spatial domain.) He greatly enjoys the rides in his carriage. He likes to stand up while the carriage is in motion, and likes also to watch the motion of cars, boats, animals and other objects. He shows a new awareness of twilight and dark corners and closets. During vigorous play, he often lowers his lids and blinks. He seems to enjoy the exercise of this protective blinking, as he noisily bangs his playthings. He likes to participate in repetitive nursery games such as "Where is the baby"? All these behavior patterns have visual connotations.

Thus the child steadily builds his spatial world through progressive elaborations of his action system. The gradualness of the development of his sense of depths is neatly reflected in his reaction to test objects which invite discriminating tridimensional responses—the cup and cube, ring and string, and formboard. At 40 weeks, the baby thrusts his hand into the cup and fingers a cube at the bottom, as though he were oblivious to the possibility of extracting the cube and unaware of the relationship between container and contained. But in another month he shows a new tendency to elevate his arms during playful manipulation of objects, and accordingly he seizes the cube, withdraws it, and re-thrusts his hand into the cup. At 1 year, he voluntarily releases a cube into the cup. The foregoing is a developmental paradigm which reflects the slow yet progressive stages by means of which the visual world of the infant undergoes tridimensional differentiation.

In the ring-and-string situation, the 40-week-old infant regards the ring and string as a single unit. At 44 weeks, he pays special regard first to the ring and then to the string. At 1 year, he secures the ring and crowns a bell with it, showing a certain realization of the permeability of space and the transposability of objects in space.

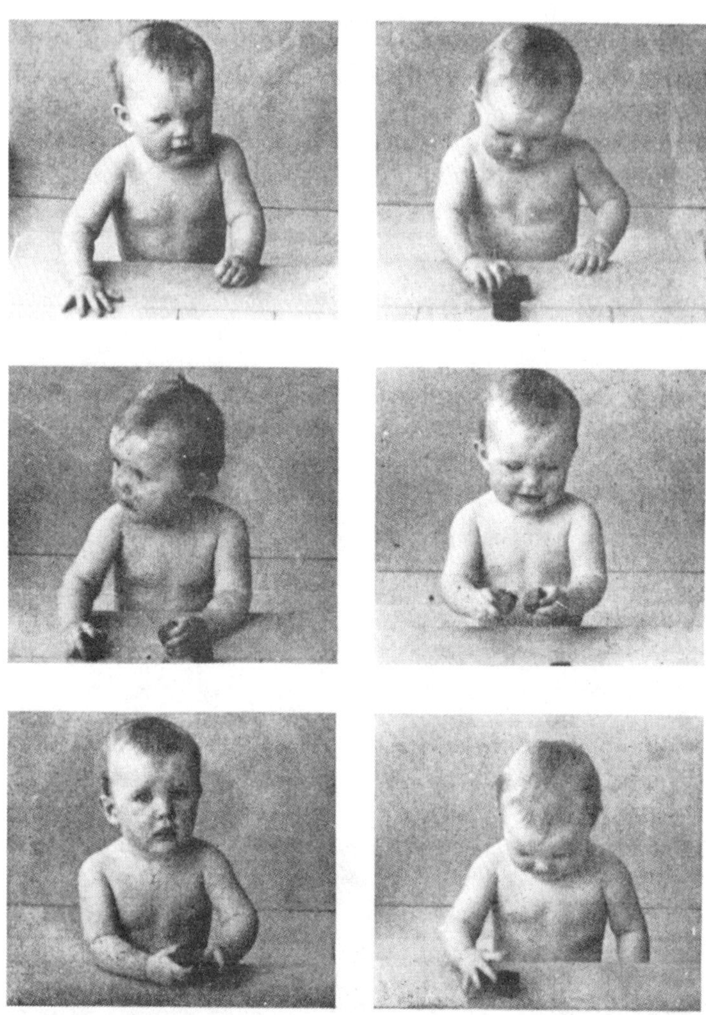

Figure 37. Visual behavior patterns at 1 year. (a) Regards incoming object with right-handed postural set, (b) Regards and manipulates at arm's length, (c) Regard diverts, but manipulation continues, (d) Pleasurable visual and manual combining, (e) Sober regard, without manual relaxation, (f) Releases cube with intensified regard and purposeful placement.

The formboard reveals a similar sequence. At 40 weeks, the infant fingers the round hole. At 44 weeks, he singles it out for selective visual regard. At 48 weeks, he brings a round block to the vicinity of the hole. At 1 year, he lifts the formboard bodily and peers through the round hole. This amusing pattern has philosophical implications. It indicates a certain awareness of the emptiness, as well as the contents of space. At any rate, the infant is no longer completely immersed in space, as he was when first he was born.

12 MONTHS

The year-old infant is in the midstream of developmental changes which come to more patterned fulfillment at about the age of 15 months. We can better interpret his behavior characteristics if we think of him as a 15-month-old child in the making. He is graduating from elementary babyhood. Simple toys do not engross him as much as they did formerly. He is a more social being and senses in a new way his own status in interpersonal situations. Sometimes this expresses itself in coyness.

To be sure, he usually adjusts better socially if his mother is present. But he likes to meet new people. He is rather inclined to repeat performances that are laughed at. He enjoys applause. He both imitates and reciprocates. He reciprocates in simple back-and-forth play, such as the to-and-fro rolling of a ball. He readily assumes a patterned give-and-take mood. He likes to "give" an object into a receiving hand and to have the object given right back; but he takes evident satisfaction in releasing it.

He exercises this new power of voluntary release in many different ways which involve the visual and the manual organization of his action system. Having "learned" how to grasp, he must learn how to let go. So he picks up one cube and drops it, picks up another and drops it, and picks up still another and drops that. The releases, being immature, are expulsive, but they modulate with time, and the ocular releases coordinate more smoothly with the manual.

His visual perceptions and manipulations show progress. He is much interested in buttons and buckles, in flowers and bright objects. He is aware of distinctive physical features—a wrinkled countenance, a bald head. He perceives emotional expressions. He picks up a spoon with a discriminating digital grasp of the tip of the handle. This betokens a refinement of spatial awareness.

His spatial sense of position and distance is likewise more sophisticated. In his exploitive play, he brings one object beside another or above another, or into another if the other is a hollow container. Being an experimentalist and a social imitator, he will even doff and don a cereal bowl as though it were a hat for his head. Held in lap, he raises his arms to gesture "up," he wriggles and looks down when he means "down." Such behavior patterns indicate increasing orientations in the visual domain.

Ears, as well as eyes, contribute to this orientation. The end organs of hearing are rigidly set in the sides of the head and lack the mobility which oculomotor muscles impart to the eyes. Nevertheless, hearing is a very ancient sense, and the infant

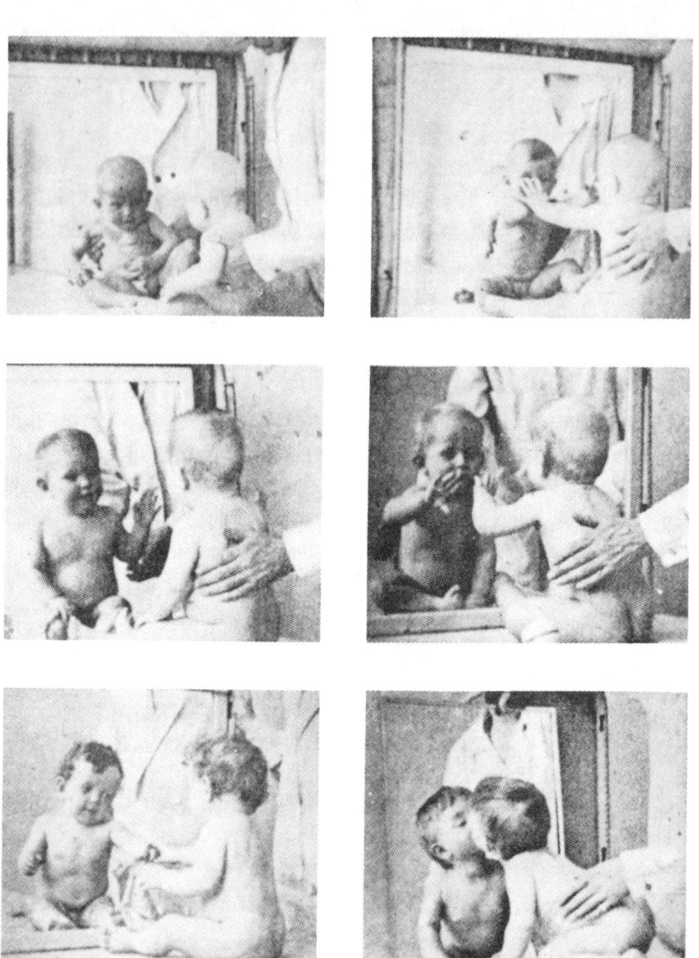

Figure 38. The infant's reactions to his mirror image at 16, 24, 32, 40, 44 and 52 weeks. (a) 16 weeks - Chiefly regards reflection of own eyes; vertical eye movements predominate, (b) 24 weeks - Regard more mobile; horizontal eye movements occur; pats mirror, (c) 32 weeks - Intently regards reflection of hand as he moves it, (d) 40 weeks - Increased experimental interest in self-induced movements, (e) 44 weeks - Contacts mirror in various exploitive ways, including poking, (f) 52 weeks - Reactions now social and playful (From Gesell and Ames: The Infant's Reactions to His Mirror Image.)

shows a new auditory wariness and also an increasing auditory awareness of distant places. He gives heightened attention to the bark of an unseen, distant dog. Vaguely, at least, he localizes a dog in far-away space.

15 MONTHS

The assumption of the erect posture came late in the history of the race. It comes by slow stages in the history of the individual. The 15-month-old child can attain the standing position unaided; he can walk alone, and usually has discarded creeping. Having attained upright steadiness on his outspread feet, one of his first and favorite exploits is to bend over and to look between his two legs. Vision will not be denied; space must be conquered!

Sitting, however, is much better established than standing at the age of 15 months. In the sitting posture, the infant shows versatility of head and eye movements. At one moment, his whole physique participates in an attitude of visual expectancy; at another moment, he looks away from a previous focus of interest, dissolving the total reaction with ease, and keeping both the visual and the manual components separately active. His eyes are not riveted to his manipulations, but shift ahead to anticipate the next move; or they fasten upon some fine detail analytically segregated from the total situation. He goes to extremes of flexion and extension, holding an object close to his eyes or at arm's length. He cannot deploy his eyes with equal ease while standing.

Seated, he enjoys following with his eyes moving objects, persons, and automobiles. He can tilt his head to the side and backward in visual pursuit. He visually pursues a moving car as far as he can, and then returns to the initial head posture to watch and to follow the next car. He likes to cast objects from the high chair and from the pen with an expectant interest in the destination of the object. When putting objects into a container, he keeps his eyes on the container. This again suggests that he is achieving an important discrimination between the movement of an object and the placement accompanied by that movement. He extends objects to a person and is visually interested in the fate of the object. He is beginning to relate objects to their remoter associations—his hat, for example, definitely suggests an excursion outdoors. Auditory awareness becomes more perceptive. He has a fear of strange and ominous sounds, like that of the vacuum cleaner.

He does much listening, and he listens with a far-away look as though eyes and ears shared in the act of distance projection. Sights and sounds become cues to one another and to life situations. If he wakens at night, he quiets as he looks at the far-away lights outside his window.

Of great psychological interest is the emergence of an awareness that other persons besides himself possess the function of vision. At about 15 months, he begins to use the words *look* and *see.* He points to an object of interest and says "See!" to invite the visual attention of another onlooker. This is a reciprocal interpersonal relationship which reminds us forcefully of the far-reaching social implications of vision. At 18 months this interpersonal relationship manifests itself in a striking way. The child pokes at the eyes of a doll or of a companion. On command, he readily points to his own eyes. They interest him. He will give them special attention again when he begins to draw the human figure.

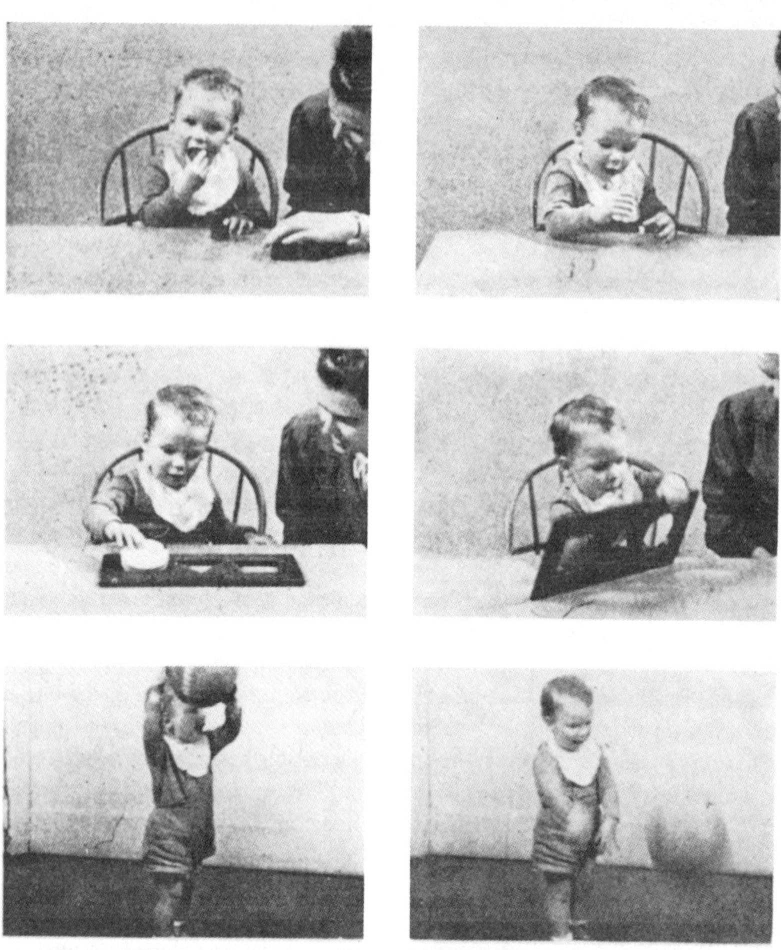

Figure 39. Visual behavior patterns at 15 months. (a) Mouths cube exploitively, as he looks forward, (b) Peers at pellet, which he has just dropped into bottle, (c) Places round block in round hole of formboard, (d) Attempts to place round block after board has been rotated, (e) Lifts ball high with two hands, preparatory to throwing, (f) Watches ball after throwing it.

The visual space world of the child is a product of growth. This perceptual world may be likened to an organism because it reflects in its every aspect the structure and the functions of the child's own action system—the child himself as an organism.

In an elementary sense, the child during the first year has acquired all the attributes of adult vision. But the development of human vision cannot be explained in terms of attributes. It must be pictured as a growing complex of structured functions which change with the advancing morphogenesis of the action system.

The 1-year-old child is only beginning to stand alone. He must learn to walk and to run, to turn corners, to turn knobs, to make vertical, horizontal, and oblique strokes with a crayon, to identify pictures and symbols. He must learn to adjust himself to the complex geography of his physical and social environment. By the age of 5, he will have performed countless acts of vision. Each act is conditioned by the maturity of his sensory-motor system at the time of performance. His visual skills and his temporary visual ineptitudes are growth phenomena.

CHAPTER 7
The Preschool Years

Growth is such a closely knit continuum that any lines drawn to subdivide age periods are necessarily arbitrary. Conventionally the period of infancy comprises the first two years. At the Yale Clinic, however, we have found that many 18-month-old children are behaviorally mature enough to join for a brief hour once or twice a week a small, well-supervised preschool nursery group. So we may reckon the preschool period as extending from 1 1/2 years to 5 years of age.

The developmental organization which takes place during this period is prodigious in amount and profound in its consequences. Vision is in the making, but not as an isolated function. The eyes are under constant necessity of coming into an effective relationship with a rapidly changing motor equipment. These changes involve the child's fine and delicate musculature, as well as far-reaching transformations in patterns of posture and locomotion. The sphincters of bladder and bowel must also come under control. Speech and respiratory mechanisms undergo intricate elaborations. Cultural demands multiply at a relentless rate, requiring countless interpersonal adjustments expressed in deportment, manners, morals, emotional controls, and adaptations to time and space.

It is easy to underestimate the intricacy of the organizing processes which take place conjointly in all fields of behavior—motor, language, adaptive, and personal-social. The correlation of visual functions with the functions of posture, locomotion, and manipulation is particularly significant. Normally these functions organize harmoniously. Visual defects and deviations express themselves not so much in failures of acuity as in discoordinations, various forms of awkwardness, faulty timing, and hesitations. Closely observed, these atypical preschool behavior patterns have significance for early diagnosis, prevention, and treatment of visual difficulties.

18 MONTHS

The 18-month run-about has graduated from mere babyhood. He is emancipating himself from the lap; he is so much on the loose that he often needs a harness more than apron strings. He is in a dart-and-dash phase of his visual-motor organization, which results in multiple invasions of an expanding environment. He is entering the preschool period of development.

He strains at the leash, lugs, tugs, pushes, drags, pounds, dumps. He wields a paint brush with bold daubs; he shifts the brush from hand to hand because he is in a bilateral phase of motor organization similar to that of the 28-week-old infant. His motor drive is so strong that his eyes often seem to follow, rather than to direct, his precipitate activities. But eyes and action system are operating in an ever-varying

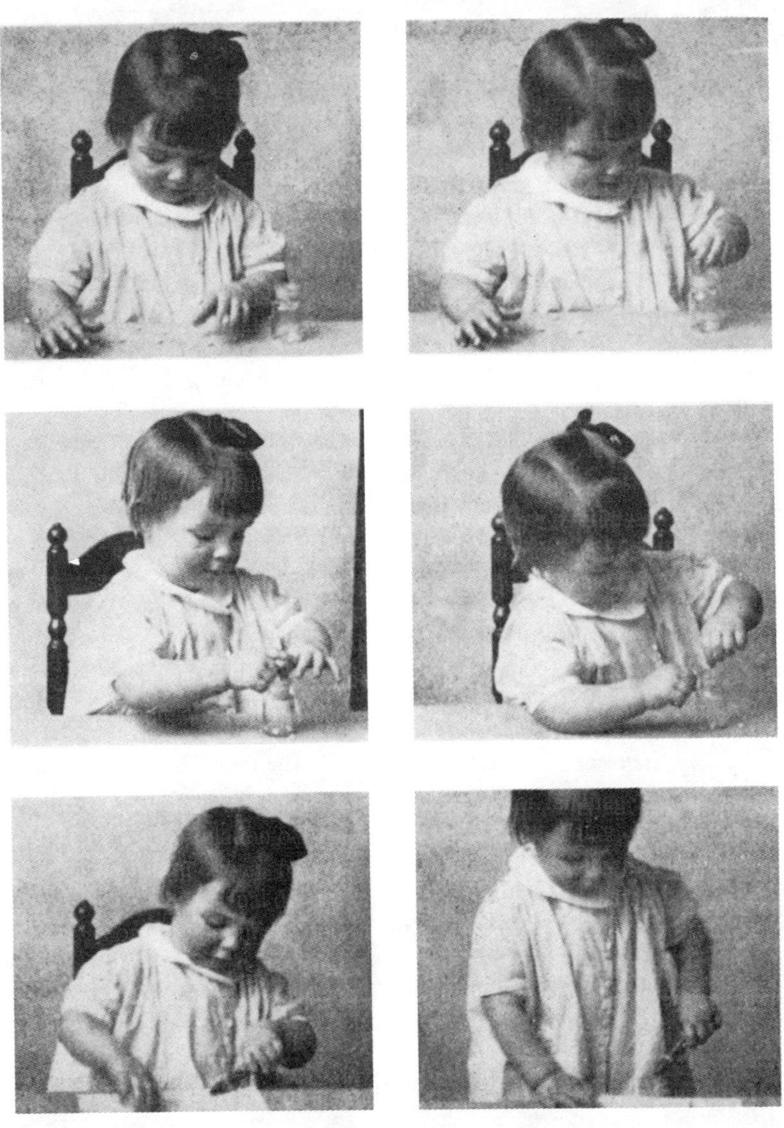

Figure 40. Visual behavior patterns at 18 months. (a) A left-handed girl (also pictured in Figure 41) approaches pellets with left hand; right hand poised to assist, (b) Picks up pellet in left hand and inserts in bottle, (c) Brings up the free hand, thus combining right and left, (d) Shifts whole body to the left to maintain a central orientation to the bottle, (e) Wields the crayon with left hand, (f) Spontaneously stands up to continue the stroking.

interaction which in time confers upon him an increasing sense of places and placements. He attends chiefly to the here and now. He wants everything he sees, but his localization of far-off objects is crude; he runs toward them headlong. He plunges uncritically into nooks and corners and byways, and goes up and down stairs. By one device or another, he carries a toy from place to place—abandons it, returns to it, and resumes with postural twists and variations, making sudden rapid turns of 180 degrees or even walking backward. It is as though he were deliberately exploring and discovering new vectors of space. He is a rather bungling explorer because he functions in an episodic and one-track manner.

Nevertheless, this extreme mobility does not exclude a predilection for specific place associations. He likes to help put groceries in their places where they belong; he knows where his father's slippers should be. He resists a strange toilet—he wishes his familiar own. Once seated in a chair, he likes to stay seated in full possession of that place. If he gets up, he wants to return. He likes to replace objects in their proper places. All this denotes a new kind of spatial manipulation which involves his whole body, as well as his oculomotors and his exploitive hands.

In his exploitations, perhaps because of his bilaterality, he shows a predilection for vertical sectors. He builds towers; he has difficulty arranging his building blocks horizontally. He piles three blocks upon a formboard, one upon another. In some measure, he even invades the unseen vertical sector behind him. He does this by a curious simultaneous bilateral upsweep of the arms which brings the hands behind his head, near shoulder level. In this manner he can lift a large ball, hurling it up, over, and behind him. This movement pattern may be a preparatory developmental step which leads ultimately to bilateral tossing and hurling, and later to unilateral throwing. In modified form, we thus see the lineaments of the tonic-neck reflex (TNR) and the symmetrotonic reflex (STR), which were so naively exhibited when the infant was in a supine stage of development. The infant is now in an upright stage on his two feet, and he must develop new visual motor coordinations which are ontogenetically linked with more primitive TNR and STR patterns.

21 MONTHS

Growth is now so rapid that by the age of 21 months the general behavior picture shows a definite change. The eyes have assumed a leading and more directive role. The 21-month-old child, therefore, is less driven, less impulsive. Indeed, he stops to stare, he freezes as though fascinated. This is the very opposite of impetuous 18-month rushing. In such opposites we glimpse a developmental logic—the reciprocal accentuation of paired but counterpoised reactions.

His increased visual appreciation of the spatial aspects of interpersonal relationships makes him timorous or suspicious at the sight of a stranger, makes him cower when the stranger approaches too suddenly. But when visiting away from home with his mother, the 21-month-old child is content to sit quietly in a chair, visually following the activities in the new surroundings.

At home, also, he does a good deal of intensive looking, especially at the household activities, which he begins to imitate sketchily, and which he will mimic more dramatically in a few more months. He also exhibits a new awareness of the fixtures

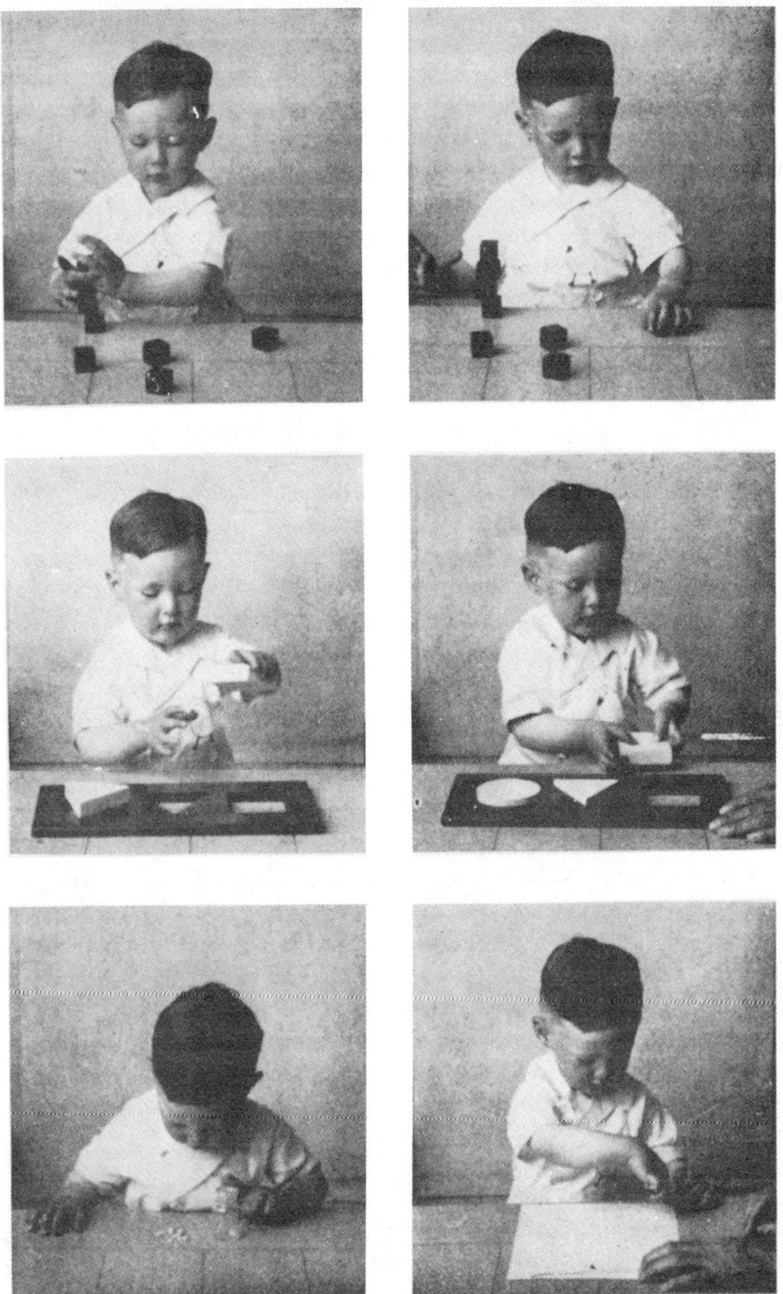

Figure 41. Visual behavior patterns at 2 years. (a) Eyes lead hands by glances to side. Builds tower to right, beyond shoulder line, (b) Eyes maintain fixation while hand grasps, (c) Eyes again lead and direct next move, (d) Finally solves the whole formboard, (e) Leans forward to sharpen regard, (f) Intently regards horizontal crayon stroke.

of a room. He exploits the electric plug, the window, the radiator, door, wallpaper, plaster, curtains. He enlarges his spatial domain by climbing upon chairs and tables and window sills, but his interpretation of intervals of space is still very imperfect. Children of this age, and during the next few months, are especially prone to accident from falling out of a window.

When out for a walk, the 21-month-old child enters byways more knowingly. He is more cautious. His spatial and personal orientations to the physical environment, however, are tender and precarious. Therefore, he shows a tendency to cling inordinately to some favorite object when he goes to bed. When he goes to nursery school, he may take such an object and cling to it throughout the whole morning. Perhaps the object has a fetish-like property to make him feel at home even though he is abroad. Emotional associations color his orientations to spaces and places.

Not having much facility in the psychological manipulation of space, he cleaves jealously to hearth and home. This is not a favorable age for a family to change its domicile. It may take a child a few months to overcome the anxieties that go with spatial dislocation and to accomplish a reorientation in a new abode. Evidently, visual functions and personality reactions are akin.

2 YEARS

The typical 2-year-old is, without doubt, a preschooler. He can run without falling; he can use words to express, to report, and to control his behavior; he can pull on a garment; he can keep a spoon right side up as he puts it into his mouth; he can turn the pages of a book singly and identify an increasing number of pictures.

He uses his eyes more flexibly. He watches what he does as he does it. He gives discriminating regard to the movement of his own scribble, for example, when he imitates a circular stroke. Eyes and hands are somewhat less closely associated. He can look and then act. He can interrupt his looking, stop his activity, and then give it full attention again. He looks at a container and then looks at an object, then shifts his regard to the container again before placing the object therein. He can fit simple sectional toys together. He can rotate his forearm to turn a doorknob. He likes to watch the movement of wheels and the whirling disk of the phonograph. He likes to look at the moon.

Increased visual discriminativeness is shown in his fondness for small objects, miniature cars, little books. At times, he evinces a dread of large formidable objects and may even refuse to enter a large hallway on account of its size. Again we glimpse a linkage between emotional and spatial reactions. He is gaining command of space words. These words come into requisition to guide his orientation and to allay his ever-ready anxieties. He now comprehends "where." He has no concept of the intervening space between *here* and *there*, but he achieves a sense of place and of security when his "where?" is answered with "home," "office," "big building," and

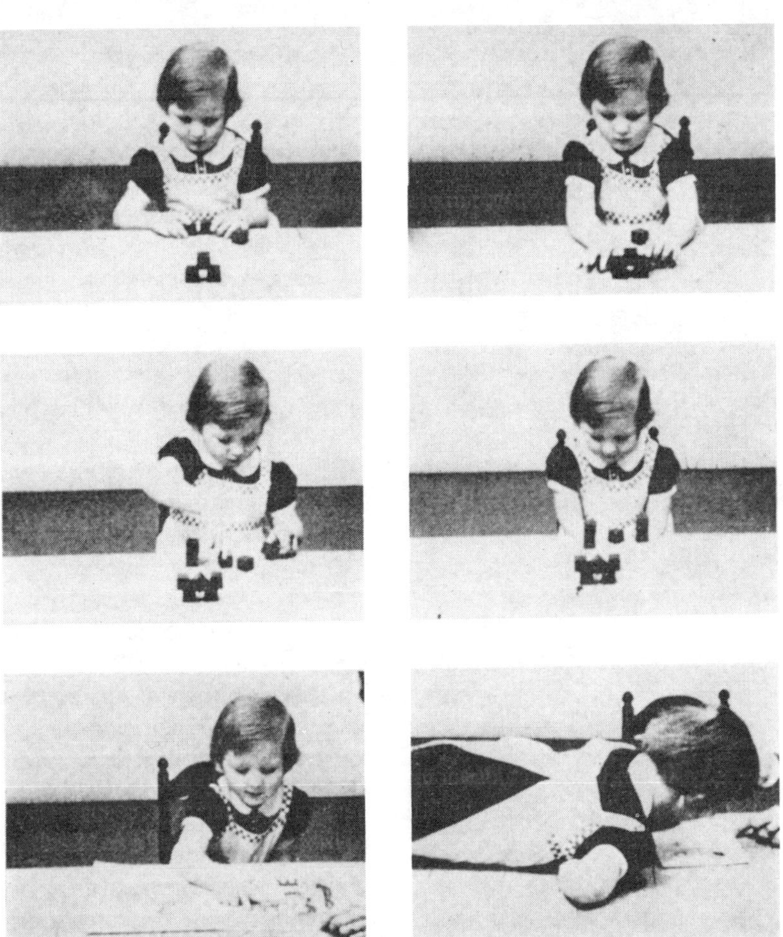

Figure 42. Visual behavior patterns at 2 1/2 years (Girl T). (a) Attempts to copy bridge in near sector, (b) When unsuccessful, builds out from body close to model, (c) Reaches over tower of two as she grasps cube in right hand, (d) Has made a partial copy of gate, (e) Points to pictures while talking about them, (f) Lies on table as tensional outlet, but continues to respond.

so on. This is an elementary but significant form of localizing projection. And yet his sense of place is more sophisticated than formerly. He looks for missing objects even in the dark and, conversely, he himself likes to hide toys. When out for a walk (and he likes to walk great distances), he can turn his head and eyes to the side to regard an object in the margins of his vision. He picks out curbings and walls to walk on, and he is beginning to respect curbs. He uses eyes and hands in more flexible association. By all these tokens, his visual behavior seems more mature.

2 1/2 YEARS

During the third year, the child makes a manifold transition out of babyhood. The complexity of that transition is manifested in the bewildering behavior traits of the

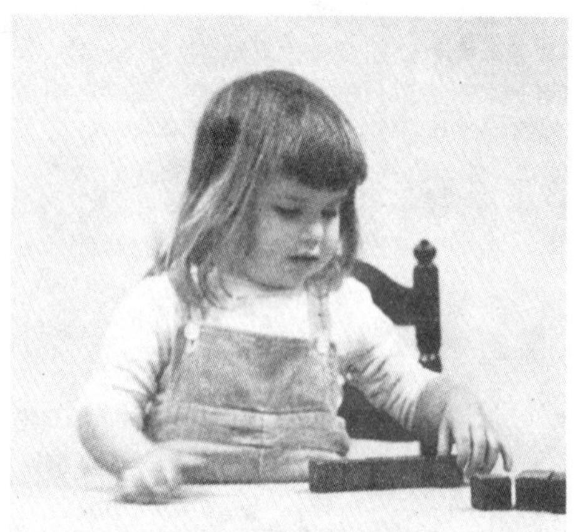

Figure 43. 2-year-old builds wall.

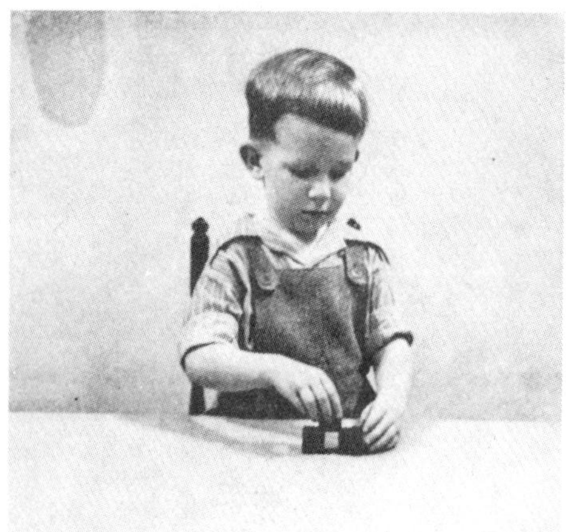

Figure 44. 3-year-old builds bridge of three blocks.

2 1/2-year-old. We shall etch these traits in sharp outline, and later contrast them with the traits of a typical 3-year-old. Our purpose is not to exaggerate a single temporary phase, but rather to indicate the developmental dynamic which organizes the child's changing visual world.

To understand the psychology of the 2 1/2-year-old, we must invoke the principle of bipolarity. He is just becoming aware of the inevitable dualisms which bisect all nature. He is confronted with a host of paired opposites which are novel to him, however axiomatic they may be to the adult. Some of these opposites pertain simply to the geometry of space: up and down, in and out, vertical and horizontal, back and forth, head and tail, top and bottom, back door and front door, on and under, high and low, far and near, front buttons and rear buttons, here and there. Facile differentiation of these simple (?) opposites requires complex developments in the field of vision. Indeed the entire action system is involved, for there is another host of opposites which concern personal-social activities and relationships: *you and I, yes and no, come and go, grab and throw, sleep and waking, give and take, fast and slow, now and then, person and object.*

In terms of development the task of the young child is first to sense these opposites, then to choose between them, and later to modulate one alternative in relation to the other. How is this accomplished? Chiefly through growth guided by experience.

When a pair of spatial opposites is barely sensed, the organism is (with respect to these opposites) in a state of neutral or indifferent equilibrium. The child is likely to get things "wrong side up;" he is susceptible to reversals; he may place a turtle on its back rather than on its feet; he may even place a wheeled toy upside down rather than on its wheels. If he perceives that the turtle in the aquarium is wrong side up, he may try to turn the whole aquarium upside down. He is orienting.

Much of the "perversity" of the 2 1/2-year-old is due to the ambiguity and confusions of a two-way street not yet under traffic control. Eyes and intelligence do not automatically tell him which direction is right and which is wrong. Eyes and hands are insufficiently coordinated, and also insufficiently emancipated. He must bring eyes and hands to a higher level of reciprocal interaction.

He resorts to peculiar devices to achieve this interaction. Picture him in a nursery group, seated at a table. He is playing with a mobile toy; he pushes the toy back and forth with rhythmic tempo, maintaining an intensely sustained regard. The repetitive pattern seems to energize his capacity to look; under the spell, he may even be able to release his regard momentarily and then bring it back to the activity in hand. But if he is even briefly interrupted by an external distraction, he loses his orientation. His eyes fail to return to the object of interest. He is so completely lost that he asks, "Where is it?" even when "it" is right before his eyes.

This behavior pattern is noteworthy because it reveals the precariousness of the visual-spatial world when it is in the 2 1/2-year zone of immaturity. At the age of 3, the foregoing pattern might almost augur a retardation of development. The 3-year-old is much more securely and flexibly oriented in his space world. He can use his eyes and hands more independently and with self-containment. He can look away and then return to the task in hand.

The 2 1/2-year-old is rather suggestible in his motor responses. He is very susceptible to marginal, peripheral, and moving stimuli. He may be heedless of verbal injunctions if you ask him to go from one place to another, but if you yourself go, he is likely to follow. He is lured by movement when it takes him into outward space. He is, however, alarmed by movement which comes toward him. He is becoming aware of the threat of a backing truck. The fear is likely to enter his dreams.

All this means that he is making an important distinction with reference to outgoing and incoming spatial dimensions. He is also sensitive to immobilization. For some peculiar reason which is bound up with the ontogenesis of vision, he often stops an activity completely in order to regard something. He is also aware of another child's immobilization and will not approach him unless he moves.

Under home or nursery school auspices, he cannot be successfully managed by direct approach. He responds instead to peripheral approach. Under visual examination, he can be enticed to project his attention to a distant target. The range of his adjustments, both near and far, however, is rather restricted, which suggests that maturation and time are essential for the further expansion of his visual world. He will modulate his orientations better when his range widens.

The 2 1/2-year-old may be highly dependent on manual contact. If he loses such contact with the object, he seems to lose sight of it. He cannot reidentify it in space by an adaptive, voluntary, visual adjustment. The fact that such an apparent "blanking out" can occur in a normal child at this stage of development confirms our thesis that vision is an act, almost a creative act, which requires total and detailed participation of the entire action system. Only through continuous motor pursuit and exploitation of objects does the child at this age acquire the fund of experience necessary for a more mature type of visual awareness. In the process of acquiring that awareness, his demeanor and adjustments vaguely suggest phyletically primitive patterns of visual behavior. It is an extraordinary fact that, as a child approaches the 2 1/2-year level of maturity, he may sometimes *look* with such overpowering intensity that his legs collapse under him.

The 2 1/2-year-old, lacking flexibility, sets up rituals to protect himself from the wear and tear conflict of opposites. Having established a going-to-bed ritual, he holds to it rigidly to insure the end result. Parents learn that if they disrupt the ritual they invite a return of the emotional conflict and of embattled opposites. Being in a paradoxical phase of growth, a child at one time overfixates in an indistractible manner, while at other times he yields to multiple foci of interest, going freely from one thing to another in a highly distractible manner. Left to his own devices in a playroom, he plays briefly with each and every toy, and in a half hour the room is in complete disarray and untidiness. Yet he has a sense of place and order, which on occasion he affirms with paradoxical intensity. He does not want the position of objects on a mantle to be changed; he may have a wave of anxiety if any of them disappears; he expects a chair to remain in a given corner; he wants it to be "right there" (a dogmatic "right" is a characteristic word in his vocabulary); he may even insist that the chair be oriented at a fixed and precise angle.

All these patterns of behavior are not as unreasonable as they seem on the surface. They are governed by a hidden logic of development which requires that the organism shall make both multiple and intensified contacts in the manipulation of space and of life situations. Modulation between extremes comes with further maturation.

3 YEARS

Three years is an organizing age period. Many of the earlier oppositions are resolved, and tangential tendencies are contained. This is shown in the personal-social attitudes of the 3-year-old, as well as in his impersonal motor behavior. He uses the pronoun "we" in a manner which signifies that he is relating himself integratively to his mother, rather than pitting himself against her as he was wont to do when he was in a more bipolar phase. His eye-hand activities, likewise, are more unified and rounded out. At 2 1/2 years, his painting went out of bounds, leaping from the paper, to the easel, to the floor. At 3 years, the painting is confined to the paper and designs are emerging. At 2 1/2, he is more interested in process

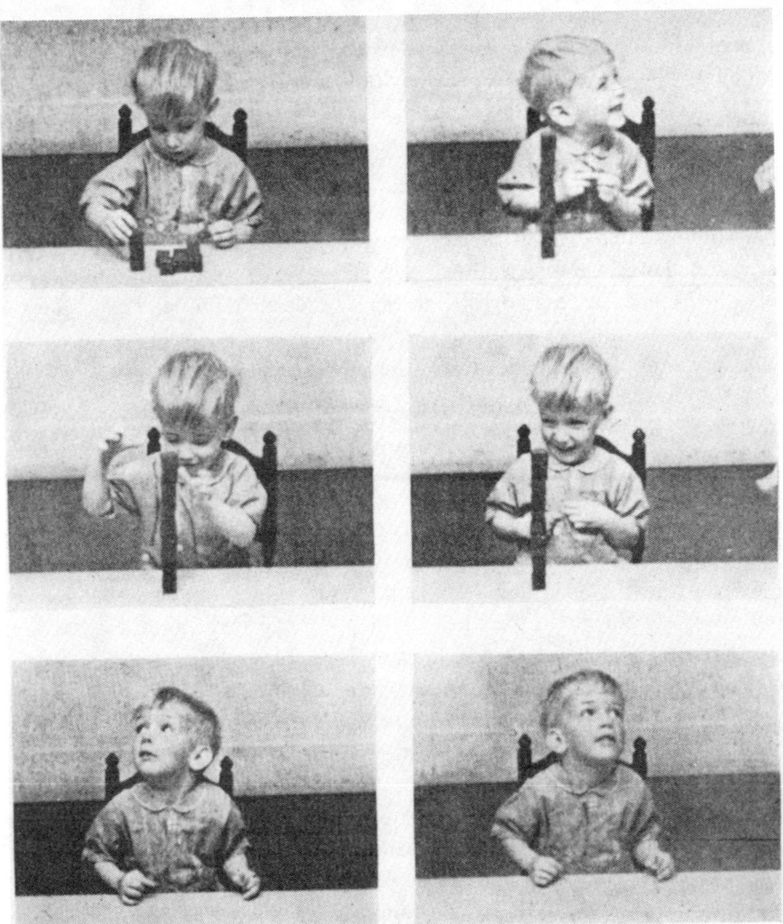

Figure 45. Visual behavior patterns at 3 years (Boy D.D.). (a) Builds tower to the right of the sagittal plane; alternates from right to left hand in placing cubes, (b) Tower has wavered; he laughs with examiner when it stands, (c) Places 10th cube successfully and withdraws hands cautiously, (d) Surveys the standing tower with delight, (e,f) Eyes sweep from left to right, and right to left, as he looks up at lights and asks questions about them.

than product when he builds with blocks, when he scrubs his hands, when he works in clay. The 3-year-old, in contrast, shows more balance and order in his block-building; he molds the clay into balls, cakes, and strips, and he names his products. And as he works at his constructions, he can deploy his hands without riveting his eyes on the task; his eyes take a more directive role, and they may rove inspectionally without associated head movements. He can plan somewhat in advance, whereas the 2 1/2-year-old often seems to go forward without a sense of destination.

The 3-year-old surveys his constructions; he casts his eyes up and down the tower which he has built; he works from the center and returns to center. When working from a model, he looks with ease from task to model to task, poising his hand expectantly for the next move. This kind of eye-hand control contrasts sharply with the often preponderating developmental draft toward periphery which is typical of the 2 1/2-year-old. But even this centrifugal drift was anchored to the central citadel of the growing action system, and in due course was counterpoised thereby.

Accordingly the 3-year-old is much more completely oriented in a space world. He displays a new interest in landmarks, recognizing and anticipating them when he is away from home, out for a walk or a ride. He may naively think that all cars going in his direction must be going also to his own destination. He shows the same naiveté in associating persons with specific places. He is bewildered if he meets his nursery school teacher downtown because she is dislocated and not in her accustomed locale. Nevertheless, we must credit him with a sense of location and of destination more sophisticated than he has hitherto shown.

He is also more interested in the wholeness of things, and in what Gestaltists would call closure. Although he likes a birthday cake, he may for a moment regret to see its symmetry broken with a carving knife. He feels it acutely when one of the wheels of a toy car is lost. This is all part of a growing esthetic sense which, of course, is based on developments in the maturity of his visual perception. He has a new awareness of light and of darkness, and may even show a trace of anxiety when he beholds a darkly colored person or a peculiarly colored object. Incidentally, it may be noted that some 3-year-olds show a new interest and preference for the color blue, whereas at 2 1/2 the preference was for yellow and at 2 for red.

Three is a nodal age, a kind of coming-of-age. There is less negativism, less vacillation. A 3-year-old rather likes to make a choice when the choice is within the realm of his experience. He is more sure of himself. Emotionally, he is less turned in on himself. He seems to fit into the culture more comfortably. His whole action system, for the time being, is in better working equilibrium—hence his good reputation; hence the approval of his elders.

3 1/2 YEARS

The action system of the growing child is continuously in process of formation and transformation—of organization, reorganization, and re-reorganization. When the rival and counterpoised components of this intricate system are in relative balance, the stream of development flows smoothly and reflects on its even surface well-configured patterns of behavior. The self-assured, self-contained, amenable 3-year-old typifies a period of relative equilibrium, during which his growth gains are consolidated—if we may manage to think of a metaphorical stream in terms both of structure and of flow.

In some children, this composed period is rather brief. In all children it gives way to a period of transition when the nascent components of higher forms of behavior stir within the growth stream, awakening new tension, new rivalries, new attractions and repulsions. The sensitive, tentative 3 1/2-year-old typifies this transition. He is beset by these growth forces, which are beneficent, even though they sometimes seem to confuse him, to freeze him into immobility, to bind him, or even to threaten him with psychologic fission. Normally he is not overcome, he is only made aware, and by cautious, experimental utilization of his multiple awarenesses, he becomes oriented at a higher level to the space-time world, and the personal-social world, both of which center in his private self. So steadily and progressively does he orient himself that at the age of 4 years he is forthright where before he was hesitant; he is decisive or defiant where before he was uncertain or anxious.

A developmental kind of anxiety is a cardinal characteristic of the 3 1/2-year-old. This anxiety has the quality of refined awareness, rather than of primitive fear. The delicately effortful play of his facial muscles betrays his inner state, which is not one of withdrawal, but which is a piquant seeking and a reaching into strange experience. The effort may be so fragile (because so new) that he may ask you not to distract him: "Don't talk," "Don't laugh," "Don't look at me!" He needs simplification of environment. He easily loses a trail; his beginnings are better than his terminations; he tends to see one side of an object or situation, to the partial exclusion of the other. He does not perceive bilateral things as a whole. It takes an insightful mother to understand his peculiar perplexities in the blended worlds of persons and things, even though he has two eyes with which to see! The implications of these behavior traits for the function of vision may well be far-reaching. Suffice it now to say that this is an important age for both the origin and the resolution of strabismus, which has a developmental basis.

The gross, the fine, and the skeletal muscles, as well as the oculomotors, are involved in the developmental transition which inevitably affects the total action system. There is a pervasive incoordination, manifested in faulty timing and poor modulation of movements. There is a definite increase in stumbling and a fear of high places. The hands often are tremulous and awkward. Dominance in handedness undergoes shifts and confusions. Stuttering, tensional chewing, nail biting, nose picking, eye blinking, increased salivation, and inexpert spitting appear on the scene, usually transiently. These symptoms exacerbate with fatigue, and the 3 1/2-year-old is given to fatigue on those days when he tries out and exercises at some length his developing capacities. His coordination difficulties are likely to bring tears when he is tired, and when he is confronted with the motor tasks of eating, of dressing, or of excessive decorum.

On close analysis, many of these difficulties prove to stem from immature visual-motor orientations in the space-time world, which are also reflected in his emotional needs at this age. This is transparently demonstrated by the performance tests of building and drawing. Consider the revealing test of building a bridge in imitation of a model. The model consists of two base cubes spanned by a third one-inch cube.

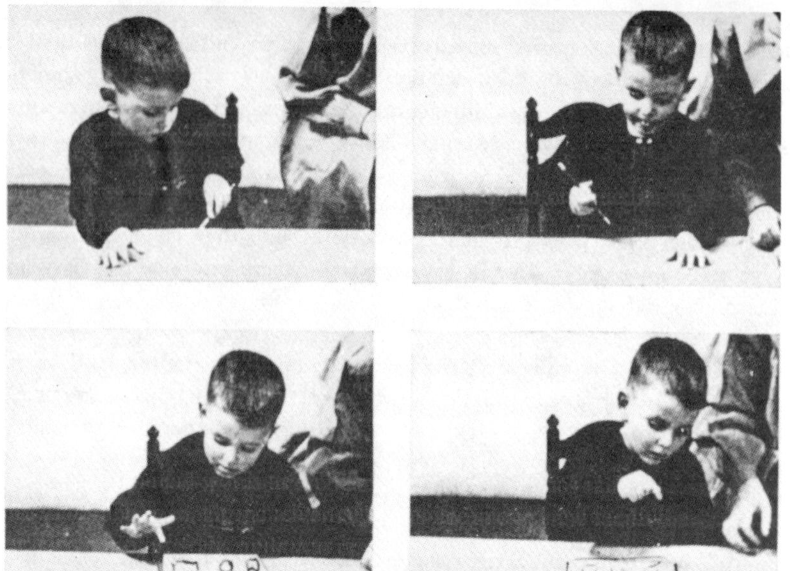

Figure 46. Visual behavior patterns at 3 1/2 years. (a) Right-handed boy wields pencil with left hand, (b) Shifts pencil to right hand, holding it awkwardly; projects tongue, (c) Fingers and tongue extend as he searches for a matching form, (d) Tongue retracts and fingers flex as he locates the matching form.

The 3-year-old takes a cube in each hand and brings the two cubes so close together that they may touch at their median surfaces. He places the spanning third cube centrally on top, then grasps the two base cubes simultaneously and tries to pull them apart to widen the gap between. This he finds difficult; sometimes he does not succeed. The set of his eye-hand coordination impels him to converge toward the midplane.

Now, the approach of the 3 1/2-year-old is typically different. It is strongly bilateral, but he is apt to place the two base cubes much too far apart; then, by one or two replacements, he brings them nearer together. The pull of the eye-hand coordination is divergent, the very opposite of what it was at the earlier maturity level. Here is an instructive reminder that the developmental organization of the space world of the child is not a simple global phenomenon, but an exquisitely minute process that leads to a multiplex occupation of what otherwise would be behaviorally empty space. The experimental manipulations and orientational "errors" characteristic of this stage of maturity show that the child is entering numerous new facets of space in his near visual field. He may arrange the three cubes in proper contiguity, but on a horizontal plane instead of on a vertical, a "flat bridge." Or he may reverse in space and attempt to place the base cubes on top, an "upside-down bridge." All this indicates that the construction of his space world is now in unstable equilibrium at a growing margin. When he seizes and manipulates an object he poises his hands in new attitudes and moves them in a forward spiraling manner, which suggests that maturational changes in his neuromotor equipment are prompting him to explore and exploit spatial relationships in a new way.

For this reason, the whole now loses some of its recent wholeness. He does not envisage a cross as a unitary design, but he constructs it piecemeal by three or four separate strokes when he copies it. The cross, as it were, falls apart into so many segments. He is aware of mutilations in persons and things. Likewise, his space world is less continuous. He sees objects effectively in the near and in the relatively distant sectors, but may lose sight of those in intermediate sectors. He often complains about not being able to see, as though he had difficulty in manipulating space. When he has a book in hand, he holds it very close to his eyes or he retracts his head for better vision. He likes to look at the book as he listens to the story which is read aloud to him.

He projects himself rather literally, or perhaps we should say kinesthetically, into the pictures of the book; he walks the pathway to the pictured house; he worms himself through the door; he becomes a rider in the pictured wagon. This projection pattern is very characteristic of the imaginative 3 1/2-year-old. It accounts for his tendency to create and adopt imaginative human companions. The companions are really projections of his expanding self. He endows them with synthetic names like Eka-a-Tuke, Bissle Bambo, Sookey and Sakey. The very names suggest the psychologic fluidity of this transitional stage of development. Indeed, the incidence of imaginary personal companions comes to a peak at about the age of 3 1/2 years. These imaginary figments are a developmental device for organizing and orienting the child in his complex personal-social world. They serve, at a fantasy level, as vehicles for defining all sorts of positive and negative interpersonal relationships. They are counterparts of the various visuomotor maneuvers which the child uses to define relationships in physical space. Inasmuch as the action system is unitary, similar developmental dynamisms operate in all fields of behavior.

4 YEARS

The 4-year-old is assertive and expansive. The key to his psychology is his high energy drive, which results in bursts of motor activity and bubbles of mental activity. He races, hops, jumps, skips, climbs with abandon. He also uses words with abandon. He enjoys imaginative antics and flights of fable and fancy. He tells tall tales, sometimes with bravado. He is lively and mobile. He has lost the tentativeness and anxiousness of the 3 1/2-year-old level. He is less entangled with his impulses and adventures. He is blithe rather than hesitant. Although he has not settled down to the compact stability which is characteristic of the 5-year-old, he has a relatively stable mental organization. Despite his tangential tendency, he does not get too detached from his moorings. But in his dramatic play, in his drawing, in his language, and in his mental imagery, he enjoys improvisations and indulges in agile variations. In comparison, the 5-year-old is deliberate, configured and self-contained.

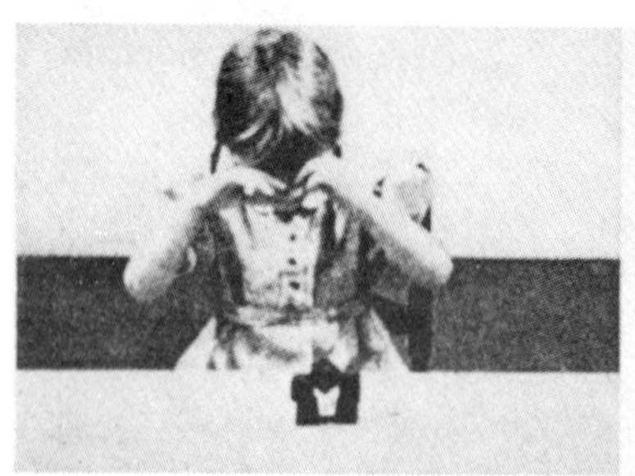
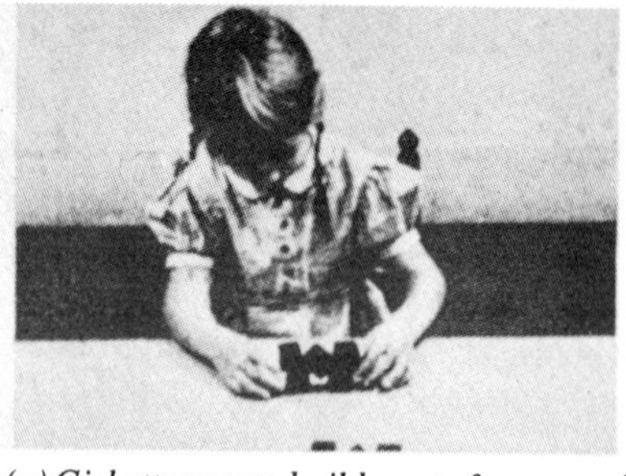

Figure 47. Visual behavior patterns at 4 years. (a) Girl attempts to build a gate from a model; recognizes structure to be inaccurate, rubs eyes as a tensional outlet, (b) Rebuilds correctly; note the characteristic symmetry of hand posture.

The visuomotor and action patterns of the 4-year-old, therefore, show a certain looseness, ranginess, and spread. His mental organization is fluid, yet he is able to take in a whole situation in a flash of perception. He is beginning to grasp large concepts like the world, the sky, the ocean. Collective nouns and generalizing phrases emerge in his speech.

His motor patterns show a tendency toward symmetry. He displays a rhythmic type of mirror posturing when he manipulates with both hands. This tendency toward symmetry gives him an awareness of two sides of a configuration. Sometimes he even sees a circle as a divided whole, made up of two semicircles. He reacts in short spurts of perception. For brief periods he manifests a strong focalized regard. But his kinesthetic memory is brief, and his energy drive easily leads to a ballooning or expansive reaction. He tends to balloon when he uses a crayon, magnifying out of proportion any detail which engages his interest.

The space world of the 4-year-old is enlarging. He makes harum-scarum thrusts to widen his horizons. Home can no longer contain him. He much prefers to play out-of-doors. Even his play yard becomes too confining, so he climbs the fence. He may wander too far and get lost, although he also respects established boundaries. He can look both ways before crossing a street, but he is apt to dart too quickly. He likes to go on excursions—to the fire station and to the dairy. He would prefer to return by a "different" route. He likes diversities that will multiply his orientations. For similar reasons, he is a great neighborhood visitor.

On all these counts, 4 impresses us as a conspicuously growthsome period of life. The transition of the 3 1/2-year stage are best understood when considered as a passage from the 3- to 4-year level. The 4-year-old characteristics, likewise, are better understood when regarded as a developmental reorganization and extension of 3 1/2-year-old traits, and as a preparation for the solid conservatism of the 5-year-old. Five is a nodal age. Four is fluid, but 5 is in focus.

CHAPTER 8
The School Years

This chapter embraces the years from 5 to 10. We begin with 5 years because it is a nodal age, a maturity level which marks both the beginning and the end of a growth epoch. The developmental changes which take place in the first five years of life are more swift and dramatic than those which take place in the remaining half of the decade. The maturity difference of twelve weeks between a 16-week-old infant and a 28-week-old infant is more evident than the difference of twelve months between a 6- and a 7-year-old child. In a sense, psychologic growth slows down during the school years, and the annual changes are not as striking as those which occur in infancy. Being less dramatic, these subtler developmental changes are easily overlooked both at home and at school. Individual differences in temperament, aptitudes, and cultural background, on the contrary, become more conspicuous, and these tend further to obscure the underlying processes of maturation.

These processes, however, operate with lawful certainty, and follow a ground plan of sequences which are characteristic of given groups of children. By systematically comparing one age group with another, it is possible to single out distinguishing maturity traits and developmental trends. On the basis of such progressive comparisons, we have drawn up a series of brief profiles, devoting a separate section to each age level.

The profiles represent behavior characteristics which are more or less typical of intelligent children of favorable socio-economic status in our American culture. A profile does not portray a statistical child, but is a composite sketch based on longitudinal studies of a various group of children at successive ages. In series, these profiles may serve as a frame of reference for the interpretation of the maturity of observed behavior. It is needless to remind the reader again that the age labels are approximate and are not to be applied too rigidly. It is, however, always profitable to inquire into the sequential order of developing behavior.

5 YEARS

Four is fluid; 5 is focus. It is not without semantic interest that we can use the visual phrase *in focus to* describe the behavior make-up of a typical 5-year-old. He is neither blurred nor diffuse. For so young a child, he has himself well in hand. He gives an impression of self-containment because he is not seriously in conflict with himself nor with his environment. Within limitations of which he himself is partially aware, he is something of a finished product.

Compared with 4 years on the one hand and 6 years on the other, his mental life is matter-of-fact and realistic. Even the emotions of the 5-year-old seem more subdued, as though they had to be subordinated to the demands of a concrete unsentimental world. He is so occupied with the organization of an inner world of concrete perceptions that he seems somewhat impersonal. Emotional projection is at a relative minimum. He does not markedly identify his ego with the external world. His mood swings are brief in span and less frequent.

Self-limitation is stronger than self-assertion. He seeks help from adults, and tends to conform to cultural demands. Indeed, within his limitations, he likes to be helpful. One of his favorite tasks is setting the table, and he often does this with a real sense of accomplishment and finish.

He is not as facile with beginnings and initiations as he was at the age of 4 years. But he has a better comprehension of the relationship between beginnings and ends. His endings are definite and clear-cut. "That's all I can do." "That's as nice as I could do it." He does not like to go beyond his limitations. He does not make harum-scarum thrusts. He prefers to finish a task and, having finished it, he readily undertakes another without carryover from the preceding experience. There is a certain discreteness in his adjustments both to the physical and to the social environment. He operates in terms of concrete entities and episodes. He takes up one thing at a time, and does not go too far beyond his depth.

This conservatism imparts an air of caution to much of his behavior. He thinks before he speaks and acts. He knows what he is going to draw before he starts to draw. He makes few projections into a distant future. Instead of venturing on innovations, he is more likely to repeat and repeat an activity in order to intensify an experience. In a novel social situation, he tends to deliberate. He is apt to stand back and stare, but within a short time he may make a confident approach to a stranger. The adjustment to a new person or a new situation is facilitated by providing familiar play materials, interesting blocks and toys, crayons, and so on. He likes to draw, to trace, to copy, and to color. He prefers colored crayons to pencil, and colored picture books to black and white.

The mental world of the 5-year old is compact rather than expansive. It centers in his home, and his mother is the center of that home. He usually knows the name of the street on which he lives and the house number. He has an overweening interest in house and home. He repetitively draws houses. Often he completes a picture with a drawing of a house. Houses figure in his dreams. It is difficult for him to think of God as not living in a house. He plays house for an hour or more at a stretch, preferably with one playmate.

He lives in the here and the now. He likes specificity of orientation. He does not like to open strange doors. He tends also to manipulate space in conventional directions. He operates with more facility in the vertical direction than in the horizontal. He is beginning to use the word "long" in preference to the word "big."

He shows a new awareness for "points" and "corners." He is more aware of longness in vertical, as opposed to oblique and horizontal directions. He lacks command of oblique strokes even when he wields a crayon. The vertical line is the easiest for him to execute. Sometimes he draws this with an upward stroke. He not only executes his strokes in a vertical direction, but tends to scan a page in a vertical meridian, from top to bottom or from bottom to top. He is sensitive to variations of form, position, and size. He likes to match form with form, size with size, and he tends to arrange visual test materials in the vertical meridians to which he is so hospitable. These perceptual predilections are doubtless associated with the current maturity status of his ocular patterns and total action system.

In his perceptual activities he displays a characteristic discreteness of response. He singles out specific details or familiar features without losing an awareness of the total entity. He picks out capital letters and numbers. He identifies letters out of books and in store signs: "That's in my name." "This one is in Daddy's name." "That's my number." He enjoys the calendar on the kitchen wall and the figures on the kitchen clock. This trait is most conspicuous in the visual sphere, but he also displays it in the field of language. As he listens, he singles out special words in a spoken sentence and asks their meaning.

The dynamic traits typical of the 5-year-old reflect themselves in postural demeanors and in motor habitudes including oculomotor patterns. His self-limitation imparts a kind of tightness to his postural sets and to the approach which he makes to new tasks. This same tightness, however, also enables him to hold fast to an adjustment which he has achieved or is in the process of achieving. In the visual examination, therefore, he is able to report and to maintain a phoria at near distance. Posturally he goes to fewer extremes than he did at 4 years. His extensor tendencies have decreased. He is more closely knit. He holds his arms near his body. His stance is narrow. He moves eyes and head almost simultaneously or in close succession as he directs his regard conservatively to a new object of interest. He climbs with more sureness and with less abandon than at the age of 4. He moves with more deliberation from one object to another. His postural demeanor gives an impression of relative finish and completeness. Ease and economy of movement are present in finer coordinations, as well as in his locomotor activity. He shows an increased precision and command in the use of tools.

Ontogenetically, he has gained a complex of behavior capacities which is vaguely reminiscent of an early stage of culture, perhaps a primitive golden age in the evolution of the race. But action system and vision are, after all, far from complete. His difficulty with oblique strokes suggests that the relationships of eyes and hands will undergo still further refinements and elaborations. With the eruption of the sixth-year molar, and even before, he is caught up in the perturbation of a new surge of growth. The race evolved beyond a primitive golden age. So must he.

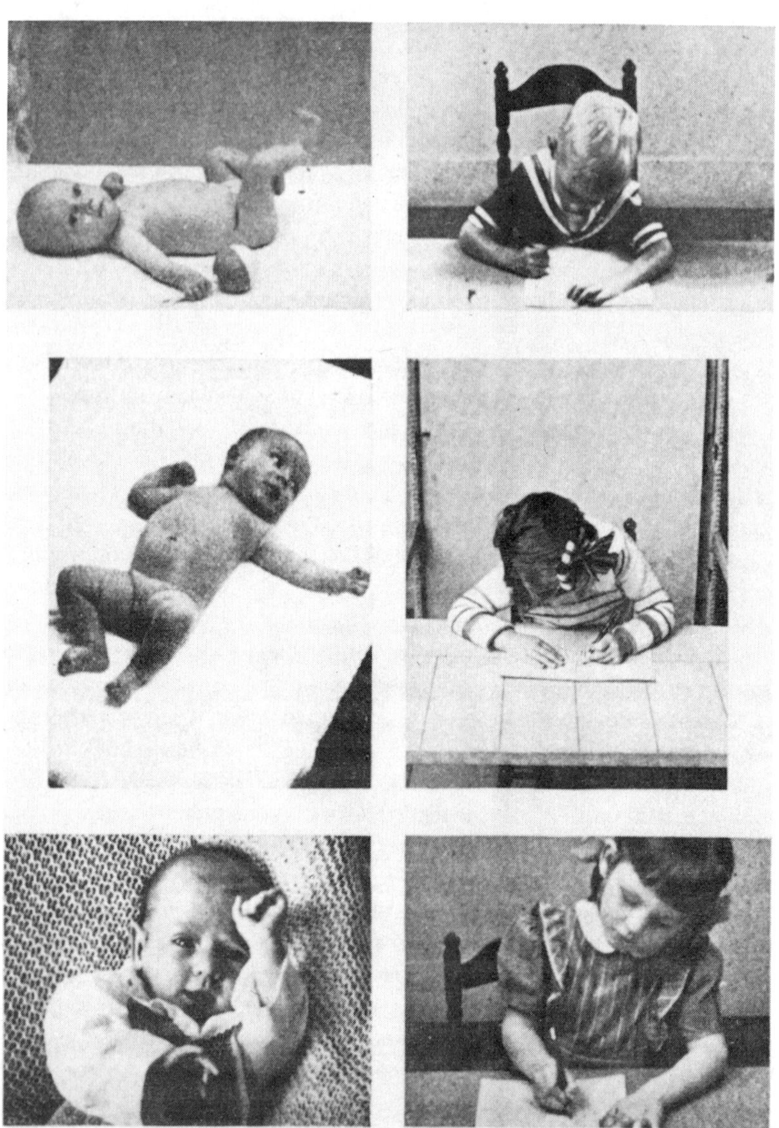

Figure 48. Visual behavior patterns at 5 years. The early tonic-neck reflex attitude of each of three children also is pictured to show individual differences in laterality. (a) A right TNR attitude (associated with a poorly defined left TNR) in infant D.D., (b) This child (D.D.) grasps and holds pencil with some awkwardness at 5 years, (c) A well-defined left TNR in Girl a, (d) This girl has shown consistent left-handedness throughout infancy and childhood; characteristic 5-year-old postural orientation and facile left-handedness at 5 years, (e) An atypical alternating TNR in infant T at 8 weeks; the extensor arm thrusts forward rather than laterally, (f) Prefers right hand at 5 years, adducts right arm to bring about central orientation.

6 YEARS

The 6-year-old presents such a wealth of behavior changes since he was 5 years old that his parents are often tempted to think he is a different child. At 5 the tides of development flow smoothly and in rather well-defined channels. A typical 5-year-old is self-contained, and on friendly and familiar terms with his environment. His very postures, the economy and precision of his motor coordinations, the directness of his approach and demeanor, and his general deportment suggest a well-adjusted action system.

But, under the pressures of growth, this golden period of relative equilibrium comes to an end, not suddenly and yet relentlessly. At about the age of 5 1/2 years new impulses, new actions, new intensities, announce that the underlying action system is undergoing revisions. There is a "loosening up" which brings about paradoxical and startling changes in behavior patterns and attitudes. During their early transition phase these changes, uninvited by the culture, may seem lawless and chaotic, but they have a developmental rationale. And they, too, have their day; for by the age of 7, the organism begins to return to more settled and more predictable modes of reaction. It would be strange indeed if the visual mechanism did not share in such deep-seated developmental transformations.

The eyes of 6 show frequent shifts in mood: they twinkle, they brighten, they glower, or become dull. Mothers have a way of detecting and reading the announcements of his eyes. When he tells tales with too much fabrication, he portrays it by "the look in his eyes." When he is immersed in serious thought, his eyes sweep conjugately from side to side or upward. From time to time, a binocular coordination momentarily lapses. One eye may deviate nasally, temporally, or upward.

It is a period of transition to a higher level. The eruption of the sixth-year molars is but one manifestation of growth changes which involve the whole organism. The child is more prone to physical "complaints;" his allergy reactions are high; he is more susceptible to infectious diseases; otitis media reaches a peak; the mucous membranes of eyes, nose, and throat also congest readily; his skin is peculiarly sensitive in head and neck regions; he tires more readily than he did at 5 years; he perspires more easily; bladder and bowel movements may become more expulsive; his motor activities are more clumsy and headlong. These instabilities and exaggerations of function—metabolic, humoral, voluntary, and autonomic—are reflected in innumerable tensional outlets, including visceral reactions.

The tensional manifestations are exacerbated by unwise pressures at home and at school, and even by such ordinary cultural demands as table manners. Under tension, the reactions may vary from wriggling, leg-swinging, grimacing, and blinking, to violent tantrums and outbursts of screaming, striking, and name-calling. He churns his fingers in his mouth, he chews his pencil, he laughs and utters an "ugh." Under the stress of getting ready for school, he often complains of a stomach ache. His fears and dreams show his new vulnerability. They concern wild animals, darkness, fire, thunder, lightning, and sometimes even the destruction of his mother.

Explosive behavior is perhaps more characteristic (on the average) of 5 1/2 years than of 6. Even at 6, there are discernible traces of modulation, and of increasing self-control. The child (from 5 1/2 to 6 1/2 years) does go to extremes, and often he exhibits extraordinary intensity at the "wrong" extreme. But he also exhibits engaging qualities to a marked degree. In fact, he goes to extremes in "goodness" as well as in his "badness." His virtues more than compensate in the end, and as he grows older he learns to modulate his behavior. Slowly, and more or less rhythmically, he builds up buffers and margins of reserve. Choices become easier and, by the same token, obedience becomes easier, for obedience represents a choice.

When choices are too hard or too numerous for him, he spontaneously resorts to various solutions of his difficulties: (a) he dawdles, (b) he refuses, (c) he vacillates, (d) he rebels. These reactions are both symptoms and adaptations. It is well to reflect on their functional meaning. They manifest the current state of the organism. Dawdling is a form of aimlessness. The child has much more capacity to start an activity than to stop, so he continues aimlessly. Contrary refusal may mean that, at the moment, he is unable to shift from one postural set to another. When the balance is more even, he oscillates between two choices, makes both rather than one. In the same afternoon—in fact, in the same hour or minute—he may give verbal expression to contradictory hate and affection. In rebellion, the emotional component is overintense, not always merely because of the limitations of the organism, but sometimes also because the demand of the culture has been excessive or ill-timed.

The behavior or 6, therefore, often appears to be unpredictable. His attention makes multiple thrusts. Nevertheless, in these thrusts he repeatedly comes back to a starting point. In this sense, he is more facile with beginnings than with completions. This same trait is displayed in his early reading patterns. He frequently loses his place as he reads. He is apt to carry down and repeat a word that will fit into the context of the story. By his very repetitions and relocations of attention, he strengthens a growing behavior pattern. He needs the benefit of repetition when given instructions. One has to repeat a direction three or four times to secure response. The delay is not due to perversity.

The growth trends of the action system of the 6-year-old can be appreciated through further comparisons with the 5-year-old characteristics. Six is losing the impersonal quality so characteristic of the 5-year-old. He seems to be more self-willed, even though he is not sure of himself. But he is aware of himself. Five is self contained; 6 is self-centered. His orientations to space have a strong self-reference. When he tries to relate himself to certain locations and dimensions in space, he reveals his difficulties by saying, "Can I fit in?" He indulges in arm-stretching and other gestures as he attempts to project himself perceptually into spatial relationships.

He shows a new interest in dimensions. He wishes to know how big, how long, and how far things are in his surroundings. Space is unquestionably widening for the 6-year-old, and he resorts to curious postural expedients while he tries to attain orientations which always proceed from his own center of reference.

This growth trend expresses itself in his efforts to gain mastery of the oblique line in his eye-hand coordination. We have already referred to the predilection for the vertical characteristic of the 5-year-old. The 6-year-old shows an interest in oblique directionality. His eyes differentiate between a vertical and an oblique stroke but, in his effort to execute an oblique stroke with his crayon, he twists his body and shifts his paper at various angles. His difficulties usually are transitory, but they may continue for a long time, and they take on diagnostic significance when found in association with reading disability.

The 6-year-old is beginning to read words as well as letters. He identifies familiar words on cereal packages and in magazine advertisements. He shows new facility in memorizing stories read to him. His ability to pick out words which he knows at random is correlated with his reading ability. In recognizing words, he makes major use of the initial letter, a trait which is characteristic of his increasing interest in beginnings. While reading, he has difficulty in holding to a horizontal line. This difficulty is another symptom of his immature but growing orientations to structured space, in minute as well as in gross aspects.

Because of his motor ineptitudes and conduct difficulties, it is easy for one to overlook some of the subtler manifestations of his growing action system. He is showing some sensitiveness to the beauties of nature, to sunsets, clouds and rainbows. He often displays a passion for flowers; picking flowers is a favorite activity. He is becoming aware of different shades of color. (Girls like to match hair ribbon and socks.) His drawings are embellished with blue for sky, green for grass, and red for flowers. If he is in a fiery mood, the red become a very active color in his drawing; or the mood may shift toward the glowering end of the spectrum and express itself in gross and heavy pressures with a black crayon.

The temporary limitations of the organism are most clearly and impersonally displayed in the field of sensory-motor coordination—in a new kind of awkwardness in his motor tasks. Sometimes there seems to be an actual decline in skill. In building a tower with small blocks, he works with less speed and accuracy than he did at 5 years of age. Eye and hand function in looser coordination. He overextends and overabducts in much of his motor behavior: he tends to approach with too much abandon or too much deliberation. Often there is more activity than accomplishment. Impetuosity may cause him to stutter, or may even impede his utterance. Nevertheless, at 6 years his behavior is more fluent and dynamic than it was at 5 years. The behavior of 5 is relatively more static, more episodic. At 5 1/2, his behavior tends to gather continuity of flow. At 5, ocular fixation is superior to ocular pursuit. At 6, pursuit tends to be superior. Thus, normally in the natural course of maturation, psychomotor difficulties tend to resolve, preparing the way for further increments at the 7- and 8-year age levels. The eyes share, and sometimes lead the way, in this process of progressive elaboration and reorganization.

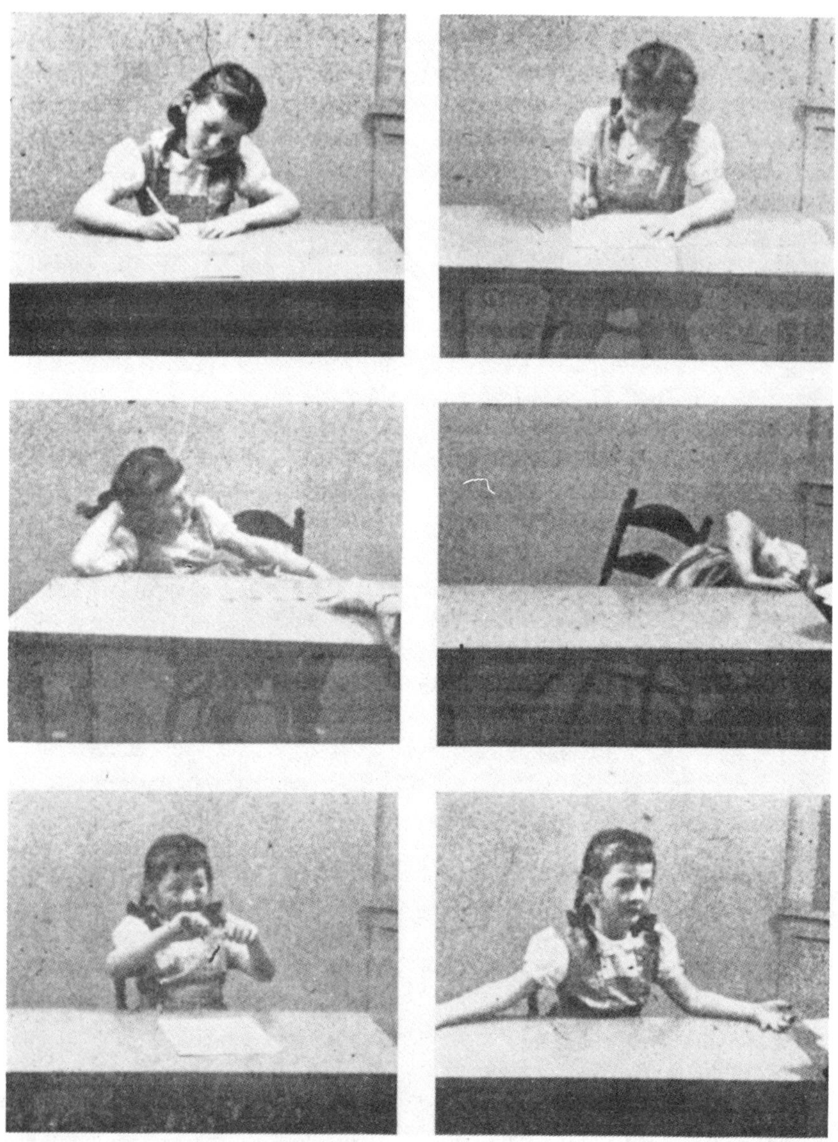

Figure 49. Visual behavior patterns at 6 years (Girl T). (a,b) Girl T shifts total body posture, including arms and legs, (c,d) Sprawls and spreads posturally in a manner typical of the 6-year-old, and in contrast to the poised orientation of the 5-year-old, (e) Screws up face when asked to write with left hand, (f) Spreads arms widely in typical abduction.

7 YEARS

At 7, there is a kind of quieting down. It is as though the more turbulent 6th year had accomplished its developmental mission and prepared the way for a calmer period of assimilation and consolidation. The child is not so often caught in conflicts with himself and with the outside world. Despite the earlier conflicts and, in part, because of them, the 7-year-old has a firmer and more organized self into which he can withdraw.

Seven lives in a thought world. He likes to think things through, communing with himself. He may even talk to his image in a mirror. Given a problem in oral arithmetic, he immobilizes. His eyes dart laterally and obliquely upward, and he comes through with an answer. Asked how he secured his answer, he says, "Oh, I figured it out." He may even say that he has a special counting place in his brain. He is unquestionably more subjective than he was a year ago.

This is an age of withdrawal. Where, before, the child made brash and unthinking thrusts into his environment, he now goes into lengthening periods of self-absorption and meditation, in which he apparently works over impressions and experiences. Of course, this change in demeanor does not come suddenly, and yet it may be so pronounced that he seems like a different child, even to his mother. She knew him when he was 6! We underline the contrast in this thumbnail sketch in order to indicate the trend of development and to point to a rhythm which belongs to the logic of development.

The introversive tendency of the 7-year-old, therefore, is normal unless it goes to a depressed extreme of excessive withdrawal, as happens on rare occasions. If the developmental deviation is in the opposite direction, the child is hyperactive, making repeated thrusts with poorly sustained attention. If pushed too hard, such a child may exhibit pseudochoreiform movements. Ordinary withdrawal leads to constructive imagery, inner speech, soliloquy, and reflective phantasy—mechanisms by which the mind works over its psychological grist. The cerebrum is, after all, a thinking machine. The cortex is undergoing growth changes and, if there was reason in infancy to manipulate two cubes with eyes and fingertips, why should not this child of larger growth manipulate memories, feelings, and meanings acquired through deepening powers of perception?

These psychological materials are not ineffably occult; they all have a sensory-motor genesis and motor components which are traceable in large measure to speech, to sight, and to ocular movements. If there is something brooding and pensive about the mental life of the 7-year-old, it is because he has a new awareness of the whole furniture of life—himself, the attitudes of others, and his orientation in time and space. Inner tensions are the key to his psychology, whereas gross outward thrusts were more characteristic of the 6-year-old. The sensitivities of the 7-year-old are not unlike those which he will experience on a higher level in adolescence.

Seven is something of a perfectionist. He is developing a sense of self-control. He can pull himself together to ward off a cry. Sometimes his striving goes to excess, expressing itself in dread of failure, anxiousness lest he be late for school, and fear that he will not attain the grade of 100 in his school work. Six is good at beginnings; 7 likes to carry through to a finish when it lies within his power. He often pushes himself to the limit. He endeavors so successfully that it is easy to forget that he is exercising new and immature powers and, therefore, is vulnerable to fatigue. He holds up well at school, but he may collapse with relaxation as soon as he reaches home. Sometimes he is not equal to an afternoon session at school. He does not have the robust rebound of the more mature 8-year-old, who is facile with both beginnings and endings.

Lacking rebound, but retaining a measure of self-appraisal, 7 tends to withdraw from situations which are likely to overtax him. If he gets into a tough mix-up on the playground, he may deliberately leave the group, muttering as he secedes. He may rush into a room and slam the door. He may even threaten to run away from home, but he has a much broader capacity of self-recovery than he had at 6 years.

As a matter of fact, he gravitates to his own home and he has a new interest in places—his own individual place in the household, the places of other persons and also of things. He identifies himself personally with places. This awareness is bound up with his increasing sense of self and of his position in home and community. He feels uncomfortable if he loses his assigned place at the table or his accustomed location in the automobile. He also displays a new interest in maps, but the interest is for discrete places with boundaries. He does not comprehend the earth as a unit. Again, the 8-year-old is more fluid and global.

Perseveration is a maturity trait characteristic of this age period. The 7-year-old tends to repeat a behavior which affords satisfaction. He does this in his drawings, his play, his games. Interminably, he bounces his ball against the side of the house. He listens endlessly to reading and to radio. He puts his hands over his ears to shut out distracting noise. It is part of his self-absorption. Sometimes his parents think he must be deaf, but under test his hearing may prove acute. The perseveration and perfectionist tendencies of 7 often carry him to extremes. However, he is less inept motorwise than at the age of 6. He shows a growing interest in skills which require unilateral posturing of the TNR type—management of gun, bat, bow and arrow. He spontaneously tilts his head to the non-dominant side. Frequently he rests his hand on his free arm as he writes, reads, or listens, occluding one eye and tensing one side of his body as though he were organizing a complex behavior which required functional asymmetry.

Seven is serious about himself, about his responsibilities. He is cautious rather than headlong in his approach to a new task, a strange social situation, or a novel physical activity. He is very fond of pencil crayons, but self-critical of his productions. He has a new awareness of irregularities in size and outline, and he uses his eraser with amazing frequency in his efforts at self-improvement. He recognizes and corrects reversals which he may make when printing his letters. He has a new inclination to print them smaller, perhaps because of his inwardizing propensity. Sometimes he mutters words of self-disparagement.

8 YEARS

Eight is an interesting age, particularly when one looks at this zone of maturity in the perspective of the outgrown past and the prospect of the approaching future. The 8-year-old is in an intermediate expansive phase of development. He is no longer a young child; his own individuality, physical and psychological, is becoming more defined, foreshadowing adult patterns. When he dramatizes, as he often does, you can almost see him stretching out toward maturity. More obviously than ever before, he seems to be governed by a growing impulsion which brings him into positive contact with his playmates and his elders.

The seeking of contacts is an outgoing propensity different from the inwardizing pensiveness of the 7-year-old. It is a form of expansion which projects the self into manifold relations with other selves. It is a somewhat naive and impulsive process. The consequent judgments may be callow and flashy. The burgeoning 8-year-old, however, uses his eyes and ears intentively to catch cues in the facial expressions, the words, and the actions of the grown-ups. He likes to form clubby organizations and to join in group and community activities. He gets along better in groups. He really enjoys the wrangling and the problems of adjustment which grow out of association with his equals. He maintains an alert relation to his widening frontiers.

As a 6-year-old, he was likewise in a spreading stage, contacting a multitude of new facets on a frontier, but then he could detect only beginnings. He saw in fragments or in opposites. He acted on impulsions of approach and reversal. At 7, his reactions became less piecemeal, and were incorporated into a steadily organizing sense of self. Now at 8 he is more ready to see conclusions, contexts, and implications. He is laying the basis for firmer evaluations in another year. By the same token he has a gift of making swift and serviceable generalizations. He likes to reassemble the separated parts of his toy gadgets. He exclaims with a delighted "Oh" when he suddenly comprehends the wholeness of a task or problem. Although he conceives the whole he does not have the sustaining power of 9 years and he is apt to leave projections incomplete.

There is less need for brooding and rumination. His action system is well geared for speedy performance and perception. Postures, walk, and motor demeanor are well formed. Often they are unconsciously graceful and poised. His flexors and extensors are in better balance. He finds a new enjoyment in swimming, skating, jumping rope, climbing, and playing baseball. He shows increased speed and smoothness in fine motor tasks. Tensional outlets are minimal. He shifts eyes and postures adaptively. His eyes now roll in a sweeping arc when he thinks hard. His manual approach and grasp and release of a pencil are rapid and facile. He writes with more uniformity of size, slant, and alignment. He is beginning to draw in perspective.

This heightening awareness of perspective is in some way correlated with certain developments in his visual functions. The awareness suggests an improved orientation in time and space. Near and far vision are in better balance and interplay, as shown by the greater ease with which he handles both blackboard and seat work. A year ago, his adjustment was limited to either blackboard or desk alone. Now he can shift from one locus to the other, and can even transfer the written materials from the blackboard to the nearby paper on his desk.

For similar reasons, the 8-year-old has a fairly clear notion of the points of the compass and the relationship of roads and pathways in his neighborhood, including shortcuts. He can distinguish right and left on the person of others, as well as on his own person. He has a new interest in remote places, in museums, zoos, and trips afield. He draws maps with zeal and imagination. Eight is truly interested in geography. It satisfies his expanding appetite. Somehow he grasps, at least dimly, a sense of the world as a whole, the awareness of a continent, and the oneness of the universe. At 7 years, it will be recalled, his mind had to set limits for itself within which to operate.

A mail-order catalogue is a magic carpet which takes the child to new realms, satisfying at one stroke his cardinal maturity traits of speediness and expansiveness. He likes new adventure. He likes to take a novel shortcut, even though his impulsiveness and overconfidence may lead him astray. At times, he tends to spread too far beyond his limits in his reading of a mystery story or his listening to the radio. So he ends up too far afield, with fears and bad dreams. Impulsiveness in physical activity makes him especially prone to accidents.

These hazards and excesses, however, are counterbalanced by a certain deep-seated capacity of recovery and rebound. He knows how to turn off the radio when it gets too fearsome. When in difficulties, he wants only a hint by way of help for he likes to work things out by himself. He likes to grapple with obstacles, to conquer. If he is afraid of the dark, he likes to go out with an adult at night in order to conquer his timidity. He puts himself on his mettle.

All in all, 8 is more seasoned than 7. He makes a more secure adjustment to school and does not tire as easily as he used to. Home and school are in better balance and mutual understanding. Parents can now place more reliance on the child's report of his school activities. Teachers are better able to appraise the child in terms of his home life. The visual interests of the 8-year-old are in themselves indications of a decided developmental advance. He likes to look on and observe, as never before.

He takes an enlarging interest in books and pictures. He delights in comics; he buys, collects, barters, borrows, and hoards them. He has sufficient visual and emotional stamina to enjoy motion pictures and to select favorites among them. He may even have a movie projector of his own. He takes to television. The voluble comments which he makes as the images play upon the screen, and on his receiving retina, indicate that he is coming into the visual inheritance of the culture into which he was born.

9 AND 10 YEARS

At 9 and 10 years, the abundant promise of year 8 comes to realization in a more integrated and solidly organized complex of behavior traits. The 8-year-old characteristics of speed and expansiveness and evaluativeness are still present, but they function at a higher level and are more deeply identified with the central self. The 9-year-old is less influenced by the contingencies of the environment. His adaptations are engendered more from within; they are less sketchy, less episodic. Through growth and experience he has built up reserves of self-reliance. He is capable of new reaches of self-motivation.

Self-motivation is the key to his psychology. Accordingly, he is more realistic, more businesslike, and more self-dependent. He wants to be "on his own," he likes to test and to tax his skill. He accepts responsibilities and even takes over responsibilities on his own personal initiative. He can shake hands spontaneously, without coaching from the sidelines. He does not like pointed directions or condescension. He is reasonable and seeks help when he needs it, but instinctively he wishes to have his status and individuality respected.

A typical 9-year-old is interested in proving his skills, whether in throwing darts or dividing by one digit. He will practice endlessly, once he is motivated—a trait which is valuable for visual training, but which might be over-used. Eye-hand coordinations seem to have a special appeal. He enjoys watching athletic performances with a more or less critical eye for detail. He uses a pencil to sketch still life, maps and designs. He likes to draw from a model. He has a growing interest in perspective, in depth, shadow, and relief, but may need considerable help in representing them. Handwriting, however, has become a facile tool and increases in volume and speed. He no longer holds a hammer near its head, but swings it with carpenter-like competence. He plays with an erector set by the hour. This gives him a wealth of eye-hand experience.

He has a new awareness of himself and of his mental processes. Reciprocal-wise, he has a clearer consciousness of what others think of him. He will not accept a compliment if he feels that he does not deserve it. He shows not only a capacity but a propensity to make a realistic appraisal of himself. Sometimes there is a note of self-depreciation: he may disparage his poor memory. He says, "Oh, this is just like me."

This inwardizing tendency reminds us of the 7-year-old. Occasionally it causes 9 to key up too tightly and to report symptoms when he is under strain: he feels "funny inside," "shaky all over," "dizzy." Such temporary symptoms should not be taken too seriously, lest he dwell upon them too long. Nevertheless, he is a fairly reliable reporter and if he complains consistently of getting tired from reading, the matter should be looked into. Likewise, he may report that colored movies tire him more than black-and-white.

He may be an omnivorous reader but, typically, he is not a recluse. On the contrary, he often shows surprising social insight, making just estimates of the conduct of his elders and of himself. He likes humor, and is beginning even to accept jokes on himself. He responds well to a compliment. He enjoys competition. He will ardently pursue a chosen activity to the point of fatigue. Although he shows a tendency to overdo, he is not given to prolonged or drastic emotional expressions. His tensional outlets are comparatively mild. He is likely to cry only when his emotions are overtaxed by fatigue or by angry protest against injustice. He has a passion for fairness. All in all, he is well-disposed toward his contemporaries. At his best, he tends to be realistic, reasonable and responsible.

His social, factual realism shows itself in a new interest in numbers and in quantitative values. He may insist on knowing the money value of his coat, a football, a house, or even his father's salary. He may be inordinately concerned in ascertaining the ages of persons whom he knows.

His cardinal maturity trait of self-motivation asserts itself in various ways. It underlies his zeal for collections, his fury if his mother unwittingly disposes of chosen treasures as trash. He sets up a goal and drives through. He renews his persistence when interrupted. He shows a creditable ability to return to the object at hand after an interruption. Having set himself a stint like mowing the lawn, he may adhere almost obsessively to his task.

All this means that the centrifugal spreading tendencies of the 8-year-old maturity level are now being counterbalanced by introjective delimitations and intensifications. The 9-year-old contracts his activities into self-set channels. He prefers to restrict his ramifying to a single nucleus of interest. Visually, he operates closer to his plane of regard. This dynamic has important implications for education and therapeutic training.

Nine, therefore, is less episodic than 8. Having a greater interest in process and skill, he is more facile and modulated. His elaborations emerge from within. No one needs to tell him to make his inventories; no one needs to tell him to notice the varying attitudes and demeanors of his companions, his teachers, and his parents. He is increasingly perceptive of social conduct and aware of the evidences of

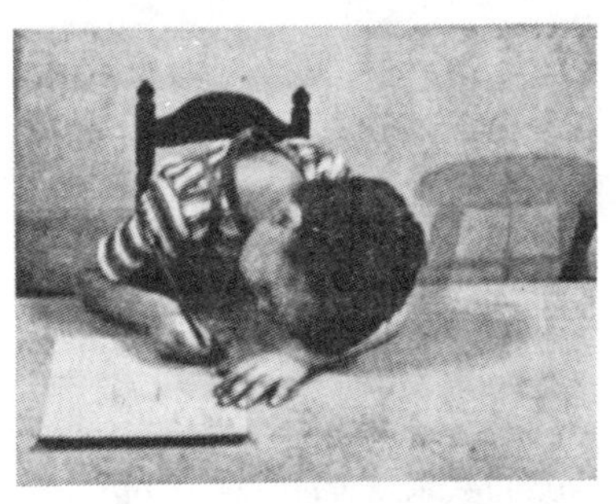
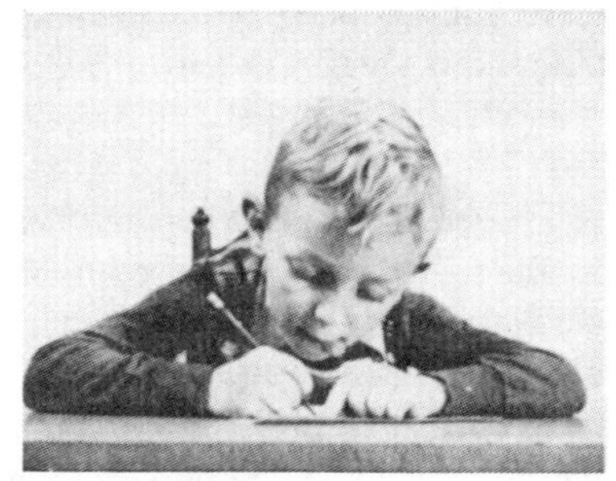
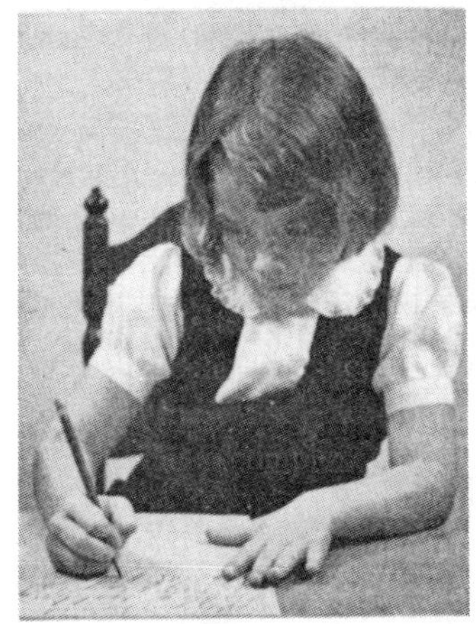
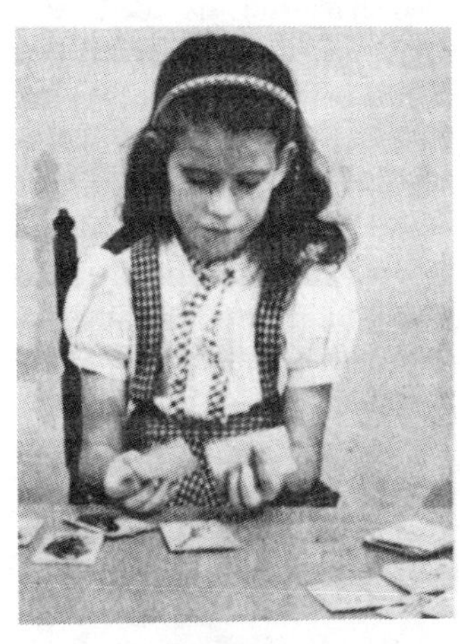
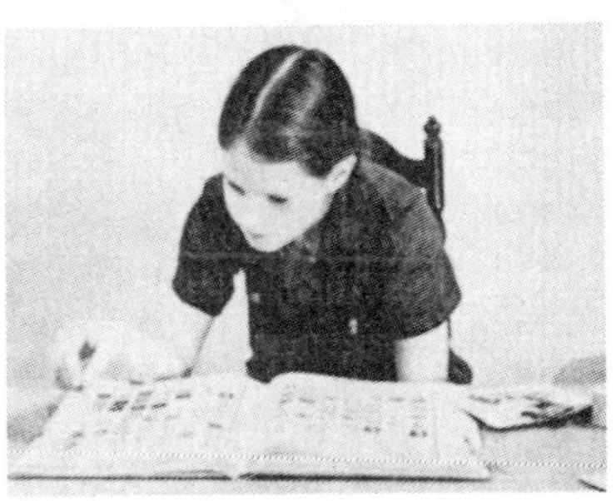
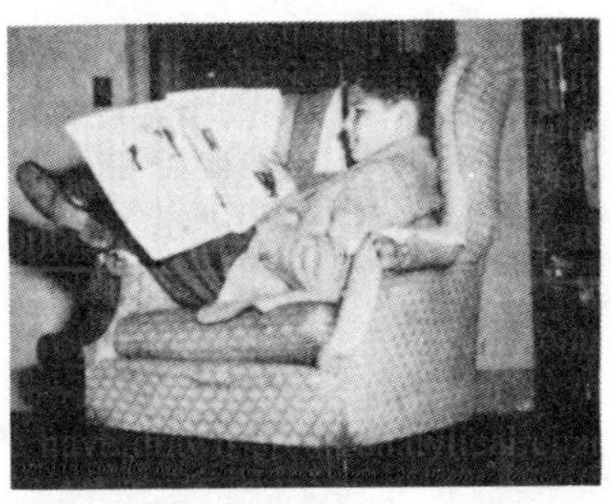

Figure 50. The child from 5 to 10. (a) 5-year-old printing a capital letter, (b) 6-year-old with characteristic tensional outlet, (c) 7-year-old writing posture, (d) 8-year-old working with card collection, (e) 9-year-old examining her stamp collection, (f) 10-year-old reading headlines.

worthiness and wrongdoing in others. This is reciprocal to his power of self-appraisal. A conscience is organizing and growing.

These developing traits are still further realized at the 10-year maturity level. The 10-year-old is in yet better equilibrium. He is somewhat less zealous and less channelized. He is more relaxed and can take things in his stride. (Girls may show impressive poise and wisdom for their age.) The 10-year-old is more casual and yet alert. He shows greater capacity to budget his time and does not, like the 9-year-old, find himself in unremitting contest with time.

These increments of maturity sum themselves up in greater self-possession and savoir faire. Behavior in general is more modulated. The 10-year-old is well oriented interpersonally. He likes to feel pride in his family. Already, at the age of 9, he displays protectiveness toward a younger brother or sister and a solicitous concern over undesirable behavior on his or her part. He feels loyalty to friends. Similarly, he shows a high capacity for hero worship and a deeper susceptibility to concepts of social justice and social welfare. There is a dawning interest in problems of war, crime, poverty, democracy. Intellectual and emotionally colored concepts are becoming an integral part of his action system.

Although he is stamped with individuality, he already foreshadows traits and trends which are universally associated with adolescence. He is a pre-adolescent. He has journeyed a long distance since the bipolarity of 2 1/2 years and the impetuousness of the 6th year. In his well oriented equilibrium, he resembles the nodal age of 5. A developmental spiral has come to full circle. Ten, like 5, is a nodal age.

PART TWO
DEVELOPMENTAL OPTICS

CHAPTER 9
The Visual Domain

In an oft-quoted phrase, the mental world of the newborn infant has been described as being a "big, blooming, buzzing confusion." This offhand characterization scarcely does justice to the visual life of the infant, even during the earliest weeks. His visual experiences may be somewhat sporadic and highly variable, but they are scarcely chaotic or disordered.

In a remarkably short time he exhibits patterns of ocular behavior which denote adaptive responsiveness and active initiative. Often, when his eyes are closed one may detect movements beneath the lids. These movements are various; they may be conjugate or unilateral, oblique or rotary, horizontal or vertical. The infant makes comparable eye movements when the lids are open and when, presumably, he is awake.

But his visual awakeness is not maintained at a uniform level. At times, his eyes rove in a lackadaisical manner, suggesting a minimal degree of visual awareness; proprioceptive awareness of such eye movement, however, may be well-defined. Recurrently, his eye movements halt with abruptness. This is an important motor ability, for it lies at the basis of fixation. He thus exercises the capacity to inhibit, as well as the capacity to execute seeking and pursuing eye movements. Head, arms and legs may be moving in an apparently incoordinate, undirected manner; suddenly he halts these grosser movements at the very moment that he halts his oculomotors. By such synchronization he further organizes his power to fixate, and to stare.

Some of his staring is very vacant, as though it served only proprioceptive and not teleceptive purposes. The stare is blank, but with increasing frequency it takes on a little luster, and for a fleeting or prolonged moment he gazes upon some capacious distant target—a window, a ceiling, a curtain. The gaze is vague and diffuse, but it represents a rudimentary type of fixation, a first look into optical infinity.

Vision does not automatically, and once and for all, tell the infant where he is. At every stage of growth during infancy, childhood, and youth, the visual mechanism undergoes changes which serve to reorient the ever-transforming individual. For him the space world is not a fixed and static absolute. It is a plastic domain, which he manipulates in terms of his nascent powers. He commands less space when he is 1 year old than when he is 5—not because he is weaker and smaller, but because his total action system has occupied less operational territory. He was born with a pair of eyes, but not with a visual world.

Newtonian physics and geometric optics cannot describe the relativities of the space world of the growing child. This world is his own private possession. He carves and constructs it out of a tenacious enveloping cosmos. He appropriates it by positive acts, reflexive, subconscious, autonomic, wished and willed. The space world thus becomes part of him. To no small degree, he is it. A description of his personality might well begin with the characteristics of this private space world of his. It is part of the "make-up" of his personality. The make-up changes with the developmental transformations of his total action system. The psychosomatic maturity of the action system influences all visual phenomena.

While the infant is awake, his eyes are constantly busy in one way or another. He has self-protective mechanisms which keep him from overtaxing a single activity. He reacts at scattered moments with varying degrees of intensity and complexity. In the course of a single day, or of a single minute, his visual attention ranges from profound vacuity to startled intentness. The infant reacts in small quantums of adjustment and, although these adjustments have no obvious arrangement, they are governed by a physiology of development which leads to specific patterned ends. Almost from the moment of birth, the infant reacts with optic nystagmus to a slowly rotating target, refixating at brief intervals as the stimulus moves across his near field of vision. Between the refixations the eyes make pursuit movements. Coordinate compensatory eye movements also occur during the first week.

Although the infant early stares into faraway space, his structured visual world begins close to his eyes, and derives its psychic essence from bodily needs and satisfactions. His visual ego, so to speak, first organizes at punctum proximum! A small object of interest, brought into a susceptible area of nearness, evokes a degree and a kind of fixation which is quite different from that of a faraway stare. One eye at least aligns itself with the stimulus object, immobilizes and brightens. Momentarily, there is a directed regard accompanied by a wrinkling of the forehead.

By this token, the infant has registered a fleeting orientation in nearby space. It is a minute experience, but it is not altogether reflex nor fragmentary. It is a manifestation of a visual-space world which grows at a prodigiously swift rate during the period of infancy. At first the orientation is mainly ocular and only sparsely related to postural sets of head and arms. As the infant matures, however, the strands of orientation multiply and become deeply incorporated into limb and body attitudes. By the age of 8 weeks, the infant achieves binocular convergence and is already adept in compensatory eye movements and in simple pursuit movements. At the age of 12 weeks, he intently fixates upon his own hand at a working plane of regard.

Throughout infancy and childhood, he is engaged in multiplying and in shifting his planes of regard and in organizing his ability to manipulate space effectively on either side of each and every plane. In number, these planes soon approach infinity. In position, permutation, dimension, and configuration, the planes are also infinitely various. Inevitably they transform as the infant keeps adding cubits to his stature and as he acquires through growth an ever-changing action system and personality.

The potential planes of regard at any given age define the boundaries and the dynamic structure of the child's visual space world at this age. This world may be vaguely pictured as a more or less globular domain, which elaborates as the child gains in visual competence. Schematic models of the domain and its planes of regard at progressive ages—4 days, 4 weeks, 40 weeks, 40 months, 10 years—would vary enormously. The supine infant, the runabout infant, the sedentary school child, each has his own space world with a distinctive set of planes of reference and regard. The world of the myope may well differ from that of the hyperope. Every individual organizes his space world in obedience to laws of development, general for the species and unique for himself.

The infant does not fill a space void by a homogeneous extension of visual projection. His visual world does not expand symmetrically like an inflating balloon. It is an organismic product of his own morphogenesis. He lives in an orderly Alice-in-Wonderland environment where relativities rather than absolutes prevail, and where three feet is infinitely far away at one age and is within familiar home ground at another age.

To comprehend the manner in which the visual domain is occupied and elaborated, one must think in terms of biological space rather than Newtonian space. Biological space is a function of the organism. Accordingly the value of any point or interval in space depends upon its position in the visual domain, and upon the developmental maturity of the organism at the given time. In last analysis, our interpretation of the child's orientation in space depends upon a knowledge of his own developmental mechanics. The prolongation of human infancy enables man to bind space in terms of time.

For this reason, the development of human vision is extremely intricate and involuted. Instead of advancing into space on a steady, even front, the organism moves forward by rhythmic thrusts and apparent retreats, invading the unknown in a complicated series of overlapping panels, consolidating all gains in near territory. Here the organism gets the footing (or shall we say the eyeing?) which gives a purchase for further projections into more distant space. These projections are not whimsical, but are governed by a developmental dynamic morphology, which stakes out and organizes various sectors of space, more or less simultaneously. The young infant, at one stage, may fixate with intent regard an object a foot away, giving only faint and sporadic glances at the same object as it retreats to a distance of two feet. But his visual mechanism is growing rapidly and very soon he gives equally sustained regard at one and at two feet, whether the object retreats or approaches. Thus he organizes in a three-step manner, going both forward and backward in the process. This is his interweaving method of organic growth. It is a morphogenetic phenomenon, and the architecture of the child's visual space world is more truly a product of intrinsic morphogenesis than of learning or conditioning.

The geometry of this growing space world can scarcely be represented by a homogeneously expanding balloon. A fabulously involuted artichoke with myriad overlapping bracts would better serve as a schematic model, each bract symbolizing an organized or organizing area of a dynamic complex.

For the organism, near space and far space—whether close or widely separated—are bipolar opposites. These opposites are alternatives, which in some way must be reconciled and balanced. The task of development is to bring opposites into effective counterpoise. The development of vision is permeated with numerous bipolar opposites and paired alternatives: near versus far, center versus periphery, monocular versus binocular, abduction versus adduction, vertical versus horizontal, incoming fusion versus outgoing fusion, "plus" versus "minus," clockwise versus counterclockwise, unilateral dominance versus bilateral symmetry, skeletal versus visceral, inhibition versus excitation, flexion versus extension, and so on. These and many other opposites beset the pathway of development. To a slight extent, the opposites have a cultural origin, but basically the seat of conflict is in the organism itself. The normal organism has the capacity both to create and to resolve counteracting forces. The resolution is brought about by a developmental mechanism, which we describe as the process of reciprocal interweaving.

This process is as pervasive as the principle of bipolarity itself. It is a key to an understanding of the fluctuations, the periodicities, and the accents of ontogenetic development. If the paired opposites grew on an even front, with simultaneous uniformity, the cycle of growth would lose much of its intricacy and variety. But the exigencies of functional organization are so complex that Nature has adopted a method of cross-stitching, or interlacing, which brings opposing muscle systems (and functions) into reciprocal relationship. This means that one member of a reciprocal pair of functions—for example, flexion and extension —may be temporarily in relative ascendancy, while its opposite is in relative subordination waiting to assume ascendancy at a later time.

Sherrington's law of reciprocal innervation describes a mode of development which provides the structural basis for the physiological mechanism of reciprocal innervation. How the organism achieves a reciprocal balance between antagonistic muscle groups is patently illustrated in the ontogenesis of prone behavior patterns which lead to crawling, creeping, and ultimately to upright walking. Over 20 stages in this ontogenesis have been identified. Some of these stages are characterized by a dominance of the flexor musculature, others by dominance of extensor musculature. Comparable developmental shifts of dominance undoubtedly occur in the motor aspects of visual behavior and in the harmonization of competing visual functions. Such shifts introduce irregularities which may seem to contradict conventional expectations, but which nevertheless are consistent with the logic of development.

The law of reciprocal interweaving has wide scope in the interpretation of the development of vision. In broad terms it may be formulated as follows: The organization of reciprocal relationships between two sets of counteracting functions or motor systems is ontogenetically manifested by more or less periodic shifting ascendancies of the component functions or systems, with progressive integration and modulation of the resultant behavior patterns.

CHAPTER 10
The Complex of Visual Functions

Vision is a complex sensory-motor response to a light stimulus mediated by the eyes, but involving the entire action system. By this definition, fixation becomes the most basic and, phyletically, the primary visual function. Fixation is the directing or orienting of the organism so that a stimulus or an image falls in optimal relation to the visual receptor. All other visual functions are in a sense subsidiary to fixation, or they are refinements of fixation. In the last analysis, every act of vision must be referred to a single unifying action system. But it is possible to distinguish several functions.

The camera concept of the eye has tended to create a stereotyped view of these visual functions and of the mechanisms of refraction. We should think of the eye and its annexa as an extremely versatile structure in which energies are transformed and patterned in a plastic manner, reconciling both inner and outer forces. Functions are characteristic, distinguishable activities, but they do not operate as separate entities. They are so closely interactive that together they constitute a unitary organic complex.

We have called vision itself an *act,* but this should not blind us to the fact that vision is also a process. The process is an instantaneous quantum-like concentration of biophysical and biochemical events which, after they occur, are ascribed to so-called functions.

Nevertheless, it is profitable to consider the several functions individually, and to analyze their specific role in an admittedly organic complex. Organic complexes grow, and it is important to inquire how the individual functions of the complex take shape, and how their interrelatedness changes throughout the long period of ontogenesis.

As an aid to such inquiry, we have drawn up an analytical chart (see page 113) which classifies the components of vision into three functional fields and four panels or modalities. The three fields, broadly interpreted, correspond in general to the conventional Fixation-Focus-Fusion triad. From the standpoint of developmental optics, these functions do not operate as specific and fixed entities. They undergo growth changes which are correlated with the three primary neuro-embryologic divisions, namely, (A) Skeletal (fixation, (B) Visceral (focus), (C) Cortical (fusion, etc.). The chart will suggest how these three fields combine to produce a great variety of visual behavior patterns and how these patterns elaborate with the advancing maturity of the visual system.

Almost from the beginning, the three functional fields develop conjointly, but by no means uniformly. They are, however, interdependent and they form an interacting triad of relationships within the total visual system. Arranged in a hierarchy, the major functions fall into the following sequence:

A. SKELETAL: The visual system seeks and holds an "image."
B. VISCERAL: The visual system discriminates and defines an "image."
C. CORTICAL: The visual system unifies and interprets an "image."

By "image" is meant any effective optical stimulus or optical cue. The visual reaction thereto results in ascending degrees and modes of attention, identification, localization, apperception, and mental synthesis. The highest acts of vision are so interfused with cortical influences that they belong to the supreme realm of abstract thought.

The foregoing hierarchy is not as simple as a ladder. In the course of development, gradients of performance are built up concurrently in all three fields, and the various levels of these multiplying gradients are interwoven in an intricate but progressive manner. Accordingly, each age of infancy and childhood affords a distinctive picture of visual behavior, characteristic of its stage of maturity. The trends of organization are regulated by deep-seated growth factors and by the sheer mechanics of the visual system.

The factors which enter into this organization are indicated in four panels as follows:

1. COORDINATION refers to the correlation of the two eyes, conjugately and disjunctively: I. one eye alone functions, II. right or left, alternately, III. right and left in combination, IV. right and left as an integrated team.
2. REACH refers to the distances at which the visual system operates, whether diffusely indeterminate (I), near (N), medium (M), or far (F).
3. SCOPE refers to the relative salience of central and peripheral areas in a plane of regard, whether highly central (C[p]), or peripheral (P[c]), or combined central and peripheral (C & P), or an integrated central and peripheral (CP).
4. DRIFT refers to the developmental drift or growth trends of the visual system as manifested in the preferred zone of regard, the duction-break relationship, the preferred zone and direction of accommodation, and the dominances and directionalities in motor attitudes, movements and perceptual organization.

The chart aims to show the multiplicity of the components which enter into vision and to suggest how these many components vary in their interrelations. It would be an oversimplification to reduce vision to the three classic functions of fixation, focus, and fusion because each of these functions is subject to morphogenetic and dynamic changes. No function matures independently, but in the process of ontogenetic organization it comes into shifting and progressive correlations with associated functions. Nor does the visual complex develop in isolation. It is pervasively influenced by the status and the growth of the total action system, of which it is but a part. Our chart, therefore, adds an over-all panel of organismic or *action system factors.* These include age, sex, maturity, metabolism. experience, education, acculturation, and constitutional traits and personality make-up.

With so many components, variants and complicating factors entering into the functional complex of the visual system, it is natural that no two individuals should see exactly alike. The chart suggests that the possible constellations of visual components—normal, atypical, and abnormal—are beyond enumeration. No method of examination is competent to gauge all the elements which enter into the functional efficiency of the visual system. Nevertheless, a panoramic view lends perspective. The chart helps to envisage the developmental drift, as well as the dynamics, of a growing visual system. It adds a developmental dimension to a frame of reference.

The functional complex is in a true sense a growing organism, in which a multitude of constituent patterns are in a process of progressive correlation and integration. This morphogenesis is inconceivably intricate. It introduces numerous variables into the task of visual examination and appraisal. During periods of rapid growth, the components of the complex are being interwoven in a reciprocal manner. Shifting in orderly sequence, now one visual behavior trend and then another comes into prominence. One form of visual behavior may seem to recede while another advances, but normally the total morphogenetic complex attains its goal. Ideal normality depends upon a developmental organization which brings into well-timed and harmonious combination the numerous functional components which are summarized in the schematic chart.

An optimal adult visual mechanism might be defined as one in which the basic skeletal, visceral and cortical functions have attained full stature and operate in balance and harmony. Child vision, however, is never merely a reduced version of its adult status. The relative strength and priority of the fundamental functions vary with the accents of development. Visual behavior patterns grow.

The skeletal components of vision are, in a sense, the more basic and primitive. Embryologically, they have their origin in the mesoderm, from which are derived the muscles that orient the vertebrate creature to its gravitational fields, and to the lures and threats of the visual fields. Mere awareness of light scarcely is vision. The biologic purpose of vision is to set the organism in effective relation to moving and to stationary objects. This is accomplished by gross postural adjustments of head and body and finer postural adjustment of the eyes, through gravitational, oriental, and vergence reflexes. These reflexes are so ancient that they are present even in fishes. In primates they are highly evolved and operate in intimate correlation with visceral functions and voluntary cortical controls. As indicated by the chart, the

COMPLEX OF THE VISUAL SYSTEM

FUNCTIONAL FIELDS	COORDINATION Teaming	REACH Distance	SCOPE Centrality	DRIFT Growth Trend	Action System Factors
A. SKELETAL *Fixation* Postural Seeking, following, immobilizing	I.one eye alone II.Right or *L*eft III.*R* and *L* IV. *RL*	*I*ndeterminate *N*ear *M*edium *F*ar	*C*entral (p) *C*(p) or *P*eripheral (c) *C* and *P* *CP*	Preferred zone of regard Duction Breaks Duction Recovery Break-recovery span	Age Sex Maturity
B. VISCERAL *Focus* Attention Discrimination Definition	I. one eye alone II. *R*ight or *L*eft III.*R* and *L* IV.*RL*	*I*ndeterminate *N*ear *M*edium *F*ar	*C*entral (p) *C*(p) or *P*eripheral(c) *C* and *P* *CP*	Preferred Accommoda-tion zone Preferred Direction of Accommodation Preferred Direction Free Accommodation	Metabolism Experience Acculturation
C. CORTICAL *Integration* Identification Localization Synthesis Interpretation	I.one eye alone II.*R*ight or *L*eft III.R and *L* IV.*RL*	I,N,M,F I,N,M,F I,N,M,F I,N,M,F	C,CorP,C&P, CP* C,CorP,C&P, CP C,CorP,C&P, CP C,CorP,C&P,CP**	Dominances and Directionality Motor attitudes Perception Gestalt	Constitut ional traits Personality make-up

development of the skeletal functions carries with it progressive pattern changes involving coordination, reach, scope, and preferences for zones of regard.

The visceral functions, likewise, are phyletically ancient. They trace back to the enteric canal, which has played an enduring role in organic evolution. To eat or to be eaten has been a basic problem both for lowly and higher creatures. Food and foe are fundamental objects of interest, and the focal mechanisms were evolved to sharpen awareness of these objects. A basic skeletal response is assumed. A visceral response may occur more or less concomitantly; this is mainly accomplished through parasympathetic nerve action, which produces a manipulation in the focusing mechanism. It has been experimentally shown that stimulation of the cervical sympathetic causes a lenticular meridional change. This strongly suggests that a functional type of astigmatism may be a normal feature of the visceral aspect of the visual act, at least at certain developmental stages and under acute stress or challenge.

Accommodative changes, furthermore, may be associated with voluntary or sub-voluntary convergence. Focus reactions, accordingly, are governed both by the autonomic and the central nervous systems, operating and interacting synchronously or in sequence. Nowhere else in human behavior do we see such intimate linkage between sympathetic and cortical reactions. This unique linkage profoundly incorporates vision into the total psychic structure.

The organ of vision is a distance receptor. There is always an interval of space between the object of regard and the seeing eye. That interval is bridged by locomotion, by prehension, and by innate motor attitudes which embrace the entire skeletal musculature including mouth, hands, and the oculomotor muscles. These innate attitudes are primarily a product of evolution and serve to project or localize the object of regard in outer space —without, however, detaching it from the eye. Even when the organism decides to run away from the object, it gives evidence that the object has been located in a practical world of space and directionality. Localization is implicit identification in space. At a primordial level in the race, and at a rudimentary level in the life history of the individual, this projection is crude, but it is instinctive, because in one form or another the evolution of vision has always been associated with movements toward and away from objects which had a position in space, or which themselves were moving in space. Sherrington, Chavasse, and Duke-Elder all emphasize the fundamental role of body and limb movements in the mechanism of vision. Franklin holds that "the very consciousness (of the organisms as a whole) of the presence or absence of an image in any given field is dependent upon, or determined by, the 'normal' body-limb motor response to a retinal stimulus."

Here we begin to glimpse the significance of the cerebral cortex in the evolution of the higher orders of visual consciousness. The capacity to project accurately in space became of increasing importance in the later stages of evolution, when one hand was used with preferred or shifting priority as in brachiation, pursuit of food, tool using, and constructive manipulation. *Tarsius,* which used both hands with simultaneous bilaterality, could do with a minimum of convergence. In more advanced species, the demands for more diversified and exact projection are achieved through a refinement of convergence, adapted to varying distances, coordinated with postural sets and movements, and based on bitemporal rather than nasotemporal retinal representation.

Fusion, on Franklin's evolutional interpretation, is the unification of projected retinal images into a single true image by the two limbs moving actually or potentially toward the images in the contralateral side of the binocular field. "With noncrossing temporal fibers, as in man, diplopia is overcome by converging visual axes for various planes of binocular fixation, by which means projected retinal images are shifted into opposite fields and the phylogenetically basic conditions for 'fusion' reestablished." The fusion function is highly developed in man, and is manifested in many different ways.

Human vision, thanks to the intrusive cerebral cortex, has advanced far beyond the mechanics of elementary fixation, focus, and fusion. Even in the early months of infancy, we see evidences of voluntary cortical participation in the patterning of visual behavior. The cortex functions as a master tool of synthesis and integrative interpretation. It organizes visual acts in terms of the optimal needs of the action system. Indeed in last analysis, the cortex becomes the seat of action for the action system. It funnels and organizes the electrodynamic forces which culminate in adaptive behavior.

The cortex is also a kind of meeting ground where the pressures of native growth and of acquired experience are reconciled and assimilated. The cortex itself as a protoplasmic organ is subject to maturational changes, which determine its capacity for learning and assimilation. With increasing age and experience, the cortex normally grows in powers of interpretation. It shows great adaptability in making use of cues, and in compensating for limitations in the subcortical mechanisms of vision. It integrates and regulates. The cortex also supplements bilateral balances with unilateral dominances; it offsets the disadvantages of rigid symmetry by eccentric but useful forms of functional asymmetry. The cortex is the true seat of handedness, eyedness, footedness, and sidedness.

Lateral dominance, therefore, is a functional trait which displays many interesting changes over a long cycle of growth. Although the physical organism, with its numerous paired organs, seems to be constructed on the basis of bilateral symmetry, it shows a consistent trend toward functional unilaterality in handedness, eyedness, footedness, and torsal sidedness. The developmental forces generally favor the right over the left; but the organization of this rightwardness requires recurrent secondary inclusion of leftwardness, and also of simultaneous right and left capacities. In the development of ocular and manual behavior, this means recurrent alternation and reciprocal interweaving of right and left components and of monocularity and binocularity. It must be an extremely complex morphogenetic process; two pairs of opposing trends are in mutual rivalry—bilaterality versus unilaterality, and right versus left. The organism solves the developmental problem by adopting temporary and mixed dominances along the way, with a basic trend which satisfies the principle of functional asymmetry.

Directionality is a functional trait allied to laterality, and indirectly related to it. It concerns the preferences which the organism exhibits in the directions of its limb-body movements and eye movements. Do they proceed from center to periphery or vice versa, up or down, clockwise or counterclockwise, or in some other direction? These directionalities are objectively observable in the drawing of simple forms, such as vertical and horizontal strokes, circle, cross, square, and triangle. Despite environmental fortuities and individual differences, the directions of movement are strongly influenced by postural sets, which are determined by maturity factors. The human infant, at one age, has a propensity for brandishing his arm in a vertical sector: he bangs. In a few weeks, he shows a comparable predilection for the horizontal sector: he brushes back and forth. Command of the oblique comes much later. The eyes, of course, are in some way involved in these directional tendencies of the action system.

The cerebral cortex thus serves a triple purpose in the organization of visual behavior. It corrects imperfections, when possible, in the primitive mechanisms; it reinforces these mechanisms through energy discharges; it introduces subtleties, substitutions, and suppressions or accentuations. For example, it can sharpen interpretation by volition and by deliberate adjustment of head posture; it may heighten an interpretation by a clench of the hand. Or it may use a pertinent cue instead of striving for a clarified image. In time, a symbolic cue in the form of a printed word replaces the immediate necessity of manipulatory cues.

The visual system, therefore, is an extremely versatile system. It may operate at a primitive level or at a sublimated level, and in countless constellations within these extremes. The problems of child vision cannot be appraised by a simple criterion of acuity. All vision is mediated by an intricate functional complex. Our task is to interpret vision in terms of actual achievement, and to analyze that achievement in terms of the components of a growing complex.

CHAPTER 11
The Young Eye in Action

In this chapter we shall attempt to come somewhat closer to the reactions of the seeing eye at the very moment of their occurrence. What is the seeing eye? It is a moist, warm, elastic organ, geared for response by a delicate arrangement of extrinsic and intrinsic muscles. It is a series of limpid chambers and transparent media which transmit waves of radiant energy propagated in an immaterial medium. It is a sensitive electrodynamic cup, carpeted with photochemical substances, whose myriad molecules are poised to transmit, to select, and to sort the energy waves which come to, and also from, the organism. It is the most direct corridor to the vast networks of the brain cortex, where billions of neurones organize and engender the energies which issue in vision. Inconceivably intricate electronic events take place when this amazing complex of structures is stirred into reaction.

We should like to know more about the nature of these events. Do they declare themselves by outward signs which are objectively detectable at the moment of occurrence? Much can be deduced by observing the postures and movements of the eyes, the facial expressions of visual attention, and other behavior patterns. But if we wish to look more directly at the eye in action, we must project a benign beam of light upon the reflecting surface of the retina and take note of the returning light. Will such a reflex of light show significant changes in relation to identifiable moments of visual reaction?

We put this question to a systematic test by a series of retinoscopic examinations of children from 30 weeks to 4 years of age, inclusive. (Seven age levels were covered in the survey as follows: two cases in the first year, five at 21 months, 11 at 24 months, 13 at 30 months, 17 at 36 months, 15 at 42 months, 10 at 48 months.) The investigation was conducted under very favorable conditions, from the standpoint of external controls. A total of 73 examinations were made on 53 children; 26 of these children, who were examined in November, were carefully checked by a reexamination in the following May, after an interval of six months. A streak type of retinoscope was employed, with a 5-watt electric bulb, and a resistance coil to step down the light intensity. To preserve optimal natural conditions, all observations were made without cycloplegia. There was no evidence that this caused an abnormal spasm of the ciliary body. There were no obvious avoidance responses, and the cooperation of the children was excellent. A stenographer recorded the observations, which were immediately reported by the examiner.

The conditions and the surrounding circumstances of this section of our study merit brief description. With the exception of the two youngest infants, all the children who were retinoscoped attended the guidance Nursery of the Yale Clinic of Child Development. These children were of high average or superior intelligence, and came from homes of comfortable socio-economic status. They were so familiar with the general surroundings of the clinic that they adjusted readily to the examinations.

Sometime during the course of a morning, while attending the nursery, the child was called for by a guidance teacher, who accompanied him to the examination room on the next floor above. The near presence of the teacher was a stabilizing factor, both in the initial adjustment and during the course of the examination. Almost no resistance was encountered and the more articulate children spontaneously expressed a desire to come back to "see the pictures," and so on. Without the control of the personality factors, the retinoscopic study could scarcely have been undertaken.

In each instance, the actual procedure was adapted to the general maturity level of the child and to his individual characteristics. A typical procedure for the younger preschool child was somewhat as follows: the guidance teacher conducted the child into the room, where her charge seated himself in an adult chair, with a footstool for his dangling feet. The guidance teacher was seated next to him. If he was timid, she might for an initial period hold his hand to reassure him. His attention was attracted to the illuminated screen on the further wall of the examining room, and a nearby assistant observer projected slides on the screen. Sometimes he viewed the slides with silent interest; at other times, he vocalized his identification.

The examiner established prompt but peripheral rapport with the child, and through words and gestures diverted his attention to the screen or to the examiner himself as the observations required. The observations were made with a retinoscope at the child's eye level at far distance (approximately 15 feet), at intermediate distance (approximately seven feet), and at near distance (approximately 20 inches). The attention of the child was sustained and renewed by intermittent projection of slides, by verbal directions and, when necessary, by intercessions on the part of the guidance teacher.

The observations were usually completed in about 10 minutes and were verbally reported as made, to a stenographer. The visual tasks were adapted opportunistically to the readiness and the competence of the child. Part of this adaptation was accomplished through variations in the target. The basic target was a rectangular aluminum screen (14" x 21" in size) on which simple pictures were projected in succession. These pictures were crude black-and-white and colored drawings of familiar objects of interest to the child. The 2-year-old child, for example, was interested in the following pictures: *kitty, shoe, train, red car, blue car, blue ball, wagon, airplane, wheelbarrow, baby, bed* and *chair*. The child of 30 months was more ready to perceive a house and to identify details such as *window, smoke* and *door*. For children of 2 years and later ages, a picture book was also used at near to instate additional visual tasks during the retinoscopy.

In all situations, first the spontaneous reactions of the child were observed, and then his attention was guided by questions and suggestions, graded with respect to their concreteness. For example: *Do you see the bow wow? Do you see the chicken?* Or the teacher might point at a picture and say, *What is that?*

Such variations in procedure proved to be of some importance because they helped to define differentials in visual responses which were concomitantly related to the retinoscopic findings. The following manifestations were reported by the examiner as they were observed:
(a) Dullness and brightness of the reflex
(b) The color of the reflex (from dull red to white)
(c) Speed, range, promptness, pick-up, and release of motion
(d) Meridional differences

When possible, comparisons were made between the two eyes on the basis of foregoing manifestations, noting whether the reactions occurred synchronously, discrepantly, or in an alternating sequence. Occasionally, pupillary changes were also noted. By the age of 7 years, and in favorable subjects as early as the age of 5, the procedures of analytic refraction make possible further measurements, and subjective reporting also becomes available.

The findings of the retinoscopic survey, up to the age of 5 years, are described in the next chapter. For a study of this complexity, the findings must be regarded as preliminary. They are, however, highly indicative because they show a significant consistency with respect to the developmental trends and associated behavior traits of the individual child. Further investigations may demonstrate that the retinoscope has important uses in defining the nature and the needs of early child vision.

The present findings call for cautious interpretation. They cannot be construed in rigid dioptric terms. It seems evident that the young eye is in a labile condition, both dynamically and developmentally. Superimposed upon a basic delimiting refractive state, there is a margin of adaptability which is manifested in the brightness, the motion, the direction, and the velocity of the retinal reflex. Such a relationship between consolidated and plastic structure would seem to be a necessary condition for growth. The variations which are observed in a single session in a single child are not random, but are correlated with variations in his visual acts. The change in these same characteristics which takes place over the longer interval of a half-year is correlated with ontogenetic transformations. It is significant that these changes increasingly involve the functional teaming of the two eyes, operating singly and as a pair.

The increase of brightness, whatever its origin, characteristically occurs at the moment when the child identifies a target. At that moment the cortex probably releases an effector impulse which influences the total dioptric apparatus, including accommodation and convergence. At that moment, the eye and the brain appropriate the object of interest.

Coincidentally, the reflex registers an *against* motion, which by the streak retinoscope indicates a *minus* refractive value—but not necessarily a fixed myopic eye—for this "minus" may increase or decrease with the stress of the task, and, at certain moments of adjustment may give way to a *with* motion, which suggests a shift in the hyperopic or *plus* direction. Superficially, such variations may seem paradoxical and contradictory; but if one thinks of the reading eye as essentially a teleceptive-prehensory organ, these patterns of response are quite understandable. The eye gropes and grasps; it does not rest with absolute stolidity. Being in a state of relative readiness—a state of constructive labile equilibrium—it projects inward as well as outward. This introjection registered by a *minus* retinoscopic reading is part of the rhythm of a cycle of response. With this general introductory statement before us, we may now describe more concretely typical retinal responses observed at advancing ages.

A well-developed 30-week-old infant was examined while he sat in his mother's lap. An assistant observer, at a distance of 15 feet, waved a rattle to attract his attention and thereby became a target of interest. The examiner first observed a uniform *dullness* in both eyes; but as the child's eyes gradually sought the target, the reflex *brightened* and showed a *with* motion. When the attention settled and held to the target, the motion became *against*. As the attention relaxed, there was a slow oscillation of *against-with-against*, until the attention withdrew entirely, when the reflex tended to revert to a basic dullness, which in turn disappeared with the next act of visual attention.

Here we have a simple paradigm, which in one form or another recurs throughout the early years. These retinoscopic manifestations repeated themselves with a significant modification when a target moved into the near region. The examiner now closely confronted the child, and the examiner's face became the object of interest. This time, the reflex showed a definite *against* motion when the child fixated the examiner's face. Similarly, the reflex brightened and showed an *against* motion when an interesting toy (the tricolored plastic rings) was proffered. As the infant's hand came in, there was a with *motion*, followed by *brightening* as the hand grasped the toy. During tactile-visual exploitation of the toy, there was a succession of *against, with,* and *against* motion. The slowness of the motion suggested a rather wide range of oculocortical manipulations.

A comparison of the retinal-reflex patterns at near and far indicates that the infant at this age is more fully organized for vision in the nearpoint areas than at distance. This preeminence of the near area is a natural and continuing condition, although there will be many developmental shifts of emphasis in the visual occupation of spatial areas and sectors throughout infancy and childhood.

The concept of projection is admittedly vague, but it is supported by a great variety of visual and psychomotor patterns of behavior. The eye, like the hand (to say nothing of the mouth), is an organ of manipulation, and in higher adjustments each is separably, and both are conjointly, governed by the cortical brain. In the last analysis, it is the brain which appropriates the outer world, whether manually, orally, or ocularly. In the last analysis, it is the brain which appropriates the outer world, whether manually, orally, or ocularly. It does so by a projective process, but this is a two-way reciprocating process—a directional process which emanates from within the self, goes out and then returns within. Thus, projection both externalizes and internalizes. These two distinguishable phases have their counterparts in the *plus-minus* and *minus-plus* adjustments of the oculomanual prehensory apparatus. Accordingly, the retinal reflex registers *against* at the very appropriative moment when the 52-week-old infant has grasped the object; but when he extends a toy to a person, the reflex registers *with*. The physiologic basis of such manifestations is, of course, beyond exact description. Skeletal, visceral, and cortical factors are simultaneously involved, but the manifestations are not fortuitous. They are lawfully correlated with the functional and maturity status of the action system.

When the child is older, his near visual tasks become more symbolic, but the retinal manifestations and the cortical demands are not profoundly different. The eye still functions as a prehensory and manipulatory organ. The preschool child's identification of a picture or a letter in a book is comparable to the infant's prehension and manipulation of a toy. The preschool child of 3 years looks for a familiar picture and, since he knows what he is looking for, the retinoscope shows a sustained *minus*. The organism is "taking in" something—a visual kind of incoming projection, i.e., introjection. Presently the child extends arm and index finger and points to the picture; thereby he moves into the reciprocal outgoing phase of a circular cycle of response. Having "taken in," he is now projecting externally. Coincidentally, the retinoscope shows a *reduced minus*. Reduction of *minus* signifies, in this instance, a *plus* directionality. An increasing *minus* generally indicates an assimilative, introjective phase, but the final interpretation of any *plus* or *minus* value must take into account the individuality and the maturity of the total action system at the time of observation.

At 21 months, for example, the organism is visually more mature, but the retinal reflex unmistakably reveals extremes of *with* and *against*, transitional to a more effective organization. The general behavior traits of the child of this age reflect similar characteristics. (Being poorly organized for near-zone activity, he is best managed at arm's length—*his* own arm's length; he does not readily accept physical contact.) He has difficulty in shifting freely from one plane of regard to another. He shows considerable visual perseveration. When he has fixated a near object of interest, there is an increase of *against* motion while he strongly sustains his regard, and when he attempts to release regard, the *against* motion is sustained.

At 2 years, a difference between the two eyes working as a team becomes manifest. The pattern of the retinal response is not crisp and clear-cut, but there is evidence of mutual interplay. For example, on an intermediate target both eyes may react with a *with* motion; presently there is less motion in the right eye, followed by less in the left; then an *against* motion in the right eye, followed by an *against* motion in the left. When both eyes are in the *against* phase, one eye may be distinctly *brighter.* A definite transition from *brightness* to *dullness* (not observed at 21 months) is now distinctly discernible. While fixation is maintained, there may be a meridional change confined to one eye, or an alternation of meridional change from one eye to the other, the vertical meridian being usually associated with an against motion, the horizontal with a *with* motion.

These observations should not be over generalized; individual differences are apparent at every age, but it is significant that the short interval between 21 and 24 months should show a new trend in the developmental organization of the visual complex. The 2-year-old child is emerging from babyhood. He can give visual attention to a book and name a few pictures. His retinal reflex is steadier during fixation on a book and he shows a dioptric range from -1.00 to -2.00 D, with a discrepancy between the two eyes. Verbalization and pointing do not effect the reflex.

At 30 months his visual projection, at both far and near, is closely bound up with motor projection. On the book he may register a -.75 D while searching, and a -1.50 D when he "pins down" by pointing and exclaiming, "Here it is!"

The motion responses are now more clear-cut. The motion factor has become as conspicuous as the brightness factor. On a far and on an intermediate target, one eye brightens immediately and takes the lead. On far fixation, the motion is fast, suggesting good localization, but the eyes cleave close to the target because of restricted projection flexibility. In the near sector of the book, the 2 1/2-year-old shows a more appreciable advance over 2 years. There is more equivalence of the two eyes, and his inspection roves more easily over a page.

The 3-year-old has still more command of the near areas. This is partly shown in the fact that his eyes and hands are less closely bound as one than they were some six months earlier. Accordingly, there is an interesting reversal of the *minus* findings on the book. When the 2 1/2-year-old "pinned down" by naming or pointing, his minus increased; at 3 years, the *minus* decreases (for example, it may be -2.00 D on searching and -1.50 D on pointing or naming).

The 3-year-old is also less space-bound in far sectors. He projects into distances by a diversity of visual adaptations. He entertains a fuller visual awareness of situations in far space, but it is a participant awareness; he does not disengage as well as the

3 1/2-year-old child, who sometimes maintains both detachment and projection while contemplating a far-off scene.

At 3 years, the eyes retinoscopically show a high degree of variability. They seem to be more sensitive, in a double sense: they are more sensitive to light, and also more minutely responsive to changing facets of space. Both in far and in intermediate areas, pupillary and brightness differences and changes of alignment in the two eyes were noted. Motion changes are less prominent; but brightening, fading, and color changes become more discernible in actual process. During fixation of a far target, these manifestations were so active as to suggest that the eyes were exercising a new-found ability, which is merely a figurative description of a heightened functional reactivity characteristic of this stage of maturity. The visual system is growing and the retinal reflex is simply telling us something about the growth status of that system.

By the age of 4 years, the lively variability of the retinal reflex takes on a more positive and patterned character. There is more equivalence of the two eyes and the variability is obviously a more robust, adaptive flexibility. These developmental changes are already foreshadowed at the age of 41 months, when there are better defined transitions from *dull* to *bright* and from *with* to *against*, both at far and at intermediate sectors. For the first time, motion is clearly manifested during the *dull* phase. A more effective hyperopia seems to be in process of building and is becoming measurable both at far and at near. At far, a range of from Plano to +.75 D was found; at near, a range of +.50 D to +1.00 D.

The trend toward a more advanced teaming of the two eyes is particularly interesting at the 42-month age zone, which, incidentally, is a developmental period conducive to temporary and permanent strabismic symptoms. It is also a time when previously manifest squints may begin to resolve. A new kind of inequivalence is manifested, both at far and on the book. One eye may show variability in brightness and motion, while the other is relatively constant and set. A more consistent *with* motion is now evident at far.

At the 42-month age level, the book situation evoked a variety of reactions suggestive of reorganizations in interocular teaming. For example, one child with high *plus* and inequivalence at far showed -1.00 D with a definite meridional difference in one eye. Another child, with measurable equivalence at near and far, showed inequivalence on the book. Still another child, with meridional differences at far and near, showed high variability with a marked *minus* response, but no meridional difference on the book.

Despite these apparent inconsistencies, the developmental drift is toward greater equivalence and more effective hyperopia. Two children 44 months of age showed a very pretty example of rapid brightness alternation from one eye to the other. This may well represent a growth transition to the more sustained near-equivalence characteristic of the 4-year level of maturity. The typical 4-year-old is somewhat loosely organized, but not too loosely. His visual system operates with a new facility and flexibility. It is not as tightly bound by near book tasks as it will be at 5 years, but it moves with increased ease in the less exacting sectors of near, intermediate, and far space. His accommodation apparatus also moves freely, but not with the refinements which will become evident in another year. The 4-year-old is *fluid*; the 5-year-old is *focal.*

If not pushed too far, these two contrastive adjectives suggest a valid difference in the developmental optics of the 4- and 5-year age levels. But the fluidity of 4 has normally a fairly solid basis; and it is more highly organized and integrated than the variability of the 3 1/2-year stage of maturity. It is significant that the visual behavior patterns at advancing stages are dynamically comparable to the over-all patterns of the total action system. Cautiously interpreted, the retinal reflex is a useful indicator of the maturity of the young eye in action.

With more complete studies, it is possible that the interpretation of the retinal reflex can be placed upon a more objective basis. Even now, the factors of motion, brightness, quality and general pattern of the responses lend themselves to discriminating clinical appraisal. It is very significant that there should be quality differences, susceptible to graded assessment. These are particularly evidenced in gradations of color, as well as in changes of motion. Schematically, at least, these color values can be arranged in a five-step gradient, with three degrees of variation within each of the following categories: A. Dull red, B. Bright pink, B'. Dull pink, C. White-pink, D. White. A color in itself does not have absolute definitive significance; the functional contexts vary. For example, a dull (brickish) red may be associated with: 1. A high plus or high minus finding, 2. Low awareness and weak recognition, 3. Very meager or floppy effector set. Bright pink is associated with a low minus. There is more awareness and interpretation, but the "set" does not accurately strike the point of regard and it is, moreover, episodic rather than sustained.

White is at the summit of the gradient. It is characteristically linked with a low amount of plus in children. It denotes a higher grade of cortical control, with more sustained set for the visual task, and effortless modulation of spatial loci.

Arranged in orderly sequence, the COLOR SCHEMA OF THE RETINAL REFLEX is as follows:

A. DULL RED (brick)
   1. High *plus* (or *minus*)
   2. Low recognition or awareness
   3. "Flop" period (neither good quantity nor good quality of "effector set")

B. BRIGHT PINK
   1. *Low minus*

2. Higher recognition or awareness than A, but not "spatially on" point of regard, though interpretively "at" point of regard
3. A quantity of set, but only of periodic or episodic quality

B. DULL PINK
1. *Low plus*
2. Refractory period that follows B', but not the "flop" of A
3. First indications of quality development

C. WHITE-PINK (Bright and still pinkish, but not white)
1. Plano
2. Neither *plus* nor *minus*, because the effector set is now approximating point of regard without the apparent movement "around" point of regard, as in B and B'
3. Better quality than ever before, but still with minute periodic refractor shifts

D. WHITE
1. *Plus* (+.50 D or +.75 D)
2. Higher-grade cortical control of C. In more constant and "effortless" control of total spatial loci, and more constant "set" for task.
3. Now "set" with good quality and consistency

Although the foregoing is a schematic summary, it may serve as a frame of reference. It strongly suggests the presence of a developmental drift which pervasively affects the manifestations of the young eye when it is subjected to visual tasks.

It is impossible to appraise all the factors which enter into the color and brightness phenomena of the retinal reflex—to say nothing of the gleaming, the flashing, and the sparkling of eyes, which figure so prominently in fiction! Some of these phenomena are extremely esoteric and beyond demonstration. The nature of light itself is not known. Einstein conceives all light to be constituted of individual particles of energy, called photons, which travel through space in separate, discontinuous quanta. Assuming that the intensification of the fundus glow is primarily due to a readjustment of the accommodative apparatus, in response to a nervous stimulus, a complete description (if the knowledge were available) might include associated photochemical events which are far too subtle for separate identification by the retinoscope.

The absorption of light by the retina must bear some lawful relations to the emission of light. When light is largely absorbed, the fundus reflex will be dull. If there is a gradient of absorption, there is probably a critical point in this gradient which is favorable to neuronic firing. When little light is absorbed, more is reflected and the reflex will be bright. The brightening may mount in a wavelike manner, reaching a peak and then waning. Maturity and individual differences will influence the definiteness of these wax-wane patterns. In any case, the ocular system contains within itself self-regulatory chemical arrangements for the liberation and transfer of energy in the form of small discrete units.

These speculations have little bearing on the value of the retinoscope as an investigatory of diagnostic instrument. It is enough to say that the evidence now available strongly indicates that the brightening and the dulling of the retinal reflex are directly correlated with the activity of the higher nerve centers in the visual system. According to the concept of electrotonic integration, every neurone is a small chemical system whose metabolism sets up an inherent, rhythmic electrotonic current. This centrogenic current may be reinforced by reflexogenic currents, which have their origin in outlying receptors and in other neurones. When the resultant current is strong enough to rise above the threshold, the neurone fires. When the reflexogenic signals mount, the rate of discharge increases; when the signals slacken, the discharge diminishes. An optical end result of such discharges may well be evidenced in the retinal reflex. With the possibility of photo-electric instrumentation capable of making a comprehensive, objective record of retinocortical responses, the retinoscope may take on added significance as a diagnostic device and as an aid in child-vision research.

CHAPTER 12
The Ontogenesis of Visual Behavior

The science of developmental optics is concerned with the organization of visual functions in their dynamic relation to the action system. The dynamic relationships and the consequent organization are outwardly manifested in patterns of visual behavior. These patterns are evident in individual acts of vision. They undergo lawful changes throughout the whole cycle of growth. Especially significant are the developmental changes which occur in the first 10 years of the ontogenetic cycle. At no other stage of life do visual changes occur so swiftly and so elaborately.

The present chapter undertakes to summarize these ontogenetic transformations for a score of age levels, from birth to age 10. For convenience of reference, typical behavior patterns are also listed, age by age, in tabular form in Appendix B under the heading *Ontogenetic Gradients of Visual Behavior.* It will be understood that the age assignments in these gradients are approximate and suggestive. They represent maturity trends within a relatively homogeneous population and are, of course, subject to wide individual variations.

Individual variations, however, can be more readily identified and described with the aid of a frame of reference, which the gradients and the descriptive summaries of the present chapter aim to supply. The order of a gradient sequence is less subject to individual variation than the age values because the sequence is based upon a fundamental ontogenetic ground plan of maturation. This ground plan may be envisaged in terms of the growth trends for five distinguishable functional fields, namely: (1) Eye-hand coordination, (2) Postural orientation, (3) Fixation, (4) Retinal response, (5) Projection. A separate gradient has been drawn up for each of the foregoing fields. (See Appendix B.)

With due caution, the gradients and the summary characterizations of the progressive age levels can be used to interpret the visual maturity level of a given child under examination or training. It is desirable to estimate this maturity in terms of both the child's action system and the "developmental drift" of his visual functions. In Part One of this volume, we sketched the ascending stages in the development of the action system, with incidental reference to visual characteristics. In the pages which immediately follow, we retraverse this ontogenetic cycle, but with more specific reference to the visual system, as such, even though it will always prove impossible to separate the visual from the total action system.

A series of summaries of the visual functions is presented for 11 age levels, beginning with 21 months. These age summaries afford a cross-sectional approach but, when read in sequence and in association with the gradients, they also afford a longitudinal approach. The Functional Summaries should not be regarded as rigid age norms, but as orientational characterizations. No sharp line can, of course, be drawn between adjacent age periods. Nevertheless, it is always pertinent to consider whether any given child is functioning below or above his chronological age or atypically therefrom. It is hoped that the sequential growth gradients and the functional summaries of visual behavior, which also fall into longitudinal sequence, will assist in the appraisal of developmental trends and hygienic needs.

The data presented indicate the presence of significant growth trends. It should be emphasized that, in a field of such complexity, our present information must be considered merely preliminary and indicative, and should not be regarded in terms of rigid standardization.

The procedures used in making the functional tests for the age levels from 21 months to 10 years are described in Appendix A. For the period from 21 months to 5 years, the visual behavior is summarized under the following headings:

- Adjustment to the examination
- Reactions to the dangled bell
- Retinoscopy
  - Far estimate
  - Intermediate estimate
  - Far measure
  - Near measure
  - Book
- Projection

For the period from 5 to 10 years, the following headings are used:

- Skeletal
  - Phorias
  - Fusion range
- Visceral
  - Retinoscopy
  - Subjectives
  - Accommodative range
- Skills
  - Stereograph
  - Visual resolution
  - Depth perception
  - Pursuit fixation

In the formulation of the functional summaries, the developmental stages are differentiated according to the child's visual manipulation of space. Since, in retinoscopy, *against* motion is measurable with an amount of minus lens power, it is assumed that the visual mechanism is posturing and operating at or around an area within the actual position of the target in space. Likewise, if a *with* motion, which is measurable by a plus lens amount, is present, it is assumed that the visual mechanism is operating beyond the target. The age periods are classified as follows: beginning with birth to 4 weeks, 4 to 16 weeks, 16 to 28 weeks, 28 weeks to 40 weeks, 40 to 52 weeks, 12 months, 18 months, 2 years, 2 1/2 years, 3 years, 3 1/2 years, 4 years, 5 years, 6 years, 7 years, 8 years, 9 years.

BIRTH TO 4 WEEKS

Birth marks the arrival, but not the beginning, of an individual. In an earlier chapter we noted how extensively fetal eyes and brain were organized in anticipation of the act of seeing. The fetal eyes begin to move beneath their sealed lids a full half-year prior to birth.

During the first postnatal month, the functional and somatic development of the eyes proceeds at an extremely rapid pace, even during the long periods when the eyes are closed in sleep and drowsing. Variable and fitful but lengthening moments of visual awareness occur during the wakeful interludes.

Philosophers have not been able to penetrate the mysteries of this early organization of human vision. It is idle to ask whether the newly born baby brings with him an innate sense of space. If he does, that sense is far from complete. Accordingly, the baby begins at once to deploy his eyes, to move and to halt them, in a manner which denotes an active adaptation to the voidless world into which he is born. Promptly he embarks upon the long protracted developmental task of spatial manipulation.

Conjugate eye movements and optic nystagmus are present at or near the time of birth. Coordinate compensatory eye movements occur during the first week, and are efficacious by the end of the first month. In these movements, the eyes shift in a direction opposite to that of the head, simultaneously and coextensively with the head movements. Rudimentary ocular pursuit is readily elicited in the first day of life by moving fluttering fingers slowly across the field of vision, within a distance of several inches from the eyes. The pursuit is responsive to peripheral rather than central stimulation.

The tonic-neck-reflex attitude keeps the head averted. This position tends to limit the field and the direction of regard. Sustained fixation of a near object of interest undergoes rapid development. In the first stage, the fixation is typically monocular. The active eye immobilizes, except for minute lateral and vertical movements, which cause the fovea to traverse a stimulus area. The inactive eye is variously closed, deviated, or wandering but, at a later stage, when monocular fixation is still more defined, the subordinate eye becomes relatively immobile and postures cooperatively.

The hands are predominantly fisted; they clench when the palm is stimulated. Spontaneous arm movements have no readily discernible relations to head and eye postures, but such relations may be operative.

Infants generally prefer the supine position during periods of awakeness. Many infants elect the prone position during sleep. A few resist the prone orientation altogether. These marked postural preferences must have an influence on the structure of the visual domain. The head may be prevailingly rotated to a preferred side while the infant is awake and in the supine position. When this preference is marked in degree and consistently manifested, it is predictive of later handedness. Deep-seated, hereditary left-handedness is likely to show itself early in a predilection for a left tonic-neck-reflex attitude. The eye contralateral to the extended arm tends to be used in monocular fixation.

The spontaneous regard of the neonate is, in general, vague and tends to be highly variable in duration and intensity. The prevailing averted position of the head serves to delimit the field and the direction of regard. The neonate does not move his head freely for exploratory regard. His stare tends to be vacant and passive; occasionally, it is active or transfixed.

His eyes follow the movement of the dangling ring when it is brought into the periphery of his vision, pursuing it through a short arc or even through a whole quadrant.

He also regards the stationary dangling ring when it is suspended within the near zone of vision, at a distance of from four to 10 inches. He registers optimal regard by opening his mouth and by other evidences of pleasant excitement, a fact which suggests that the visual experience is already closely identified with his bodily economy and total action system.

In the course of his daily (and nightly) life, the neonate does not encounter many situations which make demands on his visual capacities. However, when he is brought to the breast, or when a bottle is offered to him, or when his mother's face or hand comes within close range, he begins to "catch" sight. That is, he reacts with fixational responses.

The nature and extent of these earliest fixational capacities have been fruitfully explored by Dr. Bing Chung Ling, with the aid of an experimental crib and cinema recording. The crib was located in the center of a cylinder (36" x 48") encased in one-way-vision screen. The inner surface of the cylinder served as a uniform white background for a two-inch black stimulus disk, which was made to recede and to approach slowly in front of the infant's eyes, within a distance of 36 inches.

Under the conditions of this investigation, fixation appeared in rudimentary form a few hours after birth and reached a high peak of definition at the end of the neonatal period (about 4 weeks). The presence of fixation was evidenced by several behavior signs as follows: quieting of body activity and of fussing, raising of upper eyelids and eyebrows, widening of eye slits, wrinkling of forehead, alignment of eye or eyes with disk, and immobilization of one eye or both.

In this early stage of development, the infant fixates definitely when the stimulus disk is a few inches from his eyes. He gives only brief, feeble glances when it moves farther away. Manipulation of the area of regard is first organized within a near and narrow working range, but the glances beyond the near plane would seem to denote a prospective occupation of a more distant sector. The visual mechanisms of the new-born infant grow at an extremely rapid rate. In a day or two, the range of sustained near fixation may extend outward several inches. In time, the fixation remains sustained while the experimental disk recedes to a farpoint of 36 inches.

The infant fixates a near plane of regard with greater facility than a far plane. If the approaching disk is brought too near (less than three inches), he retracts his head as though to increase the distance between the eyes and the disk to secure better vision. He builds up the range of fixation from the near zone outward and fixates the stimulus object at a greater distance during its retreat than during its approach. These reactions suggest again that his visual world grows in an outward direction, and that perceptual space is built up by a thatch-like series of extensions which emanate from a near region of organization. In last analysis, of course, this near region resides in the cerebral cortex and the total action system.

4-16 WEEKS

Sustained visual fixation, as demonstrated by the Ling experiment and by the cinema records of the Yale Clinic, reaches its first peak of efficiency at about the age of 4 weeks. Fixation implies an adaptive immobilization of one eye, but the fixating eye is never absolutely still. It makes minute side-to-side and up-and-down excursions. Early near fixation is monocular. The active eye is poised in line with the stimulus (e.g., two-inch dark disk against a neutral background). The non-fixating eye may be closed or partly open, resting or wandering willy-nilly. At a later stage this subordinate eye is open and shifts to its nasal corner to be at least partly in line with the stimulus. The leading eye fixates singly. In the next stage, the monocular fixation alternates rapidly from one eye to the other, the shifts being accompanied by a rhythmic left-to-right-to-left rotation of the head.

This interesting transitional stage of monocular alternation of dominance leads directly into binocular convergence, which makes its appearance in the second month. The convergence is at first accomplished by a series of short, globus jerks. With increasing age, the jerks are reduced and the act of convergence becomes smooth and gliding. But in the early phases of convergence, the infant often blinks; and under stress of too near or too long fixation, temporary strabismus sets in. From the beginning, Nature's ontogenetic problem seems to be to achieve a nice balance and linkage of monocular and binocular functions.

Conjugate deviations and coordinate compensatory eye movements, in common with fixation, are functional soon after birth. They are, of course, closely associated with fixation and, like fixation, they become more defined with age and more adaptive as a result of experience. The conjugate teaming of the eyes is not absolutely rigid. In the abversion-adversion type of deviation, the eye that is nearer the object of interest deviates to a lesser extent than the eye which is farther away. In up-and-down movements, however, there is remarkably close correspondence in the degrees of elevation and depression. This difference has interesting evolutionary implications. Ling calls attention to a significant type of conjugate deviation which is brought into requisition to explore the contour of a near object of interest. These conjugate deviations are minute, and they occur in rapid succession in lateral, vertical and oblique directions. "The extent of these movements seems to be in strict conformity with the contour of the disk."

The movements drop out as the object of interest recedes beyond the near plane of regard. This fact indicates that—even in early infancy—fixation, accommodation, and convergence develop in close correlation. It is remarkable that the basic components of human vision are present to this extent at such an early age. The infant takes hold of the physical world with his eyes long before he takes hold of it with his prehensory hands—another fact with far-reaching implications.

The visual domain of the infant undergoes numerous elaborations during the first quarter. At 4 weeks, his discrimination is episodically limited to near objects of interest and to the massive stimuli of his more distant surroundings. During the course of a half-hour, his visual responses are transient and fluctuating. At the age of 12 weeks, his visual activity is prolonged and his regard has become more selective. In the dangling-ring situation, he attends to the examiner's hand as well as to the ring—a significant achievement in visual discrimination. At the test table, he detects a one-inch cube, even regards it more than momentarily. There is also a diminution in the diverted regards which formerly went to the examiner and to the surroundings. This growing capacity to cancel out rival stimuli and to focus upon a pertinent and novel object of interest in the working zone is a major growth phenomenon. It is a reminder that acts of vision are inseparably bound up with the cortical developments which organize perceptual trends.

16-28 WEEKS

The fixation capacities of the 16-week-old infant have reached a high level or organization. This is shown in the versatility of his regard behavior, displayed in his spontaneous activity and in his reaction to objects placed on the text table. Although he will not pick up a test cube manually on sight, he will pick it up rather promptly with his eyes. He will regard it prolongedly, with augmented breathing and intensified straining. He will also shift his regard to his own hand, back to the cube, and then to his hand again, making several shifts in the course of a minute. He does this with relative facility, but his shift to a far plane is not as smooth or penetrating. He is capable, however, of a crude roving type of inspection of surroundings.

The 20-week-old infant displays more visual interest in the distant environs of a room. Whereas, a month earlier he apprehended his mother's presence within a radius of about three feet, he now perceives her at remoter distances and is disturbed if she disappears too suddenly. He is achieving new planes of regard and, perhaps for that very reason, he is not skillful in shifting from one plane to another. He holds a regard tenaciously, and releases it abruptly. He may even seem to have lost some of the facility of release and refixation in near sectors, which he had exhibited at 16 weeks. This suggests that a process of developmental organization is going on. Nevertheless, he gives much more definite and prolonged regard to the pellet. He also bestows a recurrent regard on it.

This recurrent type of regard has interesting developmental implications, and it is manifested very frequently at this stage of maturity. It is a method of growth, which prevents excessively prolonged stimulation, and yet deepens and defines experience through repetition. The automaticity of the recurrent regard indicates that it is a very basic mechanism.

At 24 weeks, regard behavior already has a more mature aspect. He gives immediate regard to a single and to a second cube, and shifts regard from one cube to another. Although he picks up the first cube on sight, he drops it to seize the second. In another month he will retain the first even while he secures the second. His grasp is crude, but he has achieved one of the most fundamental interadjustments in his whole behavior equipment—the coordination of eye and hand.

28-40 WEEKS

With the achievement of closer coordination of eyes and hands, vision takes on an enlarged role in the second half of the first year. Concurrent changes in the size and structure of lens, cornea, optic nerve, and fovea support this role, and permit the infant to exercise his new powers of vision almost continuously and tirelessly. Binocular fixation, conjugate deviations, and coordinate compensatory eye movements not only are well established but become increasingly expert with the refinement of the total motor system, including head, fingers and oculorotators.

As already noted, the infant employs minute conjugate deviation movements astonishingly early to explore the contours of objects. As early as the age of 28 weeks, he is able to discriminate in a primitive manner between simple geometric forms, including circle, square, triangle, oval, and cross (overall dimensions of individual forms ranging from 1 1/2 inches to 3 inches). With the aid of one-way-vision screen and a modified Yale clinical crib arrangement, Ling demonstrated experimentally that at this age level the normal human infant can use fine geometric form discrimination per se as a learning cue which sets up reactions of choice and avoidance.

The stimulus value of the geometric blocks was supercharged by previously soaking them in a strong saccharine solution, but the adaptive reactions of the infant depended upon the visible contours. The geographic arrangements of a total stimulus pattern were apparently less consequential. Changes in the relative position, spatial orientation, and size of the forms had very little effect on the discrimination performance. The infant evidently has a primitive, absolute sense of form which enables him to recognize a distinctive shape, irrespective of its orientation in space. This amazing sense may hark back to an ancient phyletic stage which is superseded and overlaid in later ontogenesis. Nevertheless, this "abstract," absolute sense of form does not seem to be a product of training or conditioning, but is instead an innate capacity which is intrinsic in the behavioral constitution. Therefore the capacity varies significantly with individuality. Individual differences in form discrimination and abstraction are marked and consistently evident, from age to age, during this period of infancy.

With his new visual capacities, the infant displays an increasing interest in details, in entities, and in the context and continuation of entities. All this is transparently disclosed in the changing patterns of his cube behavior. His inveterate shifting of a single cube from hand to hand (28-32 weeks), his holding of a cube in each hand with shifts of regard from one to the other (32 weeks), his pushing of one cube with a second cube (36 weeks), all denote a progressive ability to manipulate closely juxtaposed spatial relationships. This ability is a topographic discrimination, an elementary form of projicience. Or shall we call it a morphogenetic process—stereopsis in the making?

Vision takes on increasingly complex emotional qualities and concomitants. The infant accordingly is more "sensitive." He shows a rather remarkable ability to detect facial expressions. This ability is related to the discriminativeness of geometric form, which we have described. The delicate reconfigurations of physiognomy, which are facial expressions, are readily sensed because they have great importance for the economy of the organism. Cortical factors are already in operation. It is literally true that a baby can read visible signs which are more subtle than those of the printed page.

The infant also manifests an increased ability to shift from one plane of regard to another. The 28-week-old infant is not as tightly bound by near planes; he tends to extend his arms forward when exploiting an object of interest (e.g., a cube), looking on as he does so. This is an obvious outward extension of the radius of regard. At 32 weeks he persistently reaches for toys out of reach, another method of stretching the radius. Previously he "disregarded" the outlying object because he did not identify or localize it in space. Now he can move more freely into outer space; he shifts his regard from cube to examiner with new ease. He attends visually with deeper absorption, as though the visual component of his sensory-motor experience were taking on a new significance.

ILLUSTRATIVE FUNCTIONAL TEST AT 30 WEEKS

An exploratory functional test was made on one infant at 30 weeks of age. He was held in his mother's arms and his attention was attracted to a person standing at the far screen. From this distance, the examiner observed the changes of the retinal response, summarized in present tense as follows:

The infant shows a definite tendency to go out to the target, visually, although his approach is slow and rather vague. It is neither brisk nor precise. (The retinoscope registers a uniform dullness during such slow approach.) In this outward seeking, he overreaches this target (slow *with* motion), but presently he intensifies his effort to localize the target (*against* motion). In his effort to discriminate and to hold it, the retinoscope registers an *against* motion and then *against* in the vertical meridian. He cannot maintain a firm hold indefinitely, but he does adhere to the general area of the target with wide fluctuations (slow oscillating *with* to *against*). He is out there, but does not stay precisely on the spot.

In near areas, he displays intensified interest for the toy rings or the examiner's face. He reacts with a heightened visual response. As he reaches toward the toy, fixation relaxes but regard is maintained and, as the toy is grasped, vision again heightens and intensifies. Manual manipulation ensues, accompanied by visual manipulation.

At near, he regards the examiner's face with interest (the retinoscope registers a definite *against*). As a toy (tricolored rings) is brought near him, he regards it intently and there is increased *against* motion and brightening. He brings his hand toward the toy (the retinoscope registers a *with* motion). As he grasps the toy, the response brightens and there is an *against* motion. Now he manipulates the toy and the motion changes, with wide fluctuations of *with* to *against*.

He is intrigued by the dangled bell as it comes to within about six inches of his eyes. Both eyes respond with equal facility, but with a series of reposturings rather than with a smooth, fluent convergence. The eyes, however, are nimble enough to pursue the string in an upward direction toward the examiner's hand. There may be a preferential regard for the approaching hand, preceding fixation of the smaller, suspended target. His ocular posturing and ocular release are restricted in their boundaries. He releases at the plane of his regard. When he brings both hands to the target, eyes and hands operate more in unison, and then eye movements become smoother.

40-52 WEEKS

The last quarter of the first year is characterized by a general increase in mobility of regard and in awareness of depth and movement. This gain in awareness is not purely sensory, but is the product of growing insight. The behavior patterns displayed when the infant confronts a mirror are highly significant of new visual developments. Even at 40 weeks, he seems to take in the whole situation. His behavior becomes quietly experimental, and he shows a strong interest in his reflected movements. In another month, he may wave his hands to induce imaged movement. He is soberly interested in watching the retreating image of his withdrawing hand.

A similar heightened awareness of movement is shown in his daily life; in his responsiveness to dramatic nursery games and increased imitativeness. He can, however, imitate only those movements which are already in his motor repertoire. His ability to see these movements rests on his ability to make them.

He is aware of small movements and small displacements in spatial relationships. He perceives the dropping and disappearance of the pellet from the bottle. He is more discriminatingly regardful of the movement of the ring as he pulls the string. His extended index finger becomes an auxiliary to vision; he pries (with his eyes) as he probes; and by so doing he multiplies in sequence minutely spaced planes of regard in a manner which builds up a sense of depth. Not without reason, he is coordinately interested in spatial depth and in movement sensed through eyes and fingers.

His visual domain, therefore, is much more tridimensional, both in relation to things and in interpersonal relations. His back-and-forth nursery games, his waving of bye bye, his mirror play, his tendency to extend a toy in hand toward the examiner, his postural tendency to pivot and to shift his focus of manipulation from one place to another—all this represents greater freedom and flexibility in visual activity. The infant's eyes seem more mobile. He uses them more nimbly to pursue a ball as it rolls away, to watch the moving trees, to scan the examiner from head to foot with facile shift of regard. These new visual abilities serve to contribute to his still very embryonic, but growing, sense of self.

His appreciation of certain spatial relations is amazingly refined. He plucks a pellet with artistic precision. With a neatly posed oblique approach, he selectively grasps the top of the handle of a bell with his finger tips. This delicate, untaught maneuver, which contrasts so sharply with the grossness of his earlier prehension, indicates that his visual domain has undergone remarkable refinement in its spatial structure.

This refinement is correlated with a maturational advance in the visceral components of vision. The skeletal components are also developing, but during this period the infant seems to be particularly bent upon bringing his visceral mechanism into effective coordination with manual and body posturing. His auditory and visual orientation to far areas is fairly satisfactory, but at near sectors he constantly seeks new clarities through ceaseless exploitive activity. He will play for an amazingly long stretch with a single toy, subjecting it to ever-varying visual manipulations. Thereby, he organizes his space world and satisfies his visceral needs. Should skeletal trends be excessive, this organization may go somewhat awry.

The developmental problem is to bring visceral and skeletal components into reciprocal harmony. Under stress or under imbalanced skeletal predominance, the teaming of the two eyes may be more or less disrupted. Transitory strabismus occurs not infrequently. The strabismus may be benign or prodromal. In any event, this is a period when functional relationships between TNR and STR attitudes and monocularity and binocularity are actively in the making.

12 MONTHS

Toward the end of the first year, the infant definitely displays a "placement propensity" in which eyes and hands both participate. In some way, this placement propensity is bound up with the maturing voluntary capacity to release, to let go, to inhibit. The child exercises this release capacity in his cube play somewhat crudely at the age of 48 weeks, and in a more ordered way at 52 and 56 weeks when he sequentially picks up and releases one cube after another. This serial behavior simulates counting; indeed, it is the developmental matrix of counting if, by counting, we mean the identification of the members of an ordinal series. This placement pattern manifests itself in various ways. At 1 year, the child spontaneously brings the crayon to bear upon paper, making a few linear marks, which at 15 months are readily converted into an imitative back-and-forth scribble. At 15 months, he is able also to identify a picture, registering his identification in a pronate patting. In these three behaviors—the picture recognition, the crayon scribble, and the serial cube play—we already see the genetic germs of the three R's, which are destined to make such heavy demands upon the functions of vision in later childhood.

The placement propensity may involve the eyes alone, as well as the eyes and hands in association. Accordingly, we see the infant indulging the increasing agility of his eyes. He may manipulate an object in the near area, and then he may extend his arms full length and visually pounce upon the object of interest as though he were playing tag with shifting planes of regard. Sometimes he leans forward in pursuit of an object after he has made an outward thrust. Still more typically, he casts an object from his high chair or through the railings of the pen, then fixates on the object after it has landed or sometimes follows in close pursuit. We may designate this visual behavior pattern as a form of saltatory regard. He exercises this regard with greater skill when he is in the sitting position. When he is standing or walking, this type of regard is more difficult and a comparable skill awaits the future.

It is needless to say that, with these growing skills the infant enjoys watching the passing show. From his vantage point, he follows the moving pedestrian, the moving tree tops, and the automobile in transit. He is now so simultaneously alert to both place and movement that he adaptively fixates the round hole of the formboard after the board is rotated, and correctly inserts the round block. If the reader will reflect on all the implications of this one visual behavior pattern, he will appreciate the developmental advance which the child has made prior to the age of 18 months.

ILLUSTRATIVE FUNCTIONAL TEST AT 1 YEAR

A brief report of a retinoscopic observation of a year-old infant will serve to indicate the general status of visual performance at that age.

The infant gives attentive regard to a person across the room; when observed by retinoscope from this distance, the retinal reflex of both eyes is bright; one eye is brighter than the other, but no motion is evident.

However, when the examiner is within the infant's near range, motion becomes observable. As the infant reaches out and grasps a toy, the motion is a rapid *against*. During manipulation, the *against* motion occasionally changes to *with*. Give-and-take play with his mother is registered by shifts of motion: *against* while taking, and *with* while giving. When the infant holds the toy at his mouth and regards the examiner, the motion is *against*. The brighter reflex of one eye is evident at near, as well as at far. When the infant is walking with one hand held, the retinoscope shows a *with* motion.

The infant easily fixates a *dangled bell,* and pursues it ocularly as it moves toward his nose. Both eyes converge with about equal facility, and he then releases his regard to the examiner.

18 MONTHS

The activity of the 18-month-old is on a touch-and-go and a look-and-go basis. His attention typically works in brief swift strokes. His locomotor drive is so strong that it seems to dominate his visual behavior, but sight and action function with close interplay. His runabout tendencies yield him innumerable visual experiences. He sees an object; with headlong directness he makes for it, seizes it, drags it, drops it in a moment, goes somewhere else, goes back to it, and so on, and so on. His previous orientations to space and distance were formerly limited by a sedentary position and by creeping; now he has to revise and to elaborate his adjustments in terms of an upright walking. His new postural attitudes open up a new world with countless new visual problems.

From a sheer spatial standpoint,he is not altogether at home in this world. Note the way in which he meets the problem of seating himself in a small chair a few feet away. He cannot confront this problem with eyes front, so he resorts to various devices: he backs up deviously and corrects his bearings, he spreads his legs apart and leans over and peers through them to direct his aim; or he squats down beside the chair, and then sidles or straddles. A normal infant solves this and similar problems in a comparatively brief space of time. (An ament may require a year or more.)

The run-about propensities of this age serve to project him into spatial situations which he has never experienced before. In his gross bodily activity, he assumes versatile postural attitudes; he bends over and sideways, he squats, he twists his shoulders, he flings his arms in a manner which opens up new spatial facets. He even walks backward, as though he had to become aware of unseen territory in the rear. If he pulls a wheeled toy, he does not take it for granted that the toy follows. So either he is heedless or turns backward to see. From a developmental standpoint, vision comprises insight into those aspects of the unseen which are closely related to the seen.

By means of his busy brief strokes of attention, his daubs of paint, his ceaseless strokes of exploitational play, he familiarizes himself with the furniture of his physical world. When he walks abroad, even though on a leash, he busily explores byways. At home, he shows an embryonic sense of place despite his apparently mercurial journeyings. He begins to identify shoe, spoon, and other familiar objects in terms of the places where they ought to be. This is no insignificant achievement if we consider the immaturity of the child and the complexity of the spatial world.

21 MONTHS

At 21 months, this same child may show a rather amazing fetish-like attachment to an object of interest. The object itself may have simply visual and tactile interest, but somehow it is also charged with emotional values because, in clinging to the object, he feels a tranquilizing sense of orientation which he would otherwise lack. All this reminds us that vision always involves the child's ego and that the detailed structure of the visuospatial world is part and parcel of that ego.

The active run-about is under compulsion to go directly to an object of interest to establish contact. The contact punctuates his performance. This repeats endlessly, but at times the child also pauses to watch; and at 21 months he will sit and gaze transfixedly at objects beyond near range. He does not, however, release his fixation readily from near to far. He may change his body and eye postures and stare into space, as though aware that something is there, but without making an effort to localize the object in space.

The 21-month-old infant shows considerable perseveration. He reacts with sustained emphasis after he has achieved an adjustment to a near object of interest. But he has difficulty in moving freely from one plane of regard to another. He is poorly organized in the near zone and shows difficulty in projecting to variable planes even within the near zone.

FUNCTIONAL TESTS

Beginning with the age of 21 months, functional tests were administered in an examining room located near the Guidance Nursery, in surroundings with which the children were accustomed. As previously described, and as detailed elsewhere (Appendix A), each preschool child was accompanied by a guidance teacher, who was an important factor in adjusting the child to the novel examination situation. Fixation, the retinal reflex, and projection were tested in that order. The following informal description of the child's reactions to the tests will give concrete indications of the general level at which he is visually functioning.

Adjustment

As the 21-monther enters the examining room holding the teacher's hand, his expression is somewhat vague and starey. He is led to the examining chair and is helped to seat himself. The examiner approaches cautiously and, without directing immediate attention to himself or to the child, he brings the dangled bell into position.

Dangled Bell

The child is slow to fixate the bell and now prefers to stare through it to regard the examiner. If the bell is jingled, it helps him to localize it but he fails to converge as it is brought in toward his nose. On repetition of the test, he holds fixation and changes posture of the eyes, but then has difficulty in release. And when the bell is again moved in, one eye may reposture *inward* (nasally) while the other eye remains directed forward. As soon as the hand comes to the target, the lagging eye also repostures.

When reaching toward the dangled bell, he is apt to overreach, but his hand helps to form a plane of regard and thereby fixation improves. He may keep his hand near the target without accompanying regard.

Retinoscopy

Far Estimate. The child's attention is now diverted to a picture on the far screen and the examiner observes the retinal reflex from this distance. It is helpful in this situation to have the child on the lap of the teacher in order that she may direct his attention by saying, "See the kitty." If attention is undefined, it is difficult to secure a reflex and the reflex is dull.

Upon the child's recognition of a target, such as a *baby* or a *kitty*, the reflex briefly brightens. Attention may again be held by a target picture of *shoes* and, with the reflex brightening, a slight *against* or *with* motion is detectable. Brightness changes from monocular to binocular. The reflex becomes dull between the brightening responses. At this age, the child may name a few pictures: *boy, shoe, kitty, plane, light, car.* Or he may simply smile or point, saying "uh."

Intermediate Estimate. At an intermediate distance, more motion is perceptible and it is, as at far, slightly *with* or *against.*

Near and Far Measure. Attempts to secure measurement through a lens are unsuccessful. The child either reaches for the lens or tries to look at it as it is held before one eye or both eyes. As he tries to grasp or regard it, an *against* motion is seen; as he looks up at the examiner, the *against* motion is held. However, he finally releases to examiner and the motion is a slow *with*; while his regard is sustained, the *with* motion reduces. When he is holding a toy, without manipulation, the motion is *with*. There is a rather wide fluctuation between the motions of *with* and *against*, indicating high *plus* or high *minus*. No differences in the two eyes are noted at near.

Book. Despite strong lens interference, the child with the aid of the teacher can identify a few pictures in a book, pictures of animals of chief interest. While attention is thus held, a measurement can be swiftly made. Measurements usually range from about -.75 D to -1.25 D.

Projection

The stereoscope is a complicated instrument for use with a child of this age. He does not like to have a strange object touch him, and he keeps his distance from the lens-well, only briefly peering into it. He stands before the instrument and may put his hands on the sides of the well. He responds more readily to the picture on one side than on the other. When he is asked to touch the picture of the *piggy* or the *lady* he moves his hand at the appropriate side without extending it.

FUNCTIONAL SUMMARY

At 21 months, the child has become aware of new areas in space—areas outside of his own familiar intimate realm. Vaguely he senses space between himself and an object of interest out there. (At 18 months, he went headlong to the object.) Now, without going to the object, he appreciates that there is an intervening space. Under retinoscopic examination, it becomes evident that he visually works around a given area with fumbling uncertainty, a non-specific manipulation. He does not tie down to the area. He wobbles. The retinoscopic reflex registers some amount of with and against.

When an object of regard such as the interposed lens or the picture book is within his area of ocular or manual manipulation, we begin to see the nature of his visual performance. He is slow in shifting from one area to another. This is not due to overholding, but is actually a nascent effort to invade a further area. Hands may assist him to make this invasion. They help him to initiate the visual response, although the manual activity is not part and parcel of the visual act.

In near areas there is a primitive, loose type of binocularity: retinoscopically the eyes are quite equal. (The terms monocularity and binocularity are somewhat flexibly used to define the prevailing mode of teaming. This mode changes from time to time, and from age to age, in accordance with the developmental principle of reciprocal interweaving.) In intermediate areas, there is a little more evidence of monocularity, as if the child wanted to adapt and practice with one eye before doing so with two eyes. At far areas, there is neither a clearly definable monocularity nor binocularity; the brightening is brief and indifferently monocular and binocular; motion of the reflex is present, but indefinite.

The child appears to have a vague notion of visually determined space. The spatial domain extends beyond his manual reach. He visually contacts a distant object and tries to manipulate with eyes alone.

2 YEARS

At 2 years of age, the child shows a wider range of eye-hand coordination in the near region of manipulation. A few months earlier, the cracker on the table had to be at arm's length to be picked up with ease. Now he reaches and grasps it at nearer distances. His eyes also take a more directive role when he shifts an object from one location to another. However, in reaching for a distant object, his trunk and arm show a lack of continuity of function. He twists and lists to one side in an awkward manner, which suggests that the organization of the upright posture entails continuing difficulties for the growing organism.

Nevertheless, his eyes are reaching out into more distant space. He can fixate on a screen across the room without feeling a compulsion to walk to it. He can shift from a near to an intermediate plane of regard, intentionally and with increased smoothness, often performing better with one eye than with the other.

FUNCTIONAL TESTS

Adjustment

The 2-year-old enters the room with more assurance and directness than at the age of 21 months. He makes for the footstool in front of the examining chair, but the teacher intervenes and places him on the examining chair instead. There is a picture on the far screen but he is apt to shift his regard to the observers present. However, he responds in some manner to the examiner, repeats a "Hi" addressed to him, scowls or smiles, says "Mommie," or puts fingers in his mouth as he regards the examiner. When the dangled bell is presented, he may verbalize, naming it *ball* or asking "Wha's at?"

Dangled Bell

The dangled bell is picked up with a quick glance and, if it is then moved in toward his nose, both eyes converge; but one eye moves more jerkily than the other. There follows a fairly spontaneous release out beyond the examiner. The eye which moved jerkily may be the slower to release. On repetition, one eye either may have difficulty turning in, or may turn in excessively. Some children withdraw the head slightly as the target is brought in. When thc hand comes to the target, it scoops and pulls target inward or flips at it.

Retinoscopy

Far Estimate. With attention on a picture on the far screen, and with the examiner observing at the same far distance, the retinoscope registers a dull reflex, but presently both eyes brighten equally, varying from dull to bright. On occasion, one eye is the brighter. Motion is not easily observable but when the reflex is bright, an *against* motion may be seen.

The child smiles at the pictures, looks at the operator. He is interested in the light on the screen, and may name the background of the picture *light, ball, paper*. He also looks at the examiner's light, and from this to the room light. He names the color of the ball or the car, though not always correctly. He says, "Dere," "Uh," "Wha's at?"

He likes to have familiar pictures repeatedly projected, and may persist in naming a favorite picture, rather than the one on the screen. He identifies: *car, ball* or *moon, boy* or *baby, wow-wow* or *kitty, choo-choo, plane, chair, cup, mit* (mitten). Although he adjusts to the procedures, it often happens that he seeks the teacher's lap during this part of the examination.

Intermediate Estimate. At an *intermediate* distance, the findings at this age are extremely variable. The child divides his attention between the screen and the examiner, and it is difficult to differentiate the responses. A sequence somewhat as follows illustrates the changes which may occur: (1) Both eyes *with,* (2) Right less *with* than left, (3) Right *against*, (4) Left *against*, so both are *against*, (5) Meridional difference in right eye. It is usual to note a better reflex in one eye than in the other.

Far Measure. Attention to the *far* screen can be held only briefly while a lens is put before an eye; but, with dispatch, a measurement can be made. There is a definite difference between the two eyes, the measurement showing +.25 D in one eye and -.50 D in the other.

Near Measure. There is somewhat less concern when lenses are put before both eyes while the child looks at the examiner. There is a measurable but reduced difference in the two eyes. As the child selectively regards parts of the examiner's face, the measurement is about +.50 D or +1.00 D.

Book. The child glances at the pictures of the book as the teacher attracts his attention to appropriate subjects. He may look for certain pictures which are his favorites, such as *baby* or *red car*, but he needs verbal encouragement: "See the wow-wow," "Point to wow-wow." He still objects somewhat to an interposed lens, but he can call it a "winnow" (window) and inhibit reaching for it. He is slow to go into *minus*, but shows anywhere from a -1.00 D to -2.00 D when he is regarding and/or identifying in some way. There is a discrepancy between the two eyes. When he points or verbalizes, there is no change in the amount of *minus*.

Projection

He likes to stand at the stereoscope, and he peers in to regard the picture. He may name "de wow-wow" or "de kitty." Asked to touch "it," he moves his arms simultaneously, and one hand leads and goes down to the surface of the picture. He recognizes that it is away from him somewhere in space. He slaps at the picture, looks over the eyepiece for it. Whether the picture is before either eye, he extends right hand, left hand, and also both hands toward it.

FUNCTIONAL SUMMARY

At 2 years the child is more aware of distant areas in space, but does not apprehend the continuity of the areas. He can shift from one area to another, though with some difficulty, as if he were experimentally selecting an area in which to deploy his growing manipulative ability. He does not separate intermediate and far loci, but shows a good response to either, independently, without relating one to the other. The hand serves as a procurer, but not as a localizer. Vision locates and prompts the appropriation.

In far areas, he is beginning to respond on a monocular basis, but the monocularity is incipient and meager. His orientation to a far area is vague. Both eyes succeed in shifting to a far area, and both brighten somewhat, but one eye brightens more markedly than the other. At intermediate areas, the response is prevailingly monocular, but occasionally it may be binocular. He is now more definitely oriented within a given spatial area. At near range, his response is still monocular, but there is an increase in binocular response. With a specific object of interest, like a picture in a book, the response becomes measurably monocular. At near to intermediate distance, he can discriminate between two loci, keeping them visually separate. This may be considered a first step in the development of planes of regard within an area.

2 1/2 YEARS

At 2 1/2 years, his eyes are more evenly matched, and he shifts with greater directness from near to far fixation. Convergence and refixation (release) are not equally developed. When one is strong the other is likely to be weak. Since this is a pronounced bipolar stage of development, the child tends to overhold and to overrelease. He shows this trait not only in manual prehension but in ocular fixation. The mechanisms of reciprocal innervation and interweaving are in the making. In another half-year, the two opposing functions will be in better balance and the visual patterns will, to that extent, be more modulated. Elsewhere, we have shown how this temporary period of labile bipolarity leads to reversals in the spatial manipulation of objects and to symptomatic disorientations.

The eyes are, however, capable of very active fixation, as though they were exploring the contours and depth of the object to a searching degree. They cleave closely to the clay which the child molds. He takes pleasure in naming the animals in his picture book. He is beginning to enjoy looking at books by himself—a genuine visual pastime.

FUNCTIONAL TESTS

Adjustment

The 2 1/2-year-old enters the room somewhat cautiously and may be aware both of persons and objects in the room. He climbs onto the chair, where his attention can be attracted to the picture on the far screen.

Dangled Bell

The dangled bell is then presented. He may make an initial manual approach, placing the left hand on the bell. Visually, however, he locates the bell in space and maintains ocular fixation rather rapaciously. As the bell moves toward his nose, he fights to hold it visually and both eyes turn in with equivalent performance. Now that his eyes have taken hold, he does not want to relinquish the target and the examiner may have to urge him several times to "Look at me." When the child finally releases, the eyes may shift to the right or left, and then to the examiner, or he may blink and a moment later release to the examiner. On repetition of the test, one eye may be slower to release. The hand is sometimes spontaneously brought in to help him to release. He likes to watch the bell swing or to have it jingle.

Retinoscopy

Far Estimate. He is quite promptly interested in the pictures on the far screen. He now names more than one object in a picture, e.g., *house, moon, star;* or *house, chimney, bird.* Pictures of vehicles and transportation are of special interest and he is prone to describe them in terms of action: "It pulls, it's flying, coming down, puffing." *Dolly* is also a favorite screen subject. He may ask, "Wha's this?" and then name it. *Man* is his response for *mitten.*

Although a child of this age is able to sit by himself, he may suddenly slump in his chair. The teacher is then likely to take him onto her lap. He may, however, stand up while regarding the screen. Boys, especially, may raise their voices to a loud pitch. Occasionally the tongue is mouthed or extended by way of tensional outlet.

While the child's attention is on the *far* screen, the examiner observes the retinal reflex. Brightness is first noticeable in one eye, then both brighten and, with the brightening, a fast motion appears. In one child, the motion is consistently a fast *with*, in another a fast *against*. The manifested specific plane of regard is not fluctuating nor variable.

Intermediate Estimate. At the *intermediate* distance, while the child is looking at the screen, there is a similar response but motion is more readily detected. While looking at the examiner, however, both eyes are *against*, then left brightens, right brightens, and both show a *with* motion. Both the target (that is, the examiner) and the distance are more acceptable to him.

Far Measure. Measurement with a lens is more readily obtainable because he accepts the idea of looking through a "window." On the *far* measure, the majority of the children show a +.25 D in one eye and a -.25 D in the other. However, two of the children showed a good amount of *plus*, and four of them showed a slight difference in meridians in either eye or both.

Near Measure. The *near* measure is approximately +1.00 D and meridional differences no longer appear. One child with a high *plus* at far continued to be higher than the other children at near; another child, also high *plus* at far, reduced to the usual finding of +1.00 D at near.

Book. While looking at the book through the "window" the child may even ask to "see it again" when lenses are removed. He names several animals and spontaneously picks out pictures of *car, birdie, bee,* and *flower*. When asked to find a picture, he searches for it and there is a measurable -.75 D; but when he finds it, the *minus* increases to -1.50 D. Hand and/or verbalization are so much a part of his visual response that they are associated with the increase in *minus*.

Projection

The 2 1/2-year-old makes a ready transition to the stereoscope and is now seated on the chair instead of standing in front of the instrument as is characteristic of earlier ages. He names the *piggy* or *bow-wow* and the *girl*. Initially, he responds with the hand opposite to the picture presented by pointing upon the lens or at the side of the lens-well. The examiner then places the child's hand before the lens. The child moves his hand down to the surface and manipulates it grossly, or pushes against the surface. On retrial, he again points at the lens, but with a clue he gets out to the surface, and may even use the index finger to point. If he is asked to point to a detail of the picture, he becomes confused and asks, "Where is it?" After the initial response, he uses either hand, irrespective of which eye is stimulated by the picture.

FUNCTIONAL SUMMARY

At 2 1/2 years, the child is beginning to carve out various broad areas in his spatial domain. The *far* area is beginning to take on meaning; it attracts him and helps him in his general orientation. He makes a distinction between the *near* area within easy reach and the *intermediate* area which is beyond his manual reach, but which is nevertheless within his visual manipulative realm. These various areas are undefined and may overlap, but he occupies them in a preliminary manner. His hand now serves as a releaser and can assist his eyes in projecting out to a far area. His hands function also as obtainers.

His visual system permits him to establish a single locus of regard in a given area. He is therefore confined by this locus. He occupies discrete loci, but his immaturity prevents him from moving freely from one locus to another. Therefore his visual responses take on a rigid, staccato character. There are evidences of increasing binocularity, but this binocularity is episodic rather than organized and purposeful. He is, however, more definitely binocular in the book situation, and does not show the monocular difference characteristic of the 2-year level. The book makes him aware of a specific near-regard area. The retinoscope reveals his searching visual response (registered in -.75 D); when he connects visually with the locus of regard and recognizes the picture object of interest, the retinoscope registers an increase in *minus* up to approximately -1.25 D. This increase may indicate a more interpretive visual manipulation.

The eyes are beginning to be used more deliberately as implements for gross spatial orientation. Motion in his personal environment has almost a magnetic attraction. A moving object of interest tends to be followed up by a total body response. The eyes also may take the lead. Having visually grasped an object in a distant area, he goes to the place and puts his hand upon the object to complete or to confirm his response.

3 YEARS

The 3-year-old is more at home in the world, spatially speaking. At 2 1/2 years he was able to shift his plane of regard from near to far, but had more difficulty in the reverse direction. The 3-year-old releases readily at far sectors and promptly picks up at near. He is also able to project farther into space. Accordingly he is more completely oriented. His demeanors and his interpersonal adjustments reflect an increase of poise, as described in an earlier chapter. Whole body responses characteristic of 18 months are no longer prominent. The eyes have gained a greater measure of independence; they sweep up and down the tower which the child has built with relatively steady hands.

We see all these characteristics displayed in the course of the visual examination. His organism is so responsive that he more than meets the visual challenge. He intensifies his regard, and reacts with spontaneous verbalization and various forms of expressive behavior, such as smiling, mouthing and pointing. With the mounting of self-engendered interest, he may rise from his chair and stand on his feet, thus completing a cephalo-caudad cycle of response. Then he may sit down and, in due course, repeat a similar cycle.

FUNCTIONAL TESTS

Adjustment

The 3-year-old complies with the verbal request to sit on the big chair, but he is slow to approach it and the teacher takes his hand to lead him to it. He is aware of the persons present and of nearby equipment. He notes with interest the picture on the screen and often smiles as he names it.

Dangled Bell

The dangled bell is presented, and is promptly and easily fixated. He smiles and reaches for it or hangs his head and covers his eyes. Presently he looks from bell to the examiner's hand and, when asked to watch the bell, he adjusts his head slightly to one side as both eyes turn in. One eye moves slowly, and the other jerkily. He spontaneously releases in a step-by-step manner to the examiner. The eye which moved in jerkily is the slower to release. When the bell is suspended close to his eyes, he withdraws his head or brings his hand to the bell; but he can also release his regard and then refixate. On retrial, both convergence and release are smoother. He enjoys this fixation test as a game—may even like to have the bell touch his nose; and he brings his hand in playfully to explore the bell. The hand helps him in convergence, but he can inhibit a hand approach if he wishes. When he is fixating the stationary bell and is asked to touch it with his finger, he is not always accurate.

Retinoscopy

Far Estimate. He is interested in following the examiner, and he even questions him about what he is doing, but the pictures on the screen have a greater fascination for him. The *doll* is now designated as *a boy* or *a girl.* He can give multiple responses to a picture. He can further describe a picture by naming *window, buttons, hat* on request. He notes a *little fish* and *a big fish* or *another fish.*

With the child's attention on the screen and the examiner at *far*, the retinoscope reveals a new pattern of visual performance. The reflex gradually brightens and fades, though unequally in the two eyes. This occurs with frequency as though the child were practicing the performance. The motion is not, however, consistent and changes with such frequency that it is not easy to follow. There are binocular changes in the teamed eyes, as well as monocular differences. One eye shows *with* or *against,* while no motion is seen in the other; then both are *with* or *against.* Changes occur in meridians which give a scissors-like motion. Again there is a difference in the pupillary size or in the alignment of the two eyes. Despite this variability, there is now more *with* motion while the reflex is bright, but this is not steady, and the *against* motion seems to help in maintaining the visual grasp.

Intermediate Estimate. At the *intermediate* distance, the change in pupils or in alignment does not occur. Otherwise the findings are similar to those at far.

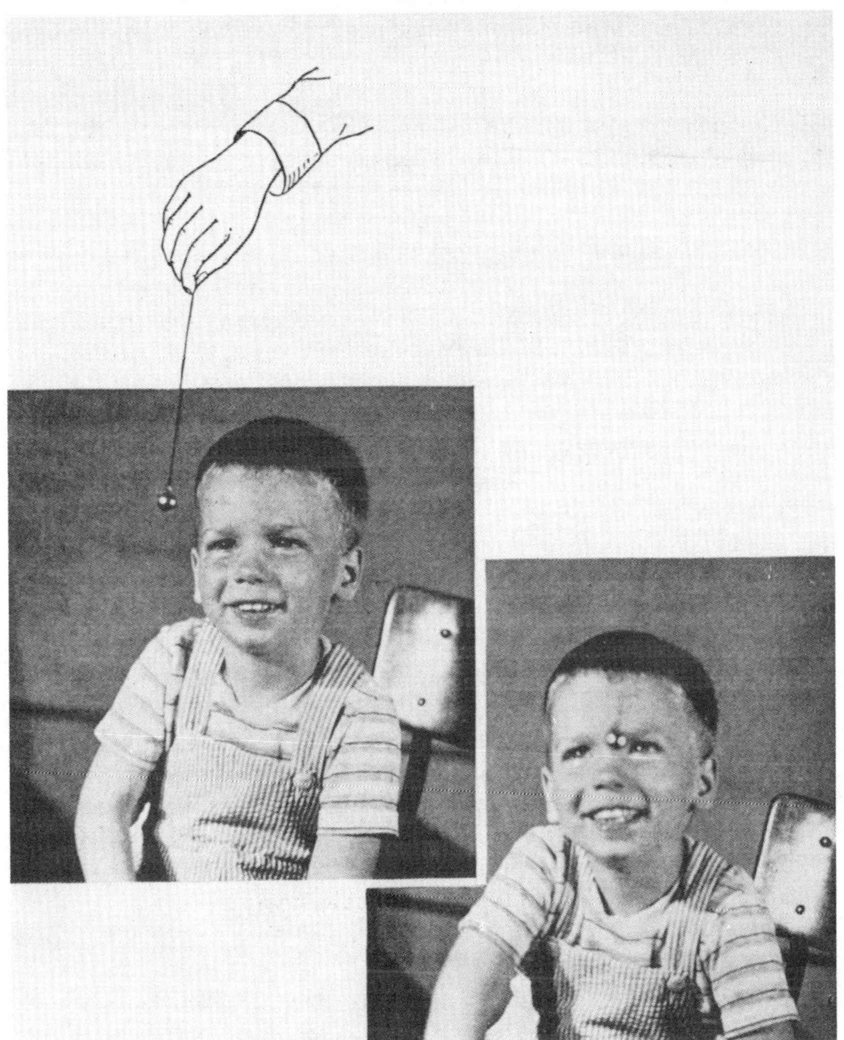

Figure 51. Fixation test: The dangled bell. A nickel bell 12 mm. in diameter, suspended by a thread, is slowly brought into the field of vision of a 3-year-old boy to elicit fixation, monocular and binocular convergence, and release. As the target approaches, the eyes converge. They release at near distance.

Far Measure. Looking through the "window" (lens) becomes a game at 3 years. Even those children who have shown initial shyness, respond to peeking at the pictures through the lens. On the far measurement, there is greater equality of the two eyes than on far at 2 1/2 years and than on the far estimate at 3 years. The measurement ranges from -.50 D to + .50 D. Two children showed the meridional difference observed at the far estimate, and one child showed a marked inequivalence in the two eyes.

Near Measure. The *near* measure is about +.75 D with the two eyes nearly alike. In one child, the inequivalence persisted; another child, who measured a higher *plus* at far, reduced the *plus* on the near measure.

Book. The 3-year-old spontaneously names several pictures in the book, such as: *bird, ball, boy, girl, flowers, fish, boat, mouse, big ball, little ball,* and so on. The measurable response is not consistent for the entire group. There are three subgroups corresponding to various types of responses (see Appendix B). However, the amounts of *minus* are not fluctuating; and the increase in *minus* with searching, and the decrease with finding, naming, or pointing, are in marked contrast to 2 1/2 years, when the reverse was true.

Projection

The 3-year-old sits before the stereoscope and easily names the pictures of the dog and the girl. Either hand responds to the picture in front of either eye, but he is more apt to point to the homolateral lens. He comments, "She's right there," "She's inside," "Over there." The hand then moves out, goes to the outside of the lens, to midspace, and then to surface. After touching the surface, he brings the hand back to the outside of the lens, or withdraws the head to peer around in outer space, searching for the picture. If allowed to see the picture, he goes back to the lens again and says, "two doggies." When he is looking through the lens and points to the picture before the corresponding eye, the pointing is accurate; but when using the other hand and projecting through the opposite eye, he places the hand around in the vicinity of picture in a groping manner. He also extends his hand underneath the septum and crosses over from right to left or left to right.

FUNCTIONAL SUMMARY

The child is now, at the age of 3 years, more comprehensively oriented in space. His visual rapport with a total spatial situation is now so fluent that he can easily move visually from one locus to another, apparently seeking an awareness of the whole. His visual awareness flows readily from far to near and from near to far. He no longer reacts diffusely to an area, but perceives specific objects, animate and inanimate, within an area. He begins to apprehend them in their relationships to each other. He is aware of both stable and mobile relationships.

He now uses his hand in various ways to direct, to confirm, and to complete his visual responses. The total visual act is a cycle of response which is intensified by incorporating various non-ocular motor reactions. He seems to energize his response by means of fine and gross expressional behavior.

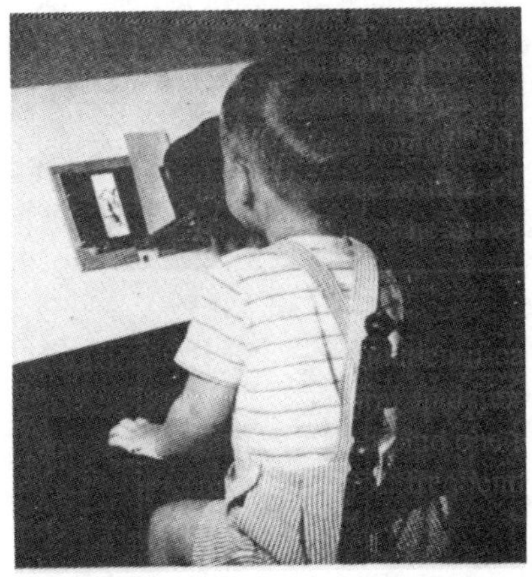
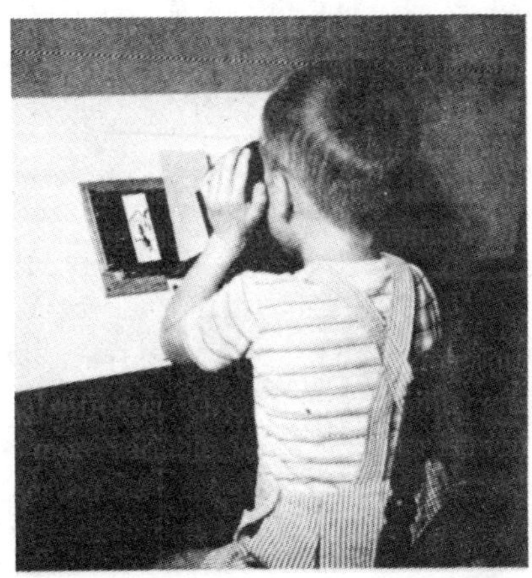

Figure 52. Projection test. The child is seated in a small chair in front of a child-size table. He confronts a stereoscope mounted on a white, sloping board. If he prefers, the child may stand to view the target.

There is more binocularity, but it is neither consistent nor well-established. The child shifts from monocular to binocular and then back to monocular adjustment. The eyes are teaming, but are not fully teamed.

His spatial manipulations have become more discriminating. The retinoscopic manifestations suggest a new kind of spatial manipulation. The visual mechanism operates on and around an object of interest, as if it were caressing contour and relief. Thereby the foundation for kinesthetic projicience is deepened.

3 1/2 YEARS

At 3 1/2 years, there are new behavior symptoms of unsteadiness, tension, and tentativeness—transitional to more complex developments in the visual sphere. The child seems to encounter new difficulties in combining eyes and hands. Some of the "difficulties," however, are self-imposed and really denote an experimental interest in new spatial relationships, and in the mutability of orientations produced by active manipulation. When he is spontaneously playing with cubes, improvising structures, he does not always proceed from one clear intent to another. Often he seems to be confused by his own innovations. He attempts combinations which defy the laws of gravity. This fluid state of affairs is a condition of growth. He is literally opening up new planes of regard by means of new planes of manipulation. The direction and extent of these manipulatory planes are determined primarily by maturational changes in the neuromotor system. Accordingly, the child seems to be trying out novel projections in near space, and to be especially aware of the frontier and the immediate outer margin of his working area. He displays more varied angles of approach and multiplies his points of placement. He does not even react to a geometric figure as an indivisible whole. He tends to see it as an assembly of pieces.

He is so fluid in attitude that when he manipulates materials he sometimes imparts to them a life of their own. All this represents a transitional, but constructive, phase of a growth process in which eyes and hands interact to multiply the meridians of familiar space through exploitive manipulation.

The nascent eye-hand coordinations are at first so partial and so tender that the child does not have a firm perceptual grasp even of structures as simple as a bridge or a cross. Asked to copy a cross from a model, he makes selective rather than total responses: (a) he may draw a horizontal stroke, and then separately supply an upper and then a lower vertical stroke, or (b) he draws a single vertical stroke, and then separately supplies two horizontal arms, or (c) he may make four strokes radiating from a center. He is perceptually oriented to the cross, but on a piecemeal basis.

Because of this analytic tendency, the child's near space world is not, for the time being, firmly structured; but the new interest in the minuter facets and intervals of space leads developmentally into enrichment of that world. What now seems tentative, delicate, and even confused, becomes in time, ordered and automatic. It is probable that the function of fusion is undergoing organization during this transitional period. There is evidence that the eyes alternate rapidly in maintaining fixation. This may be preparatory to a higher form of binocularity. The tendency toward resolution of an earlier periodic strabismus also suggests that there is a fusion factor in the making. With our present lack of knowledge, much must be left to speculation. But what is known of the dynamic characteristics of the total action system at this stage of development indicates that it is potentially an important period for diagnosis and for the management of visual deviations.

FUNCTIONAL TESTS

Adjustment

Individual differences are so marked at 3 1/2 years that orientation to the room is unpredictable. However, there is no problem about having the child sit in the "big" chair. He may be immediately friendly and begin to talk to the examiner, or he may refuse to respond. He is as interested in what the examiner is about to do as he is in what he himself is to do. He may ask the examiner what he is doing, or what the bell is doing. His protests are not always final and he responds when proper management techniques are used.

Dangled Bell

Throughout the entire series of performances characteristic individual differences persist. During the presentation of the dangled bell he may ask, "What do it do?" or remark, "Oh, it rings!" He can maintain fixation on the bell, and his eyes turn slowly inward as it is brought toward his nose. Later he withdraws his head slightly and then spontaneously and slowly releases to regard the examiner. Some children give quick glances at the bell and, when they release regard, they may make a slight upward reposturing of the eyes before resuming regard for the examiner. If one eye has difficulty in converging, this eye may overrelease before realignment.

He may limit his response to eyes alone or to hands alone. He likes to hold the bell with his thumb and index finger, or with a whole-hand grasp, or to touch it briefly with the index finger. Boys with strong motor drive strike at the bell vigorously. The hand may assist in the visual release or help to steady fixation, but it does not alter the act of converging.

Retinoscopy

Far Estimate. A 3 1/2-year-old names pictures on the far screen by spontaneously and quickly identifying *a moon* and *a star* and *a house*. Activity pictures, such as a girl picking flowers, though not sufficiently represented in our series of targets are of interest at this age. The child likes a car to have a driver. He can also project himself into the picture. "I want to get in it" (train). When the examiner asks, "Which car?," he replies, "I can't get in it because that's a picture." When asked what else is in the picture, he replies "Still a house," rather than further describing it. The forms of circle, triangle, and square are named as objects such as: *ball, sailboat, roof, tent, window,* or *blocks*. Letters may be called *numbers, a name,* or they may be identified as familiar initials. Stuttering "that's a, a, a," occurs. Children at this age spontaneously ask for a favorite among the pictures which they have seen. The voice often changes from a whisper to a shout. On pointing toward the picture, the arm is usually held close to the side, with the elbow bent.

While thus engaged with pictures, the examiner, with the retinoscope, notes the child's performance. The reflex changes from dull to bright and from *with* to *against*, and in this process the vertical meridian may be *against*. Both eyes may be bright, but one eye may brighter and may have a more definite reflex. Likewise, the movement of one eye may be more variable than that of its opposite. The interaction between the two eyes is so rapid that the examiner is now obliged to maintain the retinoscopic light more consistently on both eyes in order to secure adequate observations. In two of the oldest children in this group (44 months), there was a very rapid alternation of brightness, from one eye to the other. There is a more consistent with motion now, and the movement can be seen when the reflex is dull.

Intermediate Estimate. From *intermediate* distance, there is no difference from that at the *farpoint.*

Far Measure. On a distance measurement, a certain amount of *plus* is usual, ranging from Plano to +.75 D or slightly more. The difference in the two eyes is between .50 D and .75 D. In some children there is an extreme difference in the two eyes. Some show a marked meridional difference at this age.

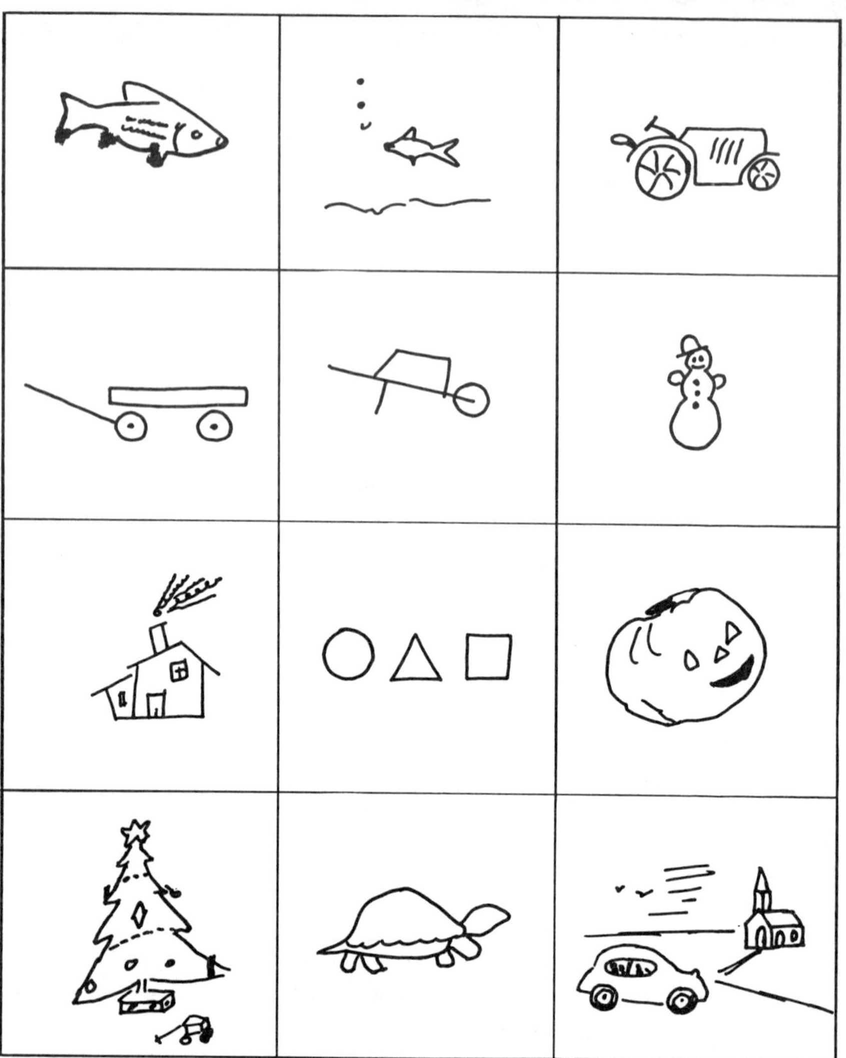

Figure 53. Targets for projection tests.

Near Measure. The *near* measure is approximately the same as at 3 years, but there is a stronger trend toward equivalence of the two eyes. When marked inequivalence is manifested on the far measure, the meridional difference tends to persist at near, but otherwise the eyes are more equivalent at near.

Book. There is less correspondence with other measures, as to equivalence and meridional difference, in the book situation. The amount of *minus* also shows meridional variations, with extremes ranging from -.75 D to -3.00 D. The inclusion of the hand/or verbalization has its individual effect, changing the response in some children, but not in others.

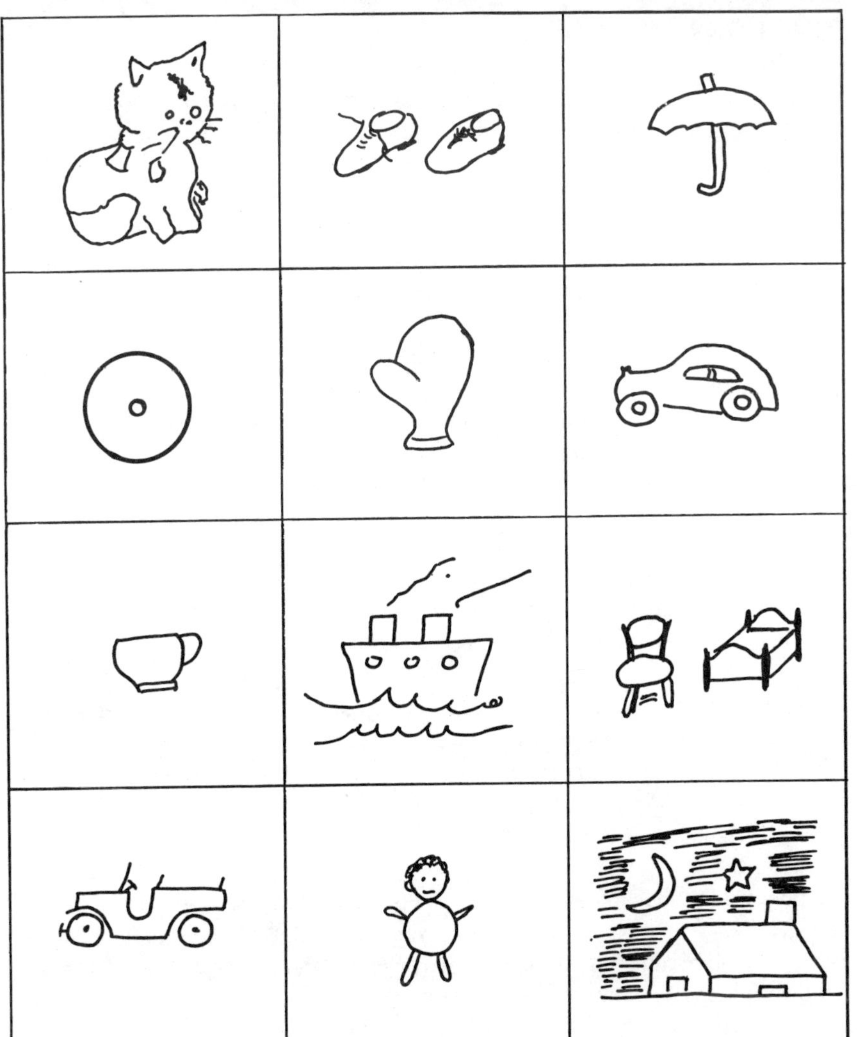

Figure 54. Targets for projection tests.

Projection

The 3 1/3-year-old identifies the picture in the stereoscope easily. He points into the lens, or fingers around the outside of the lens, querying, "Where is it? Way down there. How can we get in it? We can't." Or "Open up the drawer." Asked to touch the picture, he says, "Can't touch, it's way over," or "It's here" (lens), "I can't touch." Then he begins to reach out into midspace; poising his hand in midair, he may get down to the surface, but in vicinity and without good point localization. Or he may get to midspace toward the septum and cross over, pointing to the picture itself. Sometimes he gets to the very top of the projection board, or quite underneath the board, to reach for it.

FUNCTIONAL SUMMARY

The spatial domain in this transitional age period is somewhat disarticulated. Nevertheless, it retains a basic integrity. Developmentally, the child is in a phase of relative disequilibrium. He reacts variably to diverse sectors and aspects in space which happen to be congenial to his growth needs and his current interests. He becomes so engrossed in individual sectors and aspects that he loses his awareness of the whole. His visual organization proceeds piecemeal. He goes on a tangent. He orients to the growing outer margin of a working area in space. Ultimately, this pursuit of details and tangents results in an enrichment of the totality.

The invasion of the spatial domain is taking on a new refinement, shown in the appearance of new meridians in space. The retinoscopic findings suggest a developmental type of astigmia, now, almost measurable, as though each available visual meridian were being manipulated preparatory to a definite adaptive response. It is now more difficult for the examiner to determine a fixed plane of regard because the child is defining specific meridians in a given area of response.

The hands are used more selectively and discriminatively in the visual exploitation of an object of interest. They are more than supporters or releasers—they function constructively, even though sometimes awkwardly.

The two eyes are now teaming more rapidly; one eye is more consistently the brighter. This denotes that the two eyes are basically paired; the matrix for fusion is intact. At favorable moments of teaming, the child experiences perhaps for the first time a new tridimensionality. He is now at the threshold of higher forms of "fusion," which it will take years to bring to maturity.

The play yard at the Guidance Nursery is equipped with jumping board, rocking boat, jungle gym, tricycles, wagons, steps, slides, and sandbox—useful aids for naturalistic observation of visual-behavior patterns. The equipment releases spontaneous patterns of motor behavior significant for the interpretation of spatial orientations, postural control, and eye-hand coordinations.

4 YEARS

The 4-year-old shows expansive tendencies, both in eye movements and in his general body activity. He is rather loosely organized, but he is essentially more stable, visually and otherwise, than he was at 3 1/2 years. His ranginess and tangential tendencies are at the growing margins and usually they do not take him too far out of bounds.

His very looseness has a constructive significance in terms of growth. It leads to fluid alternatives and to multiplication of patterns of response. His mental imagery is almost mercurial and moves blithely from one configuration to another. He bravely starts out to draw a cow, which presently transforms into an elephant and, if he becomes interested in the trunk, he may draw a huge trunk all out of proportion. Indeed, he may draw more than one trunk.

Yet he has a sense of form. He can draw a cross from a copy. He can place a cube as a keystone obliquely between two other cubes; but he does not have sufficient command of oblique directionality to draw a triangle from a copy or to draw a sloping roof for his house. He also has sufficient perceptiveness of geometric form to identify, and even print, a few letters of the alphabet. In painting, he can make crude designs.

All this denotes a growing sense of form. For developmental reasons, the eye-hand relationships are not too tightly bound. His eyes enjoy a certain autonomy, if we may judge by the delight that he takes in rolling his eyes in an extravagant and expressive manner. If the eye-hand bonds were too tenacious, he would be more stereotyped. As it is, he is more unpredictable. And yet his variability is delimited; his postural patterns show a tendency to symmetry. He likes to combine cube constructions in symmetrical balance. He spontaneously makes simultaneous gestures, and moves his fingers simultaneously. He frequently orients his movements from center to periphery, but he is not equally adept in making adjustments from periphery to center.

Speaking relatively, the 5-year-old is oriented more conservatively to constricted personal space; the 4-year-old disports in loose and rangy space—he is in a growthsome stage. He tells tall tales; he boasts; he tattles; he threatens; he alibis. But his bravado should not be taken too seriously, for his attractive traits more than compensate. He is fundamentally striving to identify himself with his culture, and to penetrate both the visual and the social unknown. Sometimes he seems to be almost conscious of the growing-up process. He is much interested in becoming 5 years old; he talks about it a lot.

FUNCTIONAL TESTS

Adjustment

The 4-year-old can be quite conversational, but he conforms to the businesslike manner of the examiner. He may ask, "What is your name?" "Where do you live?" But he responds to the test situations cooperatively.

Dangled Bell

He fixates the bell easily and follows it in without resistance. The eyes, however, are somewhat wobbly, and one eye (most frequently the left) is slightly slower and staggers more than the other. Although he does not over sustain fixation at near, release is somewhat awkward and the slower eye is also the slower to release. He may even overrelease. When he takes hold of the bell with his hand, there may or may not be accompanying regard; but when he maintains regard while contacting with his hand, the eyes are steadier.

Retinoscopy

Far Estimate. He names whole pictures, rather than details, and when asked to tell more about a picture, he gives color or size. He describes the picture as *dog house* or *garage*, but he does not name *chimney, door,* or other parts. A picture may suggest, "I have one, home," "That's what we have," and he may begin to tell a story about an experience with a pumpkin, or a ride on a train. If he is asked what is on the Christmas tree, he may mention things he had on his own tree, rather than what is in the picture.

During picture identification, the reflex is changing and variable (bright, dull, with, against, neutral, and meridional differences). One eye is brighter and more definite than the other; and one is also more variable, while the other is more set. The *with* motion is most frequently observed.

Intermediate Estimate. At an intermediate distance, there are fewer changes; there is also less variability as he regards the screen, and this is even further reduced when his attention is directed, on request, to specific features of the examiner's head—namely, mouth, chin, ears, hair, and so on.

Far Measure. The *far* measure now shows a low amount of *plus* in both eyes, with only a slight difference between the two. A few children manifest a slight difference in meridians.

Near Measure. The *near* measure is typically equal in amount of *plus* (+.50 D to +1.00 D) in the two eyes. A difference in the meridians appears in some children.

Book. The 4-year-old names several pictures in the book and with *minus* reactions ranging from -1.00 D to -1.75 D. However, the *minus* varies, within a given performance, in a manner indicating a good flexibility. The meridional difference of the near measure reduces or disappears. Naming and pointing have a variable effect; at one time, the *minus* is reduced, and at another it remains the same. Two of the children showed a different amount of *minus* in the two eyes.

Projection

In the stereoscope, after identifying the picture—often elaborated by further description (*dog in house* or *girl reading book*)—he locates the target by pointing just off center between the lenses. If he gets beyond the lens, it is to the far side of the lens, or to midseptum. He may get down to surface without the assistance of a hand cue; in any event, he points toward the center. When the examiner guides his finger, he approaches the surface unsteadily, but he does contact and is able to point to the parts of the picture, always advancing toward center. In our research group, projection from left to right direction was more accurate than projection from right to left.

FUNCTIONAL SUMMARY

The 4-year-old child utilizes his command of new meridians in space to widen the boundaries of his visual domain. With the increased facility which comes with his added maturity, he combines spatial meridians into wholes and subunits without sacrificing a sense of the continuity and interrelationships between the constituent components. He senses height, width, and depth with a simultaneousness which affords him a new organic experience. His spatial domain is loosely organized, but his command of the meridians and dimensions of space is sufficiently firm so that his reactions are constructively fluid, rather than precariously instable.

He no longer needs the hands to support his visual manipulations, although the hands still have a steadying effect upon his adjustments.

The teaming of the two eyes shows some advance. Both eyes now approach a plane of regard with more unison. There is still considerable monocular freedom at a specific plane of regard, but unilateral monocularity is becoming less pronounced. With both eyes participating more equally in the total visual act, there is more evidence of a teamed response.

5 YEARS

Five is a nodal age. The 5-year-old is a mature preschooler and an immature school child. His visual maturity, therefore, can be more specifically measured.

The 5-year-old adjusts to a new situation by promptly spotting a familiar object. He shows an intial tendency to remain close to his mother, but he leaves her without protest and, as long as he is successfully occupied, makes no further demand for her presence. His attitude is impersonal and direct.

The examination is necessarily paced and limited to meet the child's demands for rapid episodic experiences. This is clearly observable in pursuit fixations; he can respond when the speed of the target is increased and when the arc is limited. Throughout the examination, the restriction of his responses is evident. He may identify only the letter at the end of a line and insist on reading the lines from top downward; or he may select certain letters in a line. The measurements also show this same quality. A phoria taken from two directions is aligned at exactly the same point; the lens of the far subjective does not change his phoria. When he refuses a situation, his refusal is final, and therefore the examination is likely to be incomplete. At 6 years, he is willing to have an interim of free play; but at 5, once he has broken away from one locale, he will not return. Occasionally, he may accept the suggestion that he stand before his chair.

The all over picture of the visual findings shows the immaturity in the organization of the visual performance. He is operating very close around his plane of regard, both at *far* and at *near*. He is more favorably disposed to changes away from him than to those toward him, both viscerally and skeletally.

FUNCTIONAL TESTS

Skeletal

Phorias. The 5-year-old gives a trigger-like response to the phoria tests. He may need a concrete demonstration to elucidate further the instructions to tell when one is above the other. Or he may need to be given a word to say, such as "Tell me NOW when one is above the other."

Phorias, at *far* and at *near*, indicate that he is interpreting around a plane of regard. When the phoria is taken from two directions, the responses are very similar and may be of the same prismatic amount. When the visceral response is changed by adding the *plus* of the far subjective, there is little or no effect on the phoria at *far*. However, at *near*, there is slightly more impact and, in some cases, the shift may be to less exophoria or more esophoria than shown without the *plus* lens.

Fusion Range. Fusion range at *far* further illustrates the characteristic developmental traits of the 5-year-old. On tolerance of base-out prisms, he maintains attention on the target as the prisms are increased, and he does not report blurring until the prisms have been moved a considerable distance, or he ignores the blur entirely. If he has noted the blur, he is unaware of the doubling, and it is necessary to cover his eyes, alternately, until he sees a target before each eye, but the prisms must be reduced before he can see the two targets without cover. He finally fuses the targets when they are within his fusional ability, which is poor at this age. When he ignores the blur, he accepts a reasonable amount of prism before doubling, and then may recover fusion somewhere around a third of the prism tolerance. His reporting is clear, and does not show the confusion of the 6-year-old. He simply tells what he sees and is not aware of the process of the performance. If he is armed with a word to use for his response, he does not need additional questioning during the movement of the prisms.

At *far*, his responses on fusion range, through base-in prisms, are decisive. He seems to enjoy the effect of prism base-in. Many children maintain a single target through a considerable amount of prism before doubling, but they do not regain a single target until the prisms are reduced almost to zero.

At *near*, base-in prism is also more acceptable than base-out. However, the comparison of measurements does not indicate a marked imbalance between the prism base-out and the prism base-in tolerances. Despite the fact that the recovery to fusion is low on both prism base-in and prism base-out, with the former the recovery is more stable and usually of greater quantity of prism.

Visceral

Retinoscopy. At *far*, the measurement is slightly *plus* or *minus* (-.50 D to +.50 D). There may be a .25 or .50 dioptric difference between the two eyes. When difference in meridians occurs, it is slight, and it is likely to be at -x90, especially in boys. (At the immediately succeeding ages, it is not usual to find the -x90.)

At *near*, the measurement exceeds the far by about +1.00 D.

Subjectives. The *far* subjective is quite consistently around +.50 D and equivalent for the two eyes; and this does not alter the naked acuity of 20/30 or 20/25. The meridional differences observed with the retinoscope are not accepted subjectively.

On the *near* subjective findings, the *plus* tolerances are low and are quite equivalent on the monocular and binocular tests. However, there is usually higher *plus* tolerance on the monocular tests. This may indicate that the 5-year-old is less adept viscerally in the binocular act.

Accommodative Range. FIVE can maintain clarity through increase of *plus* lens more easily than he can through increased *minus* lens, though it is not always of a greater measurable amount. (On all accommodative tests, larger type is used.) The amount of lens through which clarity is maintained can be excessively low for some children at this age.

SKILLS

Introductory Stereograph (Dog and Pig). The 5-year-old may approach the stereoscope by bringing the left eye to the right lens, or the right eye to the left lens. He then changes to a central position, but may still be so seated to one side that only one target is visible. It is sometimes necessary to place his head in position until he sees the two targets. Thereafter, he maintains this central position for some time, but occasionally shifts to one side, or again brings one eye to the opposite lens.

Although the fusion and phoria tests are not included here, the response to these slides illustrates rather clearly the 5-year-old's binocular-monocular adjustment to the stereoscope. When regarding the four dots on the fusion test (DB 4 and 5), even though he is centrally oriented, he occasionally reports seeing two dots (monocular) in preference to three or four dots. At later ages, the two-dots response is rarely given. On the phoria tests (DB 6 and 9), if he is asked to point to the arrow, he tries to thrust the pointer through the septum at the left side on which the arrow appears.

Visual Resolution. Directions are altered to the limitations of the 5-year-old. He is asked if he can see a dot in the top, middle, bottom, and at the same time the examiner points to these diamonds. Or he is asked if the dot is on "your side, middle, or my side." Only three positions are named at one time, and directions are repeated as often as necessary on the succeeding squares. The examiner helps him to maintain the sequence by pointing to each square. Occasionally a 5-year-old will confuse bottom and top or, if he fails to see the dot, he will persistently report it to be "top."

FIVE does not like to repeat the same performance, and it is not unusual for him to refuse to respond on the following two monocular slides. If he is willing to repeat, there is very little, if any, difference between the binocular and monocular responses. Most of the children succeed in resolving the dot through the 5th or 7th square.

Depth Perception: Form. The 5-year-old can identify the cross (10%) as standing off the page. He needs to have the forms named slowly for him and frequently he repeats "cross" directly after the examiner.

Bird in Nest. There is a variable response to these slides at this age. Some children do not see the bird on the nonstereo slide, but can see it on the slide with depth. Others who see the bird on the nonstereo slide, report seeing two birds on the slide with depth.

Pursuit Fixation: Binocular. The examiner first explains to the child what is expected of him and demonstrates how the light will be moved around. The child cooperates within the limits of his ability. His head moves with the target for a quarter of the rotation, then he maintains fixation and follows it for a quarter of the circle. He also looks toward the examiner, or stares into space, saying that he still sees the light. By limiting the excursion, he can follow with good fixation for very short periods.

Monocular. With one eye there is marked staring and almost no pursuit. The other eye follows the light by "cutting corners," as though shifting from one muscle to another.

FUNCTIONAL SUMMARY

The 5-year-old is now aware of the totality of space, but with selected spot orientations from which he makes the next move. He is freer to adjust himself in familiar space, and he is more rapid in his movement therein as soon as an initial take-off point is established. His responses are rather restricted, not on account of rigidity, but because of a preference for fast episodic manipulation of a specific space which delimits itself within total space. If, in this movement within his adopted space, he finishes with his first take-off, he does not easily return to the intial take-off point—he prefers to find another one. FIVE is a period of consolidation and of relative completion. Previous trends in total visual performance have come to a focus, thus imparting a new maturity which distinguishes this age from earlier levels.

The child's organization within space is more restricted. He visually manipulates near a plane of regard, not with indecision but with freedom of operation and without the need of defining the plane of regard accurately. The stability of his basic general orientation permits him to exercise a degree of freedom.

The skeletal and visceral components are ontogenetically relatively independent at this stage. Accordingly, an induced alteration in one component does not bring about changes in the other. The skeletal and visceral components respond in an automatic manner. The child does not show much awareness of the test demand, but he gives evidence that he visually likes to be led farther away into space.

Monocular and binocular responses alike are present, but do not conspicuously influence his orientation. His visual performance does not differentiate, for the examiner, monocular and binocular responses. On an imposed task demand, however, he will follow his monocular clues.

6 YEARS

The 6-year-old has long been known for his dramatic behavior. When we compare him with 5, there has certainly been a dramatic change. He appears to have burst forth from the restrictiveness of 5. He shows multiple new thrusts, new beginnings, new combinations. Now as he enters the room, he is somewhat bewildered, as though he were aware of the whole room as well as of his place in it. He is aware of the examiner and of the test situations. But the 6-year-old shifts readily, if not with ease. He responds fully, but not competently. His responses seem less clear; the examiner feels the insecurity of his reporting.

At 5 1/2 years, he began to dislodge objects from their set places. Form and meaning began to have new relationships. At 6 years he begins his attempts at combination. The world of the 6-year-old has expanded. He notes that there are more lights in a room than there used to be. There are so many toys that he cannot always make up his mind which to select. He imaginatively expands his drawing: "It's big, it's as big as this room, from here to here, to here, all around," as he sweepingly gestures to include the whole room. He is aware of himself as the center of this space. His area is the room, and changes from one room to another, in unfamiliar surroundings, require new orientations. When he separates from his mother, he likes to know in which room she is waiting.

The 6-year-old likes to "work," but during the visual examination he wiggles, changes position, and sighs. He may say his eyes are getting tired. The examiner shifts the instrument away at intervals, and also allows him a period to explore the room or to play with some toy. Because he is less tied to one locale, he returns to the task when he is ready.

FUNCTIONAL TESTS
Skeletal

Phorias. The "loosening" of 6 years is immediately evident. When the phoria is taken from two directions, the responses are no longer similar. When moved from one direction, the target is aligned in a position different from its position when moved from the other direction. The 6-year-old is beginning to be aware that the target is in movement. His response seems delayed. One very precise 6-year-old verbalized, "I get my voice all ready, so I can say it before they hit there, so I can say it at the right time." His phorias showed the same spread as that of the other 6-year-olds.

The *far* phoria is around the plane of regard, but at *near* several children begin to show an esophoria or an exophoria of about 5 or 6 diopters. There may be a shift evident here that will show the developmental direction the child may take in the succeeding year.

The additional *plus* lens of the subjective, at both *far* and *near*, now affects the phoria. At *far*, the direction of the shift varies in its direction from the plane of regard. At *near*, the shift is in the exophoric direction.

Fusion Range. In response to base-out prisms at *far*, most 6-year-olds recognize a blur after the prisms have been moved a considerable distance, although a few children do ignore the blur. Prism tolerance is still apt to be high and, when the child sees two targets, he may report, "Now it's on the wall," "It isn't on the paper." Or when the targets separate, the child may say they have gone way apart. There is less indication that he has lost one target completely. He apparently maintains the two targets, although, upon reduction of the prisms, the targets do not immediately move toward each other. He can fuse the targets when they are within his fusion ability, which is usually low. How secure the refusion of the targets is we did not question, but one verbal 6-year-old said, "The top one isn't fastened," (indicating that the child meant that one did not remain superimposed upon the other).

The 6-year-old is slightly more resistant to base-in prisms at *far* than he was at 5 years. He sees two targets more quickly than at 5, and he does not recover until the prisms have been reduced almost to zero.

At *near*, the 6-year-old responds to blur both on prism base-out and prism base-in. However, doubling of the target is not clear-cut. It may be necessary to occlude the eyes, alternately, to have him see two targets, but he cannot maintain the two targets until the prisms are reduced. He fuses the targets through base-in or base-out prisms at around one-third of the amount of the prisms at the doubling point.

The variability of the fusion range is great at this age. The 6-year-old does, however, respond to prism base-out, as well as prism base-in. There is no real stability in the measurements, but he can follow the targets more easily in either direction than he could at 5 years.

Visceral

Retinoscopy. The 6-year-old is aware of the light of the retinoscope. He may mention that "it goes on and off." (He may also explain the difference of type or lines with the change of lens power by saying that it is "lighter" or "blacker.")

The *far* retinoscopy shows a definite increase in *plus* (about +.50 D to +1.00 D). Those children who are closer to the plane of regard, and those who show the greatest amount of *plus*, are apt to have meridional differences of moderate amounts. In all instances, the vertical meridian is *against* (-x180).

The near retinoscopy is also increased, but still shows about +.75 D to +1.00 D more than the far retinoscopy.

If there is any difference in the amount of sphere in the two eyes, it is not greater than .25 D.

Subjectives. The *far* subjective is about .25 D more or less than the *far* retinoscopy finding. Of the group only a few children accepted a correction for the difference in meridians on the subjective, and in these children it was less than the amount of the retinoscopic finding.

There is an increase in *plus* tolerance at *near.* A few of the children have the greater change in the skeletal (phoria) findings, and a few a greater change in the visceral findings, and in these children the *plus* tolerance is outside of the usual range. It appears that the visceral functioning is more in evidence.

Accommodative Range. Amplitude is measured with the child looking at a simple word of .62M or .75M type. (A few may prefer lM.) He is not always cooperative in this test, but when he does respond, the measurement is around -4.00 D. The monocular is not in excess of the binocular, and may be slightly less.

The tolerance of *plus* and *minus* lenses is as variable as are other tests. It may be considerably higher or somewhat lower than at 5 years of age. Letters on the Snellen Chart (equivalent to 20/20 or 20/40) are used. Some children retreat to larger type as the demand is increased. There is now no more positive response to the *plus* than to the *minus*, but we find one measurement higher than the other, according to the child's individual visual performance.

Skills

Introductory Stereograph (Dog and Pig). Six is allowed to make a spontaneous approach to the instrument and is given time to discover the dog and the pig. The examiner may then ask, "What do you see?" "Can you find something else?" The child approaches with both eyes but may position the head so that it is slightly to right or to left. After he has found both the pig and the dog, he is asked if he can see both of them at once. He thereafter maintains position most of the time, but may occasionally shift with right in right lens or left in left lens.

Visual Resolution. The regular procedure is followed, except that examiner points to the dots as she designates their position and gives "your side" for left, and "my side" for right, since she is standing at the child's right. It may also be necessary to point to the squares to help him maintain sequence. In his reporting, he may substitute parts of the room—"ceiling," "floor," "wall," "door," for top, bottom, left, right; or he may simply gesture and say "side" for right or left. He may have difficulty at any square in the sequence but still be able to continue beyond this. Dots are resolved to the 6th or 7th square.

Depth Perception: Form. Many children can resolve 20% or 40%, and a few succeed through 70%.

Bird in Nest. The 6-year-old easily notices the difference between the flat and the stereoscopic slide. He reports that the "nest or bird is way in," or "it has a hole" or "hollow." A few children give the *near* as well as the *far* response, "Leaves near and bird in."

Pursuit Fixation: Binocular. He more easily responds binocularly than monocularly. There is more motility than at 5 years; fixation is less secure, but he attempts to maintain attention to the light during the full circle. He loses fixation and overshoots. In an individual child, either the lower or the upper half is better, or the clockwise or counterclockwise direction. Cooperation for pursuits in the cardinal directions is not always obtained but, when it is, the predominant pattern is to avoid the light as it reaches the central point.

Monocular. On monocular pursuits, he does not object to occlusion. The motility of one eye is fairly good, but fixation is not steady. The other eye maintains fixation more easily, but cuts corners as though moving from one muscle to another.

FUNCTIONAL SUMMARY

Space has rather suddenly taken on new import for the 6-year-old child. He is now aware of new objects and positions in space. He senses them in contextual relationship with each other and with himself. There is a functional awkwardness which arises out of a new growth tendency to realize his own relationship to the spatiality of a given situation. The 5-year-old made an adequate visual adjustment to a locus, and was quite satisfied therewith. Now he is 6 years old and he realizes that there are combinations and permutations to be considered, and that he has multiple adjustments to make in his visual repertoire.

In his general visual organization there is a loosening which enables him to project into, and to identify himself with, manifold space. This gives scope for many developmental thrusts.

The very looseness of organization permits a new and wide gamut of interplay, both at near and far, between skeletal and visceral functions. There is a new proportionality between these functions; whereas, at the age of 5, an induced visceral change did not alter skeletal performance, or vice versa. There is now a shift in one component, following a shift in the other. The resulting shift may not be as much as expected, or may even be contrary in direction. The direction of the shift, however, is not as significant as the fact that shift occurs, and that it may not occur at all at the 5-year level.

The skeletal and visceral performances do not as yet indicate a consistent direction in the development of spatial manipulation. There is variability not only among individual children, but also in the same child on repeated test performance. Although dominances may be variable, there is enough evidence of an adaptive process to indicate the emergence of a new form of binocularity. This testifies to a loosely structured matrix of binocularity which does not depend exclusively on monocular clues. Monocularity is giving way to a new binocularity.

7 YEARS

The 7-year-old at once appears more centrally oriented than the 6-year-old. He is sober and thoughtful; he wonders what is to be expected of him. So his initial adjustment has a quality of tenuousness. He may walk directly to the instrument next to the chair which has been designated for and handle and inquire about it. He may sit down and look inquiringly at the examiner. As the examination progresses, he asks, "Now what?" "How much are we going to do?"

SEVEN adjusts to the examination tolerably well. His reporting includes more details, which he notes spottily and inconsistently. The intensity of his responses is evident throughout: on retinoscopy he is slow to relax and to stabilize; on tolerance of *plus* and *minus* lenses, he may blur immediately, and then clear again. It is not surprising that he is fatigable. The examination is broken between the *far* and the *near* findings, but during this interlude he likes to do other tasks, trying out his strength on the dynamometer, or playing ball. A few children prefer a trip out of the room to the library, or ask for a ride on the elevator. SEVEN does not have the capacity to bounce back like the 8-year-old, so these changes do not lessen his fatigue. He heaves a big sigh, "Oh, eh!", especially on the doubling of the target through prisms. He yawns and may even say he feels sleepy. The examiner moves the phoropter away between tests, and also adjusts it up and down as the child changes his posture from slumping to elevation of shoulders and head-thrusting.

The child comments, "What do we have to do?" The examiner is a part of the situation, too. Seven asks, "How do you change it?" The examiner takes time to show him the lenses and how they are moved. The child's interest in this has the same intentness that is expressed in his visual performance. These interruptions are not "escapes" nor releases from the tasks at hand, but indicate an active interest in what is going on.

The "spotty" reporting of the 7-year-old is a part of his slowness to organize. The immediate reporting of blur may be followed by a report of (1) clear, (2) size change, and (3) movement change. (In the examining technique used, the children were not questioned specifically about size or movement changes.) During *far* subjective test, one child, while looking through a +.75 D lens said, "While I was looking at them, they got smaller." Also, during the *plus* tolerance test, after a report of blur, they may report that the print clears and is then smaller. These size and movement changes are not consistently reported, but occur in one or two of the tests only. The fact that the 7-year-old can sometimes observe fine details does not mean that he will not also ignore them completely; and he cannot be expected to report such refinements in all the tests.

FUNCTIONAL TESTS

Skeletal

Phorias. At *far*, he is interpreting around the plane of regard with some difference in the response, when it is taken from two directions. Several of the children have a tight response similar to that of 5 years.

At *near*, those children who are not around the plane of regard show a definite trend toward esophoria or exophoria; in a few children it is marked.

The lens of the *far* subjective will usually bring the phorias closer to the plane of regard, either at *far* or at *near.*

Fusion Range. At *far*, with prism base-out, blur may be reported either very soon or not until the prisms have been moved a considerable distance. Some children withdraw the head, but promptly reposition and maintain regard until the target doubles. The child regains fusion on an amount of prism which is slightly less than a quarter of the total prism tolerance. The awareness of doubling is especially acute in many children at this age, and a few may be slightly disturbed by it. Several children inquire how it is done. A 7-year-old may also report that one target is clear and the other one blurred.

With the increase of response to prism base-out, the prism base-in response remains approximately the same as at 6 years. The doubling of the target may occur at a lower amount of prism base-in than it did at 6 years, but the response to doubling, as well as to regaining of fusion, has more quality.

At *near*, there is increased facility in reporting blur and doubling of the target on base-out prisms, and there is now some measurable ability to regain fusion. The 7-year-old spontaneously reports doubling when it occurs (but some now suppress or lose the target before one eye). He notices blur, and there is often an additional comment that "I can't see anything," "Something's in the way," "Getting littler," "Closer."

With base-in prisms at *near*, several children ignore the blur, or some give size or movement only. Doubling may occur at a lower amount of prism diopters than it did at 6 years. If the tolerance for prism base-out has increased, there may be a lowered tolerance of prism base-in. On the whole, the response to base-in shows the greater facility.

There are more changes in fusion range at *near* than at *far*.

Visceral

Retinoscopy. At *far,* there is an increase from +.25 D to +.75 D in the majority of the children, and the *far* subjective is higher than, or the same as, the retinoscopy finding. The increase of *plus* is not the same for the two eyes, and one which was the lower at 6 years may now be the higher.

If the *plus* does not increase further at 7 years, the difference in meridians seen at 7 years may reduce or disappear. With the increase of *plus*, meridional differences appear (*against* in the vertical) or increase, and are seen in both eyes.

At *near*, the same increase of +.25 D to +.75 D can be seen, or it may remain the same. The increase is more equivalent for the two eyes than it is at *far.*

Subjectives. There is very little change in the *far* subjective from 6 to 17 years. If there is any, it is +.25 D, more or less. Most of the children now can read 20/20 letters, though a few are still reading 20/25 or 20/30.

There may be a slight increase or decrease of the *plus* acceptance at *near*, but the skeletal performance, though indicating a rather tight association with the visceral performance, still leaves an adequate working area.

There is more *plus* acceptance in the monocular findings than in the binocular.

Those children who were low in the *plus* acceptance at 6 years have a better skeletal-visceral relationship, though it is without a great deal of freedom. Likewise, those children who were higher in *plus* acceptance at 6 years than at 7 years have also this better relationship, but with the tight quality.

Accommodative Range. On amplitude test, the typical response is that it is "worser." The child may complain when one eye is tested alone: "sort of light," "strains my eyes." Sometimes the monocular response is questionable and is not recorded. The monocular tolerance is less than the binocular or one eye shows tolerance and one is less responsive. Several children prefer the 62M or 75M type.

The 7-year-old may be immediately sensitive to the *plus* or the *minus* lens changes, report a blur, and even pull his head away. He spontaneously repositions, and reports that it is clear, and a measurable finding is secured. When his responses are insecure, the fact is evident in response to both the *minus* and the *plus* lens changes. There are a considerable number of children who show increased ability to respond to the *minus* lens changes, and they may or may not be able to respond to the *plus* lens changes. If there is no increased ability to respond to the *minus* changes, this is also evident in the child's response to base-out prism tolerance.

Skills

Introductory Stereograph (Dog and Pig). The 7-year-old explores the instrument—the light control, the head rest—and he also is interested to see that the "picture" is two pictures when he sees it outside of the instrument. He cannot yet recognize, as he does at 8 years of age, that he sees it as one in the instrument. He is especially fond of the stereographic pictures, and will spend long periods looking at them by himself. He seems to derive some orientational satisfaction as he regards them, fingering them in an explorational manner.

Visual Resolution. Although many 7-year-olds can easily differentiate between right and left, it is still sufficiently confusing, under the test situation, to require that directions still be given, "your side, my side." He gestures for directions, but he also verbalizes without confusion. The only substitute offered by some children is "near you, near me."

The binocular and monocular responses may be to the same square (90%—or to the eighth square), but by many children some confusion is shown on the monocular slides. The monocular response of one eye or either eye may be lower but, after occlusion, the monocular response may surpass the binocular response.

Depth Perception: Form. Some children can resolve the 10 forms of the slide, but the more usual response is for the sixth or seventh form to be resolved.

Bird in Nest. There is an immediate response to the awareness of depth on the stereo slide. Several children express the feeling of nearness: "The leaves are closer," but most of them report that "the nest is farther away," and a very few report both. Some typical responses are: "Bird way far back. Leaves way up." "Passageway with leaves over it." "Nest is farther. I like this better, too," "Bird farther back in thicket."

The density of the leaves surrounding the nest is very often described by the 7-year-old.

Pursuit fixation: Binocular. When the flashlight and instructions are presented to the 7-year-old, to obtain the binocular pursuits he may tilt his head backward slightly, In the 60-year-old, movements seemed more mobile, but at 7 years there is more pursuit and more intent fixation. He loses fixation, but can readily pick it up again. When the target changes from one direction to another, he does not make an easy transition, but stops completely and restarts. On rotations, either the clockwise or counterclockwise direction is the smoother. In the horizontal direction, he follows either right to left or left to right more facilely. The downward direction is easier than the upward one.

Monocular. During monocular pursuits, there are gross jerking, unsteady fixation, and occasionally unstable overshooting or overrelease toward the nasal position. One eye may be better than the other, although neither performs smoothly, and often each is poor. A specific pattern appearing in the binocular pursuits may also be observed in one of the eyes during monocular following. Binocular pursuits are better than monocular pursuits.

FUNCTIONAL SUMMARY

The 7-year-old is intrigued by the interaction between his sensitive self and the tractable properties of space. This sensitivity manifests itself both in withdrawal and in intensive exertion during his visual adjustments. The exertion is often followed by self-confessed fatigue and by recognizable signs.

His visual organization is diversified, and therefore he is susceptible to varying aspects of his operational space. The lability of his organism is so great that his visual responses show a high degree of fluctuation during a single test, or a single session, or from day to day. When tests and tasks are timed to the current status of his organism, his responses are optimal. The overall character of his visual responses is also affected by basic individual differences, which relate to a predilection for either far or for near space. He utilizes vision more explicitly as a tool; subordinately, his hand comes in to further identify and to actively refine his total visual kinesthetic experience, which includes oculomotors as well as fingers.

The reciprocal relationship of skeletal and visceral components is now more firmly established, and each has also attained a more independent status. Most 7-year-olds are skeletally prone to operate around a plane of regard at *far* and at *near*. Those who do not operate around a near plane of regard show a marked esophoria or exophoria. Induced changes in skeletal performance produce a shift in visceral response which shows itself in blurriness or apparent change in target size, prior to a doubling of the target.

The skeletal component seems more advanced in its organization. Viscerally, there is more tolerance of *plus* lens power and, with it, some meridional differences appear. Although the skeletal-visceral correlation is more evident, there may be delay in associated responses.

In the continuing emergence of binocularity, the awareness of doubled targets in a test situation is frequently acute at this age. Some children may be slightly disturbed by the doubling of the target. At an earlier age, simple monocularity was the reaction of choice. At age 7, one eye leads, but the partner eye participates, a more formative evolving binocularity thus being indicated.

8 YEARS

The 8-year-old has new spatial relationships. He recognizes that another person can view a scene differently from the way he sees it, and he likes to see it from the other viewpoint, as well as from his own. During an examination, he asks many questions and becomes interested in what the examiner is doing in relation to what he sees. He may ask to operate the instrument while he watches the target change. He inquires, "What do you turn anyways?" "How do you mean?" He is also interested in his own performance. "Are my eyes good?" "Is that good?"

Fatigue is less evident at 8 years of age. Subtle voice changes give clues to the degree of surety of his responses, and fatigue may be noted in voice alone. Some children say that they are not tired, but that their eyes are tired.

The 8-year-old's awareness of speed is expressed: "You went too fast." "Go faster." He also notes the cessation of movement: "Haven't moved." "It isn't working."

He is making new differentiations and he concerns himself with many aspects of the examination, but he is responsive and the examination flows along despite his participation in the manipulation of the instrument and his verbalization. His only complaint is when the phorias are repeated, "Oh, that again!" There is usually no need to break the examination for a play period as there is earlier.

FUNCTIONAL TESTS

Skeletal

Phorias. At *far*, there is a wider spread between amounts of the phorias taken from the two directions than there was at 7 years of age. The reporting from one direction is more sure ("directly over"), and from the other it is less clear-cut ("Now; no not quite yet; now"). The *far* phoria shows no considerable change from 7 years. The wider spread of response from the two directions is around the same plane as it was at 7 years, although it may trend toward the esophoric direction. The *far* subjective changes the phoria, bringing it closer to the plane of regard. At *near*, the phoria through the *far* subjective has a shift comparable to that at *far*.

Fusion Range. At *far*, there is an increase in the ability to tolerate base-out prisms before the target is doubled. With this increased ability, the amount of base-in prism tolerance may decrease or be maintained. The regaining of a single target may be of the same prism amount as at 7 years, or may be slightly higher.

At near, a similar change is seen. The tolerance of base-in prisms is maintained or decreases while the tolerance to base-out prisms is increased. It is more usual for the 8-year-old to ignore a blur when the base-in prisms are increased.

Visceral

Retinoscopy. There is further acceptance of *plus* lens on the *far* retinoscopic finding and, with this increase, the meridional differences observed at 7 years may not appear. However, if the *plus* acceptance did not increase at 7 years, it may show considerable increase at 8 years and, in this case, meridional differences are now seen or appear in both eyes, rather than in just one.

The amount of the *far* subjective is the same as, or slightly higher than, the amount of the retinoscopic finding.

At *near*, the retinoscopic measurement is 1.00 D more than at *far.*

Subjectives. Several children show more *plus* acceptance in the *far* subjective at this age than they have shown previously, or than they do at the immediately succeeding ages. It is not unusual for many of the children to show from 1.00 D to 1.50 D of hyperopia at this age; but all the children have at least .75 D hyperopia. This increase may appear in the subjective findings without a comparable rise in the retinoscopic findings, but it usually occurs in both. Any meridional changes observed at this age are not accepted in the subjective lens unless they have been accepted at the previous ages. Even in the later instances, they may be rejected at 8 years of age.

There is a definite increase in *plus* acceptance, both monocularly and binocularly at *near*, but there is no considerable change in the skeletal performance as indicated in the phorias. There is less difference between the binocular and the monocular findings.

Accommodative Range. In amplitude, and in the tolerance of *plus* and *minus* lenses, there is an individual variation change from 7 years of age. There is a tendency to respond with more equal facility to both the *plus* and *minus* lenses. Several of the children resist the increase of *minus* lens and the target doubles. The amounts of the *plus* and the *minus* tolerance are more nearly equal at this age.

Skills

Introductory Stereograph (Dog and Pig). The 8-year-old makes an easy approach to the stereoscope.

Visual Resolution. The 8-year-old can now designate right and left. He may start giving left for right and continue to give the opposite, even if he is checked. Or he may make such a reversal during the sequence, without necessarily correcting it; and at the next left or right, he may give it correctly. There is now less difference between the monocular and binocular resolutions which are at 100%. If monocular is not as high as the binocular, after occlusion it equals or surpasses the binocular.

Depth Perception: Form. The simple test presented is easily passed, and a more refined test (Keystone SM) is given in addition to this.

Bird in Nest. The depth in the *Bird in Nest* stereoscopic picture is easily recognized. He says that it is "way far in," "more real," "deeper." A very few report the leaves nearer and, if they do, they also comment that the nest is farther away.

Pursuit Fixation: Binocular. During binocular pursuit, there is mild head tensing or overflow into the lid, neck, or body; or smiling, blinking, exaggerated lid-opening. The 8-year-old likes to take over the direction of the target and tries to move his eyes spontaneously, but he can maintain fixation and move his eyes with good motility. Patterns seen at earlier ages—i.e., overshooting, holding, or staring—may occur, but they are minimal.

There is now less discrepancy between the monocular and binocular pursuits. There may be slightly more tension, monocularly, and the spontaneous attempt to take over direction does not occur.

FUNCTIONAL SUMMARY

The 8-year-old is increasingly aware of relativities of space and of orientation. He is more conscious of his own manipulative performance. When he looks at a scene, he is beginning to realize that the scene must appear differently to another person who views it from another angle. Growing recognition of vision as a tool came at the 7-year-old level. At 8 years, the child knows more automatically the possibilities and limitations of vision. IN his visual adjustments, he does not exert himself with the former intensity. His performance shows more speed. A certain looseness and abandon replace his previous 7-year-old tension and concentration. There is a kind of resistance to repetition of an activity or of a task. Although he will allow the repetition of a visual test, he verbalizes a preference for variation.

In his skeletal visual adjustment, he localizes at and around the plane of regard. There is a somewhat increased tolerance for induced skeletal changes without disturbance of orientation to the target.

Viscerally, likewise, there is more acceptance of *plus* lens power and more facile acceptance of induced changes. The skeletal-visceral interaction, although more evident, is also more subtle. The visceral component seems to show the more advanced organization.

There is more balanced participation of each eye, and the evolving binocularity is losing its monocular characteristics.

9 YEARS

The 9-year-old approaches the examination situation in a business-like manner. He understands that his eyes are being tested. His discriminations are more refined, and he spontaneously reports size change on sphere tolerance tests, as well as the changes during the prism tests. With this finer discrimination, he is more critical of his own performance and that of the examiner. He is apt to make a mild complaint about the changing of the lenses. He reports, "Oh, goodness, I'm not so good with my left eye." He may spontaneously report visual symptoms, in some such way as, "I always rub my eyes. I don't know why." On being questioned, he can give a fair report of a specific visual symptom in relation to reading or to the movies. The typical response is that the eyes water either during prolonged reading or when changing from darkness to bright light.

He asks not only how the examiner works the instrument, but also why and what it does. "What does the glass make it do?" He may also ask, "Where did the instrument come from?" "What is that, anyway?" "Why so many cords?"

The examination is completed with dispatch and there is no sign of fatigue until the end of the test situations, when he sighs and says that the back of his neck hurts. Tests may be repeated when necessary, and there may be an increment in the performance on the second trial.

FUNCTIONAL TESTS

Skeletal

Phorias. Both at *far* and at *near*, the 9-year-old is operating near the plane of regard. Through the lens of the *far* subjective, there is very little effect upon the phoria response at *far* or at *near*. His verbal responses are more detailed or specific. He can tell the examiner that "It is going the wrong way," or "Wait a second, little farther this way."

Fusion Range. There is an increased ability to tolerate prism base-in at *far*, but there are individual differences in the response to prism base-out. He doubles the target through a reasonable amount of prism, but the ability to regain a single target may or may not show an increase.

At near, there is some change in the responses to both base-in and base-out prisms, which trend toward further organization, but which are still individually weighted so that the response to one is better than the response to the other.

Visceral

Retinoscopy. At *far*, there is a decrease (of about -.50 D) and it is now at or around the plane of regard. A few children who did not show more than a slight increase at 8 years, now show an increase.

At *near,* the shift can be either greater (+1.25 D to +1.75 D) or less (-.50 D to -.75 D) than it was at 8 years.

Subjectives. There is a decrease in the *far* subjective finding and it is closer to "average" (+.50 D to +.75 D)

At *near,* there is also a decrease but this is also nearer "average." (Visceral down, skeletal holds.) And, in the majority of children, the monocular is higher than the binocular finding.

Accommodative Range. There is a more significant change in the accommodative findings at this age. They are the supporting indicators. The change is variable and may show (1) increase in range and amplitude, (2) more positive response to the *minus* change, or to the *plus* change. There may also be a greater response to the monocular amplitude tests.

There is no significant change at 10 years, except that there is more balancing of the findings. Some slight change occurs in reorganization of both the *far* and the *near* findings.

Taking the span from 9 to 11 years, the balancing of the findings at 10 years is more noticeable in a number of the children. But we also see a gradual shift in a more specific direction from 9 to 11 years. One trend may be an increase in esophoria, a decrease in base-in tolerance, and an appearance of astigmia in the subjective finding. The *far* findings show the greatest evidence of impact, while the trend is gradually downward; the *near* findings show greater facility. Another group trends toward greater facility at *far* and gradual upward increase in *plus*, and *near* findings are also more facile.

FUNCTIONAL SUMMARY

The visual performance of the 9-year-old discloses a more precise and crisp awareness of the details of space. He is more perceptive of his manipulations in the finer discriminations needed in a given task. He is beginning to pick and choose the manipulation which is most suitable for the task or situation. He operates near the plane of regard, and his skill of operation is so well established that induced changes may have very little effect on related responses.

In skeletal visual performance there is increased tolerance to change, although there are individual differences with respect to response to specific changes, both at *far* and at *near.* Viscerally, there is greater change in performance at *near*; and for a given individual there may be either increase or decrease of *plus* acceptance, which permits him to perform close to the plane of regard. There are further individual differences in tolerance to *plus* and *minus* lenses.

Binocularity is quite well establishes but, when binocularity is disrupted, the skeletal-visceral interaction shows a resulting shift in the ratio of manipulative relationships.

At the age of 10 years, the visual reactions under systematic test show a new casualness in their facility. The 10-year-old visual mechanism takes its task more in stride. From the 9-to-11-year age levels, individualities in visual organization become more evident. Further investigation of the trends during adolescence will doubtless demonstrate ontogenetic progressions in the continuing organization of visual functions.

CHAPTER 13
Maldevelopment and Child Vision

From the STANDPOINT of vision, the total action system of the child consists mainly of two components: the ocular equipment, with all its ramifications, and the basic body-limb apparatus. Normally, these two components are closely correlated and harmonized. In extreme defects of vision, and in severe motor disabilities, the relationships are distorted and diminished. The child, therefore, fails to achieve a full measure of development. In some instances, the motor handicap is predominant; in other instances, the sensory and perceptual. These extreme forms of maldevelopment throw a revealing sidelight on the normal processes of the organization of child vision.

The types and degrees of maldevelopment are too numerous for systematic discussion in a single chapter. The developmental aspects of abnormal defects and deviations, however, can be indicated by means of brief illustrations drawn from case studies of amentia, cerebral injury, and total blindness. Amentia is a form of developmental deficiency, acquired or inborn, which reduces the capacities of adaptive behavior to such an extent that the child requires extraordinary supervision and external support. In low-grade amentia, the child is almost helpless. The amentias vary enormously in kind and degree. Cerebral injury, likewise, assumes a great diversity of forms, ranging from minimal to devastating injuries, and from slight to extensive congenital defects. Each defect leaves its distinctive impress on the developmental organization of vision. We conclude this chapter with the report of a special case of total blindness in order to establish a zero mark as a point of reference for the interpretation of the ontogenetic cycle of visual development.

AMENTIA

Consider, for a first example, the visual behavior patterns of a grossly retarded boy (GH). This boy is 4 years old, normal in conformation and physique. He bears no conspicuous physical stigmata. In a favorable moment of quiescence, he appears outwardly quite normal, even attractive—but he is rarely quiescent. Left to his own devises, he is in constant, almost aimless, activity. He wanders about the room, contacting the walls with outstretched hands, scratching the doorknob, fingering the furniture. None of this activity is purposeful. It has a fluid, compulsive character. His recurrent vocalizations, likewise, are inarticulate and devoid of meaning. In all this gross motor activity and manipulation, the eyes play a very meager role. Although normal in appearance, they seem to be almost sightless. They are restless. They move conjugately, now from side to side, now up and down. Spasmodically, the neck cranes upward or the head rotates, but there is no sustained searching, roving inspection. This boy does not look to see what he is doing, nor does he look to foresee what he will do. There is no sustained fixation, not even true staring.

When the eyes are briefly immobile, the stare is vacant. GH is equally heedless of sounds, even though he can hear. He is also heedless of gestures and commissions.

He has, however, learned to relax. When his caretaker places him in a chair, he will remain seated for an indefinite period. Under stimulation, his ocular behavior patterns now become somewhat more complex. He will occasionally hold an object, like a piece of crayon, in both hands, briefly fixating upon it as he rotates it back and forth in a mechanical manner. He spies the pellet and the bottle on the table. He plucks the pellet and inserts it with dispatch in the mouth of the bottle. It is a quick, unrestrained maneuver. It is his maximum adaptive behavior, but it is only a fragmentary episode in a stream of fortuitous behavior. Presently he resumes his aimless activity.

These behavior patterns indicate a relatively normal degree of visual acuity. It is quite probable that the ocular end-organ mechanisms in this child are intact, but all his behavior patterns, visual and other, lack normal contexts. From the standpoint of adaptive patterns, the total behavior picture is inferior to that of a 16-week-old infant—inferior in organization, purposefulness, relevance, and spontaneity. Recall the ocular behavior patterns of a normal 16-week-old infant. Such an infant fixates upon an object of interest in the field of vision. He holds the fixation for a significant period. He shifts his regard discriminatingly from his hand to a nearby object. He scans the environment with selective fixation. He holds his head steady, and relates his head posture to his visual seeking and his visual impressions. GH, in contrast, has no visual hunger. His head postures dominate, rather than obey, his ocular adjustments.

All told, this action system of this amented child is a loose confederation of quasinormal, but excessively discrete, behavior patterns such as grasping, inserting, fingering, scratching, twiddling. He has enough energy or drive to activate these patterns and to execute brief formless fugues, but the corpus of behavior is so unstructured that he does not even display well-defined stereotypy. Visual cues influence the tide of behavior, but do not impose a well-patterned design. The total behavior picture has less configuration than the smears of a preschool finger painting.

This behavior picture reminds us that, in normal child development, vision early assumes and retains a directive role. Vision also serves to integrate the total action system in its multitudinous activities. To a considerable extent, the forces of integration radiate to and from the central citadel of vision. In the low grade ament, the functions of vision are displaced, disorganized, and distorted, even when acuity, fixation, and elementary focus are relatively intact.

CEREBRAL INJURY

The term injury is here used as equivalent to any destructive lesion which produces a deficit or damage of brain structure. This would include physical traumata, infections, toxic agents, hemorrhage, anoxemia, and irradiation. The gradient of injury extends from an infinitesimal blemish to massive devastation. The sites of injury are as variant as the brain is complex. The visual mechanisms may escape harm, or they may be virtually ablated. The resultant neuromotor signs range from mild to severe forms of ptosis, strabismus, nystagmus, immobility, and randomness of eye movements. Visual defect varies from a slight, selective deficit to total cerebral blindness. The latter extreme is illustrated in the case of a girl, BY, who at the age of 3 years is unable to walk, to grasp, or to see. Like GH, she is normal in physique and of attractive countenance. Propped up, she is able to sit bent forward in a high chair. She brings her hands close to her face and activates her fingers as though to look at them. This is a defective remnant of a normal eye-hand pattern and is doubtless without visual content. The child pays no visual heed to a light in a darkened room, nor to a white enamel cup when it is brought close to her eyes.

While lying supine, she engages her hands at midline. Episodically, her eyes stop their aimless rolling and nystagmic oscillation; her head ceases its weaving, and the eyes converge for a moment on her hands. Again, this has the aspect of a motor eye-and pattern devoid of all perception because of the absence of a cortical response. This pattern partially escaped hemorrhagic injury by virtue of its subcortical localizations. But this child, at the age of 3, is so impaired that she has only the vestige of a tonic-neck reflex, and lacks the contextual patterns and neural structures for further growth. She is permanently arrested at an early infantile level, without even the organic behavior integrity of a normal 8-week-old infant. Blindness is a symptom, rather than a cause, of her retardation.

CJ, age 15 months, is a rather pretty blond infant, with wide-open, searching, uncoordinating blue eyes. She, too, has suffered from a severe cerebral injury, associated with her premature birth. The devastation, however, has not been as great as that of BY. Despite her spasticity and clenched right fist, she can grasp an object palmarwise; she sits with slight support; she feeds herself a cracker, and vocalizes single syllables. Several behavior traits are near the 28-week level of maturity.

Her visual behavior patterns, however, are below that level and show a significant developmental impairment, traceable to the cerebral injury. Her visual attention is discontinuous. At times, she is visually so heedless as to seem blind, yet her acuity is sufficient to detect a pellet; and in the ring-and-string situation, she gave exclusive regard to the string, with a curious disregard of the ring. She fixates monocularly, first with one eye and then with the other. Binocular convergence is brief, and only occasional.

This is a true instance of crippled vision. The motor components of vision are present, but they are poorly coordinated. They have not been continuously integrated as in a normal infant of comparable maturity. This child, therefore, is doubly handicapped, ocularly and manually. Her visual capacity is far below her manipulatory abilities; and she cannot, through growth, overcome the deep-seated discrepancy. She will make optimal use of visual cues, but the timing and the constituents of the growth complex were irremediably damaged by a neonatal injury.

TJ illustrates a selective rather than a devastating type of cerebral injury. Birth was apparently normal, but she was cyanotic for the first 12 hours of life. Irregular eye movements and faulty visual responses were noted early. Examination of eye grounds, at the age of 4 months, under anesthesia, showed pallor of the optic disks. In time, vision seemed to improve slightly, but the baby's developmental progress was unsatisfactory. At 44 weeks, there was marked strabismus with wandering eye movements. Sitting posture was abnormal and unsteady. The arms were tremulous, and the fingers made small athetotic movements as she groped for objects. She cocked her head in a conspicuous manner while attempting to fixate. Having seized an object, she transferred it awkwardly from hand to hand. The maturity level of her behavior, despite these visual and manual handicaps was in the neighborhood of 32 weeks.

That she retained, to a considerable degree, normal growth potentials was shown on the next examination at the age of 15 months. At that age, she crept and pulled herself to her feet. She articulated a few words and was beginning to use a soft jargon. The abnormal eye movements were no longer present, the strabismus was less pronounced. Reexamination of the eyes again revealed pallor of the disks and disclosed a defect in the central area supplied by the papillomacular bundle. This specific lesion accounted for her monocular fixation and her marked dependence on peripheral vision.

TJ thus labored under a double disadvantage—defective vision and motor disabilities. Her prehensory approach was indecisive, and disfigured by excessive hand and arm movements. Having seized an object, she swept it into her mouth in a crude "smearing" manner. Her avid mouthing and her poking and pulling at eyelids were, in part, compensations for her difficulties. But most noteworthy was the clever manner in which she utilized her peripheral vision to discover and to detect stationary objects which she could not locate by direct central vision.

A stationary object is not readily sensed peripherally, and does not obligingly move to make itself known. Accordingly, this child developed the trick of cocking her head by a sharp, quick maneuver, which caused the retina to brush across the visual beam of the stationary object. By this adaptive ruse, the equivalent of motion was induced and the object was identified in space.

A vigorously growing organism responds to a visual defect by utilizing, to the utmost, every vestige of vision which remains. We recall, for example, another infant (DI), who was blinded by congenital bilateral cataracts, but who was endowed with normal drive. In her manipulatory play with toys, she made free use of tactile and auditory cues. At the age of 18 months, one of the cataracts was successfully needled. Immediately she began to ignore these cues and adopted visual cues instead, even though for a time this resulted in poorer performance. This shows how instinctively the organism places a premium on vision.

In a similar manner, TJ is making the most of her residual peripheral vision. There is no prospect that she will overcome her sensory deficit. The motor signs, however, are already milder, and are showing a tendency to resolve. Fortunately, such motor improvement often occurs in cases of minimal cerebral injury.

In contrast, compare the case of child AC, who suffered an extreme birth injury which involved almost his entire motor system, but spared to a great extent the structures and the functions of vision. At the age of 5 years, when we first saw this boy, he presented a picture of infantile helplessness, even though he had attained full physical stature for his age. His features were well formed his countenance was normal and attractive. But his motor disability was profound. He could not hold his head up, he could not sit, stand, creep or reach. Face, tongue, arms, legs, hands, and fingers were, moreover, in almost constant, uncontrolled activity. There were movements of flexion, extension, pronation, and supination, with recurrent spasticity. Speech and ordinary gestures were impossible. Even swallowing was accomplished with difficulty. The condition was one of extreme athetosis. Cinemanalysis of the motion picture records of his supine behavior showed a well-defined tonic-neck reflex and postural patterns closely resembling those of a 4-week-old infant.

Superficially, these symptoms might well suggest mental deficiency, and this boy did come with a previous diagnosis of low-grade amentia. But he soon convinced us that he had a remarkable degree of insight, interest, drive, and social eagerness, in spite of his inability to communicate by spoken or written words or by conventional signs. Hearing, listening, and some auditory localization were evidenced. He lived to the age of 14 years. In time, he was able to sit, with support, and to register "yes" or "no" by an all-but-ambiguous head movement. With the aid of this expression, supplemented by inarticulate phonations and the devoted help of his family, he learned to "read" many words and to play a simple game of checkers. He shared the life and the humor of the household in numerous ways. We never considered him to be an ament, despite all his helplessness.

How can this amazing approximation to normality be explained in view of the far-reaching cerebral palsy? This question can be answered with some conclusiveness because necropsy showed that the cerebral damage was largely confined to the basal ganglia. The cortical cytoarchitecture of the frontal, temporal, and parts of the parietal lobes was altered by the lack of development of the ganglion cells; but few such changes were present in the cortex of the occipital lobes. The central organ of vision was not seriously damaged. The marked internal strabismus present at the age of 6 months underwent almost complete spontaneous correction during the first year. Clinical observation and cinemanalysis showed that the eyes moved and fixated in a well-coordinated manner, although sustained visual attention was impossible because of intrusive, uncontrollable jerks of the head. The eye grounds were normal. Relatively normal acuity and eye movements were inferred from reading and form perception tests.

From this well-documented case study, we draw the conclusion that the comparative fullness of the psychological development of this gravely handicapped child was due, in large measure, to the integrative influence of the ever-present, all-pervading function of vision. Most of the skeletal musculature was palsied, spastic or athetotic; but the 12 oculomotor muscles were spared. The kinesthetic experience afforded by these muscles may have supplied the main scaffolding for the orderly mental processes which were vouchsafed.

This developmental history makes an instructive contrast to the minimal type of cerebral injury associated with serious visual deficit (TJ). It also brings into relief the significance of total blindness associated with intact motor and mental abilities. Such an antithetical condition is described in a following section (Blindness).

Minimal Manifestations

The role of cerebral injury in the production of visual abnormality is not sufficiently recognized. Minimal cerebral injuries are more common than is ordinarily supposed, and in an undertermined proportion of these cases persisting visual deficits remain. A sizable number of reading disabilities and inadequacies of visual perception have their origin in circumnatal brain damage involving visual areas. Such cases fail to respond to refractive correction and to ordinary reeducation measures. In some instances, there are associated personality deviations which arise out of the developmental difficulties occasioned by the visual defect, or which are traceable to specific damage to the cortical mechanisms concerned with emotional organization. The personality symptoms are, of course, aggravated by faulty environment and by injudicious management due to erroneous interpretation.

After extensive experience with the obstetric aspects of birth injury, Ehrenfest concluded that intracranial hemorrhages are so common in the newborn that they may be regarded as normal. To a lesser extent, all children suffer from the crisis of birth, but the vast majority of normal infants make a prompt recovery. Less fortunate infants, who fall in the clinical group of minimal injury, make a slow or delayed recovery and present persisting behavior deviations with a neurological import.

Stabismus is a common symptom of minimal injury. It frequently undergoes spontaneous resolution. It may also be combined with oculomotor incoordination and atypical eye-hand patterns in which arms and fingers assume eccentric postures. This leads to bizarre patterns of exploitive behavior. The infant, for example, may poke and twiddle a cube in a restricted perseverating manner. Atypical motor patterns may persist for three years or more. These mild neurological difficulties may set up an extremely complicated interaction of developmental potentialities and dynamic forces. The mild motor disabilities may be associated with speech defects, with imperfect manual dominance, and with delayed integration. Such syndromes lie at the basis of certain school entrance problems and cases of reading disability. Vision is involved, but the total behavior equipment of the child demands searching individual study. For these reasons, eye specialists and educators must reckon with the clinical category of minimal cerebral injury and must be alert to its developmental manifestations. The early symptoms of minimal cerebral injury are often overlooked. They do not yield to the ordinary methods of clinical neurology, but they can be elicited by a systematic developmental examination of infant behavior patterns.

BLINDNESS

The causes which produce blindness in the prenatal and early post-natal periods are manifold. The underlying lesion ordinarily is not limited to the organs of sight, but involves associated neural structures. The development frequently is retarded, and behavior patterns are atypical. The resultant symptoms are difficult to interpret. Is the retardation of behavior due to blindness or to the complicating factors? Can blindness *per se* produce retardation? How does blindness, in itself, affect the shapes of the patterns of behavior? These questions have many implications for a science of vision. To answer them, we need a critical case study based on the development of a child born completely blind, but otherwise intact and potentially normal. Such a child would establish a zero line of reference for appraising the role of nonvisual factors in the ontogenesis of the action system.

The developmental career of boy MF provides us with decisive data. In this instance, Nature performed a most unwonted experiment, but one exquisitely limited to the end organs of sight. In an early stage of embryogenesis, the optic vesicles failed to bud out or, having budded, were blemished, and in consequence the child was born with clinically complete bilateral anophthalmia. Cranium and facial features are well formed; the orbits are sunken and reduced; the eyelids are small but innervated; the tissue beneath is soft and yielding; lacrimal puncta and glands are functional; the optic foramen is closed and the optic nerve lacking. An electroencephalogram at the age of 40 weeks was not unusual in any way. There was no congenital anomaly other than the anophthalmia. Except for this deficit, the child has proved to be definitely normal.

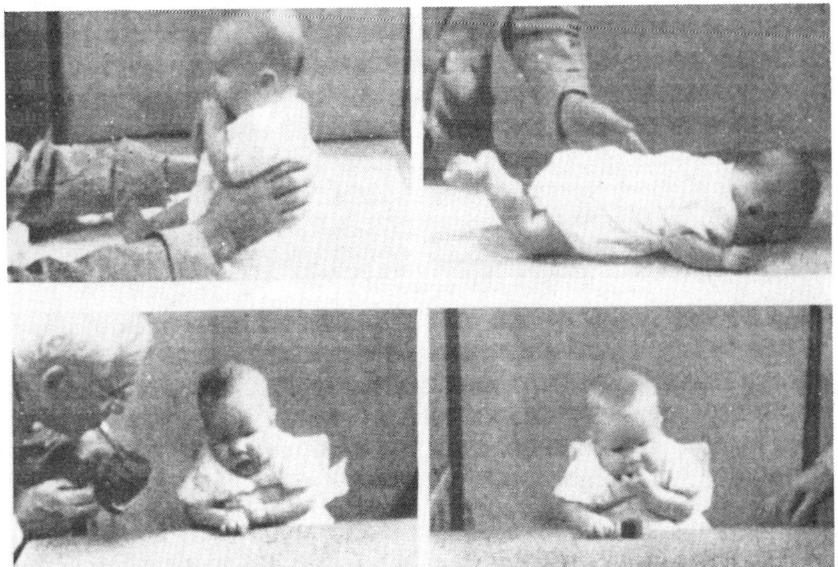

Figure 55. Blind boy, MF, age 16 weeks.
a. Holds head steady in midplane; brings hand to mouth in same manner as sighted child. Head rotation, however, is limited.
b. Placed prone, head grovels; does not lift head spontaneously as sighted child would do. Feet, however, lift.
c. Listens alertly to prolonged whistle tone. Face brightens slightly, but there is no responsive head turning.
d. Scratches table top actively on contact. Mouths free hand.

The course of his behavior development, up to the age of 4 years, has been documented with periodic cinema records. In these records, we have objective evidence of the basic role which maturation plays in the patterning of behavior. This boy has had devoted attention from an affectionate household, including an older sister. He has had all the indirect benefits of *their* surrogate sight. But the extent of these benefits has depended upon his own behavior equipment and his intrinsic growth capacities.

Vision in the sighted child develops at a remarkably rapid rate during the first months of life. We have stressed the intensity of visual hunger in normal infancy. By the age of 16 weeks, most of the infant's waking life is spent in avid looking—looking at objects, persons, lights, shadows, surroundings, and at his own hands.

Our blind infant, MF, lacked all such experience, and by the same token, he also lacked visual hunger, for he has had to develop in a world of sheer visual nothingness. Lacking the one sense most competent to take him out beyond himself, he was from the beginning pressed into his own subjective self. The psychological task of the blind infant is to overcome some of this pressure and to achieve an appreciation of realities other than his own ego. Moreover, he must locate and identify them in an ever-shifting world of persons and things. No small task! For vision is preeminently a projective as well as teleceptive sense.

If vision *per se* has a powerful retarding effect upon the growth complex, we should expect to see that effect most conspicuously in the first half-year, when vision normally plays such a prominent role. Vision, however, proves to be only one facet of a total action system, and in MF the deficit had been really limited to the mechanism of vision. On other aspects of the intact action system, the gene effects could exert their morphogenetic influence. And so they did.

At the age of 16 weeks, MF was an active child with a pleasant personality which already cast a spell on his caretakers. He could laugh and squeal; he smiled on hearing his sister's voice; he held a rattle and waved it with animation. In terms of motor performance, he met the diagnostic norms of the developmental examination almost as fully as a seeing child. He could not see the dangling ring, but he brought his hands to the midplane and spontaneously engaged in mutual fingering. By means of this pattern, he could seize an "object of interest" on tactile cue. Nature did not deny him this maturational component of the act of prehension. When he was placed in the examining chair at the test table, he immediately scratched the table with simultaneous flexion of his fingers—another maturational component of the act of prehension. He seized the handle and lifted a cup on contact. At 28 weeks, on slight tactile cue, he made an active approach upon a test object; he seized a cube, held one and grasped another, banged a cube, transferred it from hand to hand. Much of his spontaneous manipulation and exploitation of objects was indistinguishable in pattern from that of a seeing child.

Here we glimpse the manner in which maturation operates to preserve the integrity of the total action system, in spite of deficits and obstacles. Blindness profoundly alters the structure of mental life, but does not disorganize it in an otherwise normally endowed individual. And the greater the original endowment, the greater the constructive driveness to achieve integration and satisfaction.

Accordingly, MF, in his development, followed a ground plan similar to that of a sighted child. At 40 weeks, he plucked a pellet with pincer prehension (on tactile and auditory cue).

At 1 year, he cruised around his crib.

At 18 months, he released a cube in a cup. At 2 years, he combined three words; and he began to climb stairs. At 2 1/2 years, he inserted three forms in a three-hold

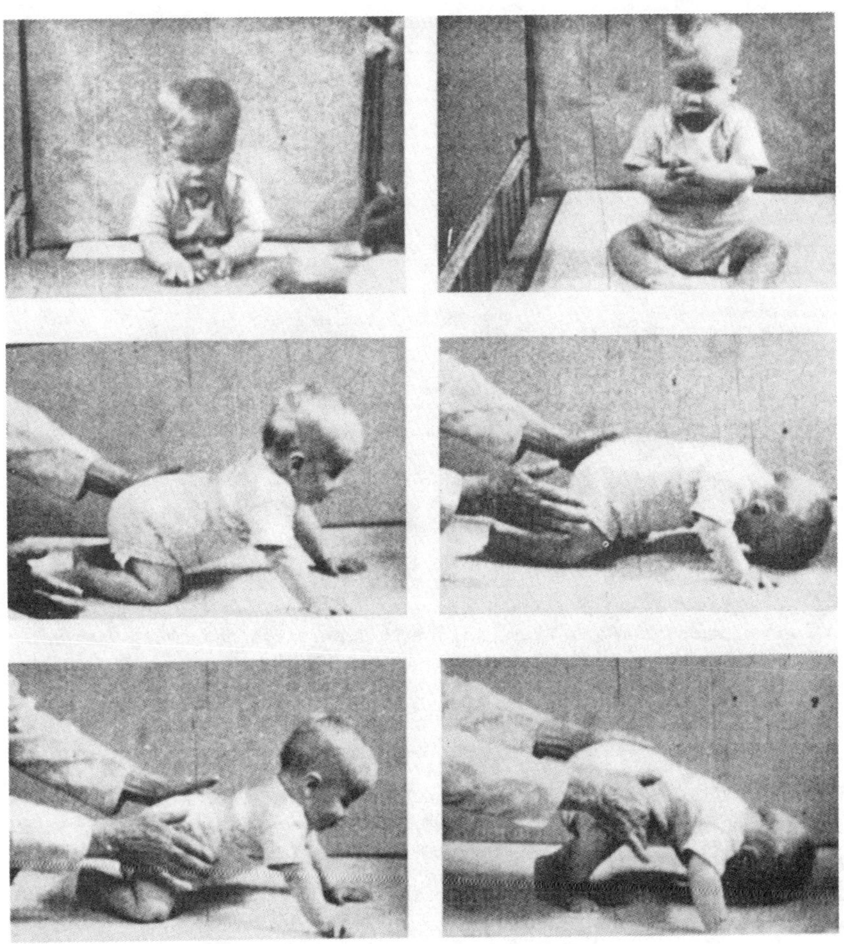

Figure 56. Age 40 weeks. a. Contacts pellets on table top with adaptive reaching. Places hand pronately, and flexes fingers conjointly. b. Pat-a-cakes amiably, on request, at close of examination. c. Momentarily assumes normal creeping stance when placed prone. d. Erect head, but presently head collapses. e. Head reerects. f. Playfully assumes wheelbarrow posture.

formboard. At 3 years, he pedaled a tricycle. At 4 years, he pours adaptively from a pitcher.

To a significant extent, the sequences of behavior development in this blind boy have been comparable to those of a seeing child. He has "learned" a great deal despite his handicap, but what he has achieved has always been delimited by the natural maturity of his growing action system. Vision, likewise, defers to matura-

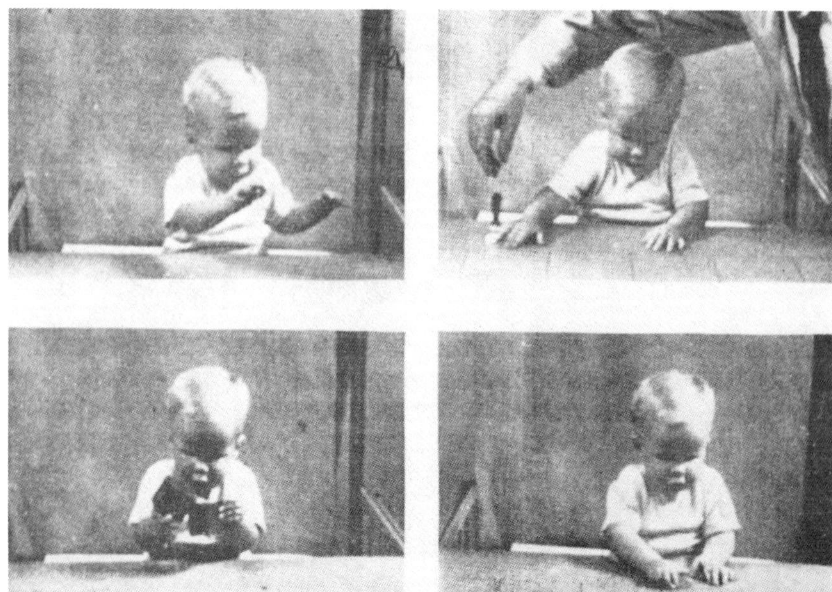

Figure 57. Age 12 months. a. Orients posturally to bell rung near left ear. Turns torso, maintaining midposition of head. Extends arms in direction of sound. b. Examiner places bell at right. Child localizes by sound, and sweeps hand toward right to contact bell. Maintains fixed central head station. c. Brings two cubes together combiningly, with intensification of interest. d. Poises hand with scissors attitude, opposing thumb and index finger on further approach.

tion. The patterns of visual behavior reflect the maturity status of the entire action system. The behavior patterns of the seeing child are pervasively influenced and guided by vision; but they are not essentially products of vision, nor of learning by looking. Even the capacity to imitate by looking is self-limited. A child can imitate only those movements which, thanks to maturation, are already in his repertoire.

Growth depends upon both specific and general potencies, which are inherent. These potencies manifest themselves in the progressive maturation of modalities and dispositions of behavior, even when normal patterns of behavior cannot be consummated. Herein lies the urgency, the almost irrepressible quality of growth. Herein lies a life tendency which works toward adjustment, harmony, and completion, even in the gravely handicapped child. Accordingly, there is an optimal utilization of impaired instrumentalities and impaired impressions. This salutary principle of growth is exemplified in the blind child. It operates in the ament, in the cerebral palsied, and in the normal child whose handicap may be limited to a strabismus or to a faulty coordination of his visual functions.

Having stressed the positive insurance role of maturation, we may now return to the deprivations imposed by blindness. Vision is normally a most ubiquitous sense. It develops not in isolation, but in close correlation with touch, kinesthesia, taste, and hearing. Congenital blindness therefore alters, by subtraction, all sensory activities, even though it may also enhance their acuteness. the blind child is not wrapped in silence; but he does not see what he hears, and this inevitably modifies the patterns of his personal-social behavior, and of his emotional reactions. To a lesser, and sometimes to a more aggravated degree, the personality traits of a seeing child are altered by defects of vision which diminish or distort his visual cues.

Vision is preeminently an orientational sense. No other sense tells us so constantly and instantaneously where we are. The blind child is entirely bereft of visual attention to cues and points of reference. He cannot use his eyes as searchlight antennae. Even when the oculomotor muscles are intact, they are of no avail without the cooperation of retina and cortex. All sense of place, space, position, distance, contour, size, solidity, substance, texture, and surface must come through the grosser muscles of locomotion, prehension, and manipulation. For this reason, even the slight vestiges of vision in the near blind are of priceless value to the groping organism.

The stone-blind infant, therefore, displays atypical orientational behavior, with reference to both his physical self and his physical surroundings. The inborn propensity of the tonic-neck reflex may cause him to avert his head, as though he were preparing to look in the direction of his extended arm. But the inspectional patterns of eye-hand coordination emerge only in fitful outline and, of course, do not come to fulfillment.

No reciprocity is established between eyes and hand. The TNR attitude dissolves and is not utilized to channelize the pathways of vision; nor can the eyes take the lead to modify the postural set. At 16 weeks, the head had adopted a midposition, which was consistently maintained. This was the most conspicuously atypical behavior pattern observed in MF during the developmental examination. Even when stimulated by the test objects at the test table, he held his head steadfast, and showed none of the free head rotation so characteristic of roving inspection in the seeing infant. At the age of 1 year, this same undeviating West Point, face-front posture was prominent. It is also characteristic of his posture at the age of 4. Whether he sits, stands, or walks, his head turns neither right nor left—why should it?

Atypical head postures were also observed at 28 and 40 weeks of age. When he was in a prone or creeping position, his head tended to collapse with the pull of gravity. In contrast, a seeing infant, under the same conditions, tends to erect the head. The seeing eyes seem to entice him to do so, for his visual fixation intensifies as he lifts his head against the pull of gravity.

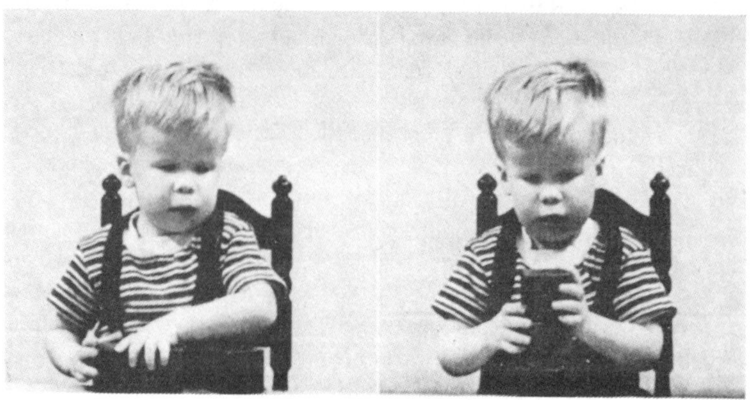

Figure 58. Blind boy, age 3 years, builds a three-cube tower on request. MF operates in a near sector optimal for tactile, kinesthetic, and manual control. Postural shifts in the action system enhance his sensory awareness.

The eyes normally play a role in the successive stages which finally lead to the upright posture. MF nevertheless passed through similar stages, in obedience to a maturational sequence. In due course, he rolled from supine to prone, assumed a creeping stance on hands and knees, pulled himself to his feet, cruised, and walked. But the absence of visual control showed itself in various ways. There seemed to be some confusion between upper and lower limbs. He brought hands and feet simultaneously toward the mouth, and used his feet for prehensory and manipulatory purposes. He showed a more than ordinary tendency to creep backward instead of forward.

With his acquisition of new powers of manipulation and locomotion, the spatial world of MF began to widen and to elaborate. For the blind, this world can never attain the vividness and the panoramic continuity which it has for the seeing eye. All spatial relations must be sensed through tactile-motor remembrance and projection. And the blind child needs constant guidance from his caretakers so that he may be brought into familiarizing contact with significant objects and locales—with floors, walls, doors, toys, spoon, chair, table, and so on. But the blind child also makes his own contribution to these contacts. When maturationally ready, he reaches out and makes forward, sideward, upward, and downward thrusts with reaching and groping hands; he pivots, he climbs, he turns corners. Thus he enlarges the scope of his space world. He builds up directional motor responses to contact cues, and begins to feel at home in an environment which, though unseen, becomes registered as latent and active attitudes in his motor make-up.

MF gave gratifying evidence of space-conquering propensities at the age of 1 year, when he made definite exploratory thrusts at the test table. At first, he contacted the table surface in an exploitive manner, and then, quite spontaneously, he reached below the surface of the table and exploited underneath with heightened attention, giving the impression that he was reacting with a sense of discovery. Later in the examination, he also made a thrust into the enamel cup, as though he dimly sensed the important relationship of container and contained. As he grew older, he made increasingly perceptive use of sounds as orientational cues; and, with the development of speech and comprehension, words became effective in establishing spatial adjustments, particularly the important adjustments essential to facile interpersonal relationships.

These relationships are of supreme significance in the psychogenesis of the spatial world of the young blind child. Words set up motor expectancies and attitudes which serve to orient the child to an environment that is spatial, as well as social. If the child's needs are too much anticipated, he is not stimulated to share in communications which challenge him to make orientations.

By the age of 27 months, MF was making excellent orientations to the human voice. He listened to a person who called to him across a long room, and he turned his steps in the appropriate direction, correcting his course as he went along, listening to the voice and even countering with the question, "Where are you?" (This is a most revealing question on the part of a blind child so young.) When he reached his goal, he stretched out his hands and established tactile contact. The foregoing behavior-event represents highly relevant behavior in the four fundamental fields—motor, language, adaptive, and personal-social. This quality of relevancy is extremely important in the appraisal of the developmental outlook of a blind child. Relevant behavior at a timely maturity level denotes a favorable outlook.

In the case history just outlined, we see, as though in a test-tube culture, the effects of uncomplicated blindness on the patterning of infant behavior. The developmental career of MF justifies the general conclusion that blindness in itself does not produce a serious degree of retardation. It profoundly alters the structure of the mental life, but not the integrity of a total growth complex. Despite congenital anophthalmia, the basic patterns of body posture, manipulation, locomotion, exploitation, language, and adaptive and personal-social behavior have taken progressive form, thus establishing conclusively the fundamental role of maturation in the mental growth of the blind infant.

PART THREE
DEVELOPMENTAL APPRAISAL

CHAPTER 14
A Developmental Hygiene of Child Vision

The concept of development adds a new dimension to all problems of visual care—diagnosis, supervision, prevention, education, training, and reeducation. This concept does not, of course, replace in any way the methods of examination and measurement which are firmly based on physical and physiological optics. But it does demand that the absolute methods will take into account the important relativities which are imposed by the sheer physiology of growth. With increased knowledge of these relativities, we shall be in a better position to protect and to promote the vision of the developing child.

The concept of development applies with equal force to the normal and to the visually-disadvantaged child. A developmental approach gives conjoint consideration both to intrinsic and to environmental factors. There is a shifting ratio between these factors from age to age, and from child to child. It is especially concerned with the interaction between the two sets of factors, so far as they are distinguishable. A developmental hygiene of child vision must naturally take into account the stages and the cycle of the growth process. In terms of systematic supervision, this would entail periodic appraisals of the child's visual economy, with special attention to the trends and the needs of his total development.

When should such appraisals begin? How often should they occur? Who should be responsible for them? To what extent can home and school cooperate in setting up safeguards, and in providing adequate experience for growing children? The mere formulation of such questions suggests the far-reaching potentialities of a comprehensive program of visual hygiene. It would be premature to attempt an outline of such a program, but it is not too early to suggest potential applications which lie within the scope of present-day knowledge of child vision and child development.

Practical possibilities in the analysis and developmental interpretation of visual functions have already been indicated in Chapter 12. Additional concrete details are assembled in the Appendix. The data show that, in many visual conditions, the child's status can be profitably explored at early age levels by means of visual skills tests, by naturalistic formalized observations of play and work behavior patterns, and direct retinoscopic examination. The present chapter, without attempting systematic clinical discussion, will illustrate how developmental factors play a role in the symptomatology and the course of visual deviations.

The great diversity of these deviations can be envisaged by reference to the chart which classifies the variables that enter into the functional complex of the visual system. These variables pertain to the *coordination*, to the *reach*, and to the *scope* of the visual functions. They are classifiable into three major fields—*skeletal, visceral* and *cortical.* These multiple variables vary as to intensity and ontogenetic timing from individual to individual. The consequent number of constellations is legion; no two children develop and see exactly alike. Many of the variations, of course, fall within a normal range. Deviations become disadvantageous and abnormal only when they seriously reduce potential efficiency. The culture sets standards of efficiency. The standards are not always valid. Often they are excessive and unreasonable; or they may be inadequate. The task of developmental hygiene is to appraise the assets and liabilities of the seeing organism in its visual adaptations at progressive stages of growth, and to bring about an optimal interaction between the child and his cultural environment.

Deviations of visual development make their appearance in various ways: (a) An essential visual trait or pattern may manifest itself with excessive or subnormal intensity. (b) It may appear too early or too late in the growth cycle. (c) It may remain too briefly or too long. The gravity of any deviation can be estimated only by observing its trend over a period of time. The problem must be appraised in the perspective of development.

Before considering specific visual deviations, it will be well to recall briefly a few general principles which apply to all developmental phenomena, whether the minutiae of vision or the totality of the unitary action system:

1. Behavior development usually tends toward an optimal realization. This general tendency applies alike to normal and to handicapped conditions. Each breach in a complex of growth is filled through regenerative, substitutive, or compensatory growth of some kind. The organism thereby makes maximal use of its reserves. Individuals, however, vary greatly with respect to the range and strength of insurance reserves.

2. Developmental organization does not advance on an even front. There is a fluctuation of dominance in counterbalanced functions—flexors versus extensors, right versus left, skeletal versus visceral, central versus peripheral, and so on. This is the principle of reciprocal interweaving.

3. The growing action system and its constituent organ systems are in a state of formative instability, combined with a progressive movement toward stability. Tension between opposite tendencies results in self-regulatory fluctuations. Stages of relatively stable equilibrium alternate more or less rhythmically with stages of relatively loose formativeness.

4. The course of development resembles a spiral more than it does a trajectory. General patterns of organization repeat themselves, in part, at ascending levels, but with increasing complexity. This is the principle of spiral reincorporation, whereby the organism consolidates its growth gains and also gives itself successive chances to attain optimal organization.

5. Every child has a distinctive ground plan of growth, determined primarily by innate, constitutional factors in interaction with extrinsic influences. His growth characteristics denote his individuality.

These general principles lose their abstractness as soon as they are applied to the concrete problems of visual hygiene, both in the normal and in the handicapped child. In a sketchy manner, we shall suggest the practical implications of developmental mechanisms as they operate in the growth cycle. The scope of these mechanisms will, of course, vary with the etiology and the pathology of underlying defects and deviations. This has been demonstrated in the previous chapter. But since the basic laws of the physiology of development are universal, we may expect to find evidence of developmental factors in all forms of child vision—normal, atypical, and abnormal. These factors conjointly involve the action system and the visual system. A developmental approach to the problems of prevention and hygiene will naturally stress age trends and maturity traits. Therefore, our discussion will deal in turn with three age periods: Infancy, the Preschool Years, and the School Years.

INFANCY

Infants reveal their visual individualities in ocular and other postural attitudes and demeanors. Virtually all infants repeatedly assume, in one form or another, the tonic-neck reflex posture and the symmetrotonic reflex posture during the first half-year of life. These postures, both quiescent and active, constitute a morphogenetic matrix for the basic patterning of the coordinations, dominances, and functional correlations of eyes and hands, singly and in pairs. The classic form of of the TNR-STR complex has already been described. Now we may note deviations which have import for the appraisal and the supervision of visual status.

Excessive hand regard, if not due to retarded development, may signify a myopic trend. Excess manifests itself in the intensity and duration of episodes, and in a marked continuation beyond the age of 12 weeks. One of our myopic subjects, now 6 years old, held the hand regard attitude so persistently and steadily in infancy that he acquired the nickname "Statue of Liberty." Delayed hand regard is a symptom of retardation, but it may also be associated with normal intelligence and atypical spatial manipulation.

Another deviation consists in a poorly defined TNR or a neutral tendency to assume indifferently either a right or a left TNR. Ordinarily, there is a defined preference for right or left which must have correlations with ocular and manual dominance, and with the organization of the functional asymmetry of the total action system. Little is known about the nature of these correlations, but we may be sure that they have predictive import for later visual patterns. The whole subject needs extensive investigation because it has significance for preventive hygiene.

Complicating clinical factors, however, must not be overlooked. If an infant is born two months prematurely, he is likely to show TNR patterns for two or three months beyond the expected time. Cerebral injuries, however slight, and possibly Rh incompatibility may cause the usual behavior picture to deviate. As just stated, there is much to learn in this important, but accessible, field of symptomatology.

Some deviations consist in an atypical relation between the TNR and STR trends. Usually, these trends interweave in normal reciprocal sequence with proper ontogenetic timing and intensity. An esophoric child, now 11 years old, showed a marked tendency to central channelization of her TNR in infancy. She held her extensor arm not at the side, but thrust forward and obliquely upward, as if in a Fascist salute. Her eyes converged extremely, though evenly. With a discrepancy in teaming, such a condition might augur strabismus. Extreme symmetric convergence tends to resolve spontaneously, within the first quarter of the first year.

Atypical inspection patterns may denote a faulty visual organization. They are especially significant when associated with atypical postural development. A very early drive to sit up, if due to a basic defect in ontogenetic timing, may be correlated with a faulty association of head and eye movements. Such a child may hold his head in central position while the eyes move independently to right and left to inspect surroundings. Headrolling may have ocular determinations which need investigation. Excessive, indiscriminate casting of objects, at the age of 15 months, if dissociated from appropriate head and eye posturing, may signify a disproportionate skeletal reaction. Eye movements, in general, should take the lead in the organization of action patterns and when the eyes follow rather than lead in the organization of such patterns, the possibility of visual complications should be considered.

Visual acuity can be conveniently examined in the early months of infancy by means of a pellet performance test. The test must be administered with careful control of a standardized procedure. The infant is seated in a supportive chair in front of the examining table. The examiner grasps a 7 mm. pellet between index finger and thumb and, holding the convexity down, he advances the pellet in a horizontal plane and places it in a standard median position. If, after 10 seconds, the infant has not reacted to the pellet, the examiner advances it to the near-median position. This white sugar pellet, at a distance of two feet, represents a visual acuity of approximately 6/288 (Chavasse).*

**(About one child out of four in our normative group of 12-week-old infants pays some kind of regard for the pellet. This regard is usually delayed, momentary, and passive. Nearly all of the infants, however, give regard to the examiner's incoming hand; the remaining regard going to the table top, to the surroundings, or to the infant's own hand. [Sometimes the examiner resorts to repeated trials to elicit objective signs of ocular fixation upon the pellet.] One-half of the 16-week-old infants regard the pellet and some of the infants now pay regard not only to the examiner's incoming hand, but also to the outgoing hand. This visual pick-up of the outgoing hand represents a growth increment in the field of visual perception. By 20 weeks, three-fourths of the children perceive the pellet in the standard median position and give definite regard, which can be readily confirmed by altering the position of the pellet on the table. With four out of 10 children, the regard is immediate. At 21 weeks, 83% of the children make a prehensory approach upon the pellet.)*

This apparently simple test, which may be applied, with adaptations, to infants from 8 weeks to 18 months of age, releases an extraordinarily rich variety of behavior responses which have significance for estimating the maturity status and functional integrity of their manifest visual acts. Such estimates, if critically made, would take into account not only the reactions of the eyes, but the total adjustments of the child to the total situation.

The clinical examination of infant behavior is essentially an examination of the central nervous system. Normative tests serve to reveal delays, deficits, and deviations in the development of motor functions. A 1-year-old infant, for example, displays a restricted and somewhat bizarre poking of the pellet; another child shows an unusual preoccupation with a single object; still another child of similar age exploits objects in a stereotyped, serial manner and fails to combine two objects productively. The diagnostic task is to determine, if possible, whether visual factors are involved in these atypical behavior patterns. This applies with special force to the problem of strabismus.

When developmental examinations are made more routinely, we shall have better understanding of the early manifestations of visual defect and deviation. Here is a field in which the pediatrician and the general practitioner play a role. Developmental Pediatrics is a form of clinical medicine which is systematically concerned with the diagnosis and supervision of child development, normal and abnormal. A developmental hygiene of vision must of necessity begin with infancy, and will therefore need, in addition to the specialists in visual care, the combined assistance of medical, public-health, and educational agencies in the early discovery of visual defects and liabilities.

THE PRESCHOOL YEARS

Visual difficulties come to somewhat franker expression in the preschool years. The child begins to leave the confines of the home and is thereby brought into more frequent comparison with his peers. If he has serious ineptitudes, he reveals them in his play activities, in postural demeanors, in his adjustments to a nursery school group, in his use of cup and spoon, of crayon and paints, and in his response to picture books. He may show a moderate amount of staring (or perhaps too little). He may show forms of caution, fear, and withdrawal which may denote visual, rather than purely emotional, factors. Indeed, even his atypical personal-social relations with his companions may have a visual basis in faulty space manipulation.

On the basis of everyday patterns, a discerning teacher may detect evidences, more or less predictive, of potential reading disabilities—specific weaknesses in drawing and in form perception, ill defined handedness, reduced acuity, atypical directionalities in movement patterns, and so on. When the norms of visual behavior are more widely known by parents and teachers, it will be possible to use naturalistic observations of spontaneous behavior for the benefit of children who need early guidance in solving their visual problems. Such observations should both precede and supplement formal visual skill tests. They become doubly important, under professional guidance, for appraising the responses of the child to lens assistance and to special vision therapy procedures. Naturalistic observation of the spontaneous child is at times more valuable than technical observation because it brings into view the total child and his unitary action system.

In considering the visual economy of a young child, one does not think only in terms of refraction and fusion. One considers the overall organization of his visual equipment, and asks whether he has the ability to meet the normal visual tasks demanded by the culture. This ability can be appraised in relation to his expected maturity level; better still, it can be appraised in terms of his progress from one age level to another. If the general trend of his organization is in accordance with a normal developmental sequence, the outlook is correspondingly favorable, even though his actual visual performance may not be altogether satisfactory. A developmental approach to his problem puts us in a better position to give him the developmental support which will benefit him more than a full refractive correction would. Indeed, in some instances, a full correction given too early and insisted upon too long may create a crutch which, in turn, becomes an impediment. The growing visual equipment then organizes about the full-strength lens, whereas a more natural and advantageous organization could have taken place with the aid of lenses of lesser strength, carefully timed to put the organism on its own best resources. The same principle applies to training procedures, and to the planning of eye-care regimes. Wise timing in small, well-spaced sessions, with interested motivation, is more efficacious than an overstrenuous practice-makes-perfect program. In all programs of visual care it is important to appraise the kind and degree of acceptance manifested by the child.

These statements are general and must, of course, be adapted to the individual child. But in the preschool years there are very few situations, whether minor or major, in which a regard for developmental trends is not a factor of safety.

The fact that myopia manifests itself at varying ages, from early infancy through adolescence, is itself indicative of the presence of developmental factors. The prior developmental history, in any given case, has a significant bearing on the ultimate outlook. Some cases are much more amenable to environmental control because less specifically determined by gene factors.

Strabismus shows similar variations as to age incidence. Developmental considerations are especially pertinent in those instances in which the strabismus is an end result of an organizational conflict between visceral and skeletal components in the visual complex. Some children solve the developmental problem by the route of myopia, others via strabismus.

The behavior symptomatology of myopia in the preschool years is a fertile field for observation. Refinement of observation will lead to an earlier recognition of the myopic trend, and to a more precise prognostication of its several varieties. The excessive hand regard of infancy has already been noted. Myopes frequently show a precocious interest in books as early as 18 months or 2 years of age. Frequently they hold the book very close to the eyes. This is one earmark; however, it should be noted, in passing, that a more occasional hyperopic preschool child will also hold a picture book at close range.

The pronounced myope shows an overconcentration on near-sector activities, which in turn may eventuate in precocious reading and verbalization and in a marked topical card-index type of memory. He shows overcentrality and overidentification. He overholds and has difficulty in making transitions. He is also reported to have a low appetite. He is overaware of color and uses it prodigiously for distant vision cues and for making fine distinctions in hue and shades. Introjective trends are uppermost. He gathers all the experience into himself, and he is in consequence better oriented within himself, but not so facilely oriented to his physical and social milieu. He is very demanding of people. A developmentally discriminating deference to this demand on the part of his elders may assist him in his problems of visual organization and personal adjustment.

The problem of strabismus assumes special importance in the preschool years in view of the Worth-Chavasse theory that the binocular reflexes are in a state of diminishing flux during this very period. The flux is held to be "coming to an end at the age of 5 years and has indeed ended at the age of 8 years in a stage of complete precipitation." It follows from this view, which is developmental in import, that abnormal reflexes which may be formed after the age of from 5 to 8 years do not assume unconditional fixity, and are therefore more amenable to correction and cure.

The causative factors and underlying pathologies of strabismus are so diversified that generalized discussion is impossible, but in what follows we shall call attention to developmental factors which are significant from the standpoint of prognosis and of early treatment. The outlook for spontaneous resolution of intermittent strabismus is, in general, more favorable than for fixed strabismus. Alternating strabismus, likewise, may have a favorable import. Even if at first the alternations are slow and crude, they signify that the developmental drift is toward ocular teaming. With an increase of speed and smoothness in the alternations, binocularity may be achieved.

There are two major types of strabismus—one predominantly visceral, the other predominantly skeletal. Developmental shifts in the ascendancy of skeletal or visceral components influence the origin and type of strabismus incurred. "Infants squint with flatulence, adults with anger." A child with poor teaming often acquires the trick of suppressing one eye or the other, at near or far, to suit his visual needs. He even practices his tricks to build up proficiency. He gives up staring. Here is an instructive suggestion that staring has a developmental function in the organization of vision. Staring may well be a growth prerequisite for binocularity. Conceivably, it may be therapeutically exploited in a training program.

Symptoms and premonitions of strabismus are prone to occur during transitional stages of readjustment in equilibrium—for example, at 21 to 24 months. At these stages, the organism is more loosely organized in order to give play to counterpoised opposites. The looseness, or morphogenetic flux, characterizes the action system as a whole and more or less evenly paired body members and paired functions, such as flexors versus extensors, abduction versus adduction, and so on. Accordingly, a liability to strabismus may declare itself in frank eye discoordination or, more indirectly, in faulty motor demeanors and awkwardness. A clumsy hand, a foot drag, or a postural slump on the "weak side" may come into evidence in a 2 1/2-year-old child as a precursor of a manifest strabismus a year or two later. Such a pre-squinter, if accurately identified, on developmental premises would be approached orthopedically first, and orthoptically later, with due consideration as to whether the condition is primarily skeletal or visceral in character. Therapy and training directed to improvement of body posture might, in some instances, be more fundamental than immediate or postponed vision therapy. Indeed, early recognition and management of pre-squint symptoms might altogether prevent the emergence of strabismus. Treatment should take into account the basic level of psychomotor integration at which the child is functioning. The treatment program should begin with reorganizations at this level, and should not be directed too specifically to the visual difficulty alone. Resistance on the part of the child can be overcome by skillfully enlisting his own interest and participation. He has a latent fund of interest and motivation based on his developmental equipment.

THE SCHOOL YEARS

The child has now reached school age and has slowly acquired some detachment from the household which has reared him during the preschool years. He is thrown more and more on his own resources, but developmental factors still prevail and play a primary role in the organization of his visual abilities as they relate to reading, spelling, arithmetic, and other fields of learning. These factors are very comparable to those which operated in the preschool period and are obedient to the same laws. Their operation, however, is somewhat concealed because the child is less naive and also at a higher level of organization. Moreover, the culture, in its sophistication, assumes too unquestioningly a sterner command over his affairs.

Five is a nodal age. The transition to age 6 is biologically complex. The culture, likewise, takes on great complexity in the eyes of the child. It assails him with new demands which lead him beyond the security of the home. He goes abroad into the community on new pathways, into new environments, and his life is suddenly complicated by the necessity of establishing a wide variety of interpersonal relationships.

The culture, as just suggested, is not too aware of the school beginner's difficulties and potentialities. Rightly construed, many of his difficulties are actually symptoms of potentialities—new abilities in the making. The culture tends to deal with him en masse, and tends to use rigid and undiscriminating procedures. If he is unfortunate enough to enter a strictly regimented school, his teacher frowns upon him even if he drops a pencil. Now, he is very likely to drop a pencil because his patterns of visual behavior are not adequate to all the demands which are made upon his seeing and interpreting equipment.

All too soon, he encounters difficulties which are due to the discrepancy of the culture and his own immature visual and manual structures. He may have trouble in adapting to the blackboard, and in making adjustments from far to near and near to far. The culture, as embodied by the schoolroom, may make unreasonable demands upon sustained attention at a stage of development when he is geared to brief and multiple adjustments that require a shifting, flexible activity program. If he began to identify letters and numerals at the age of 2 1/2, he is not likely to experience undue difficulty in responding to reading instruction, whatever method may be used. However, many children are in a phase of development, or they present individual maturity traits which make it difficult or impossible for them to profit from the prevailing method of instruction. A sizable fraction of these children in a year or two are classified as poor readers, nonreaders, and slow readers. Broadly speaking, the difficulties of these academically disadvantaged children are due to a rather clumsy disparity between the educational environment of the school and the organisms which are in attendance.

So many factors, both intrinsic and environmental, enter into this disparity, that every case of so-called reading disability needs individualized analysis and appraisal. Sometimes the disability is too blithely attributed to a "visual" defect. In other instances, the primary visual defect is unrecognized or is misdiagnosed. The importance of a visual appraisal justifies a more periodic individualized survey of the visual equipment of all school children, to say nothing of better provisions, in the preschool period, for identifying visual and associated difficulties which lead to maladjustment and failures in reading.

Periodic visual examinations during the school years should not be directed so much to the discovery of subnormal acuity as to the appraisal of the developmental factors which are responsible for visual achievement. These developmental factors are foreshadowed in the preschool period because basically even reading may be regarded as a complex task in the field of spatial manipulation. This spatial manipulation functions at four progressive, overlapping levels in the elementary school period as follows: (1) elementary spatial manipulation, (2) elementary assimilation of abstract form, (3) elementary utilization of form in relation to meaning, and (4) interpretive manipulation of the printed page—and other symbols and cues as they arise in everyday life at home, on the playground, and in the motion picture theatre.

The recognition of the ABC's and the P's and Q's of the printed page is a form of spatial manipulation. If the letters and words are apprehended at a shallow level of obviousness, and are never brought into association with the realities for which the symbols stand, the child remains nonliterate. Ordinarily, with *normal* initiation at the age of 6, he advances with each year into a succeeding stage—at 7 into the stage of *impression* and absorption which affords him elementary meanings; at the 8-year level into the stage of *expression*, in which he manifests with diversity and facility his cumulating skills; and at 9 into a period of more active *exploitation* and interpretation which is based upon a more skillful manipulation and recombination of various facets of related meanings. Even this refined process is based upon a capacity to make spatial manipulations at a more elementary kinesthetic level. Periodic examinations of the visual status at annual or other spaced intervals would serve to determine whether a retarded or visually-disadvantaged child is functioning at stage 1, 2, 3, or 4.

These stages are characteristic of an ontogenetic sequence during the school years, but they are also discernible in more limited time periods, at various ages, in relation to specific tasks. Indeed, the visual examiner who is interested in the developmental progress of his client is likely to inquire whether the condition is moving from one stage to another. Such an approach to the visual functions may well have a far-reaching effect in the resolution of learning and of reading difficulties.

All children, after the age of 5 years, undergo fundamental and more or less striking reorganizations in their visual equipment. They acquire new abilities, but not always in balanced or well-timed relationships. Often new trends become observable by the age of 5 1/2 years. Appraisal at 6 years may show a developmental direction in the nature of the interaction of the visceral and skeletal functions. At 7, there may be frank evidence of such directional trends. Typically, the visceral-skeletal inter-relation is relatively tight at the age of 7. By 8 years, this tightness gives way to a looser and more facile interplay. By 9 years, the looseness is being superseded, in turn, by a more robust consolidation of the visceral-skeletal components.

Because the ontogenetic sequence tends to proceed in this manner during the period from 6 to 9 years, 7 proves to be a crucial age in the supervision of visual development. At this age level, the visual deviate may exhibit atypical symptoms as follows: he may develop strabismus because of overindividuation of skeletal factors. This introduces a faulty organization in the teaming of his two eyes. Another child may overorganize the near visual domain: unable to shift into far, he becomes stranded in the near domain and in time he may become a confirmed myope. If the developmental hurdle from 7 to 8 years is deferred to the consolidating age of 9 years, the child may not be able to reorganize at a 10-year level of ability, and may settle into myopia.

It is difficult, with our present meager knowledge, and on the basis of a single visual appraisal at 5 years, to predict the probable course of development in the years from 5 to 10; but systematic examination and supervision of the visual functions in the preschool years will serve to identify children who present potential difficulties in learning and school tasks.

This possibility, however, should not blind us to the fact that the culture is making unreasonable demands upon many young children. The demands overburden the limited powers of spatial manipulation and, in many instances, rearrangement and amelioration of the cultural demands would be a more basic solution than a therapeutic approach to the visual handicap. In a flexible educational system, both lines of approach may be conjointly utilized; the one directed toward the environment, the other toward the organism.

CHAPTER 15
The Conservation of Child Vision

It is unnecessary to insist that the conservation of vision is a problem of vast social dimensions. The problem includes the care of the visually-handicapped; the prevention of industrial, highway, and household accidents; the reduction of illiteracy; vocational selection and training; important aspects of mental health and personality in adults; and, above all, the developmental welfare of growing children. Socially regarded, the scope of visual hygiene is so extensive that it involves several professional groups and numerous types of associated lay workers, not excluding legislators and educators.

For natural reasons, the conservation of vision began with the correction of refractive error and the treatment of ocular disease and injury. Ophthalmology is one of the most highly refined specialties of clinical medicine. In recent years, optometry has evolved techniques for the analysis of visual functions, and has greatly advanced methods of training or the amelioration of visual difficulties and the increase of visual achievement.

Both ophthalmology and optometry stem, historically, from the study of the mature adult eye. Many of the prevailing concepts in theory and practice reflect this adult orientation. It is now evident that this orientation introduces certain errors and shortcomings into visual theory which affect practical applications. We are confronted with the sobering realization that the child is never merely a miniature adult, even in his ocular equipment. He is qualitatively a *different* organism and he is always changing qualitatively at a more rapid rate than the adult. This is particularly true of his nervous system and his visual system. It should not be necessary to wait until belated adolescence and adult years to determine the efficiency of his visual functions. The developmental status of these functions should be appraised and supervised throughout the period of childhood. We need new methods of naturalistic, biometric, and diagnostic observation. New arrangements can be devised which will supply objective measurements and critical estimates of visual behavior, even in the very young.

Such child adapted procedures will not, of course, be snatched from the skies. They must be derived from a deeper knowledge of the distinctive characteristics of the developing visual equipment and the action patterns of the growing child. Because the visual system is so intimately part and parcel of the unitary action system, the social protections of vision will require attention and safeguards from many different directions. Who will participate in a continuing system of safeguards? The pediatrician, who supervises the basic stages of infancy; the parents, who manage, day in and day out, the environmental controls which affect visual welfare; nursery-school teachers, who see the child in action at his first near tasks; primary teachers, who induct him, despite his tender age, into the complicated art of reading; and the whole succession of teachers who observe his visual assets and liabilities expressed in his everyday behavior, his interpersonal adjustments, his skills in arts and crafts, and perhaps his distinctive talents based on visual giftedness.

Visual care is indeed a ubiquitous problem. It involves the public, as well as the professions, and it requires a policy of continuous general education as to the psychological meaning of sight and the far-reaching implications of visual health. Such education is, in turn, dependent upon continuous research, high professional standards, professional leadership, and cooperation between professions. General education will take care of the diffusion of knowledge; professional specialization must take care of its advancement in theory and practice.

The specialization will inevitably gravitate toward a more systematic concern for the development of vision in infants and children—normal, defective, and deviate. The social need of such specialization is exemplified in the evolution of American pediatrics. This broad specialty concentrates on a sector of life and brings development, as well as defect and disease, within its purview. A nation-wide survey has shown that well over half of the pediatric physician's time is devoted to the supervisory care of the normal infant and child. Like dentistry, pediatrics is using the method of periodic examinations for supervisory health protection. Recent movements in group medicine, industrial medicine, and community health service show similar trends toward periodic individualized care.

Comparable social forces are beginning to define the possibilities and the opportunities of professional specializations in the field of child vision. The child specialist in this area will have a basic scientific interest in the nature and needs of child development. He will relate his practice to the broader aspects of family and child welfare, as well as to specific visual difficulties; he will recognize the pervasive mechanisms of growth in his policy of periodic follow-up; he will adjust treatment and guidance to these mechanisms; he will enlist the cooperation of parents and kin through concrete homely advice; he will appreciate that vision lies close to the citadel of personality, and will so render his services that the dignity of the individual child will be respected. This he will do through deepened insight into the general dynamics of growth which underlie the patterning of individuality in vision.

APPENDIX A
Examination Sequences and Procedures

0-10 Years

The general character of the visual-behavior examination has been indicated in various chapters of the main text. These examinations were conducted as part of a research program, and were supplemented with incidental and naturalistic observations of the child's behavior on the playground, in school, and in the examining room. The developmental examinations of the child's total behavior status were made under controlled conditions, and were supplemented with detailed interviews concerning home behavior. The procedures for these developmental examinations are not here described. They require special training and clinical experience, as detailed in other publications listed here.

Gesell A, Amatruda CS. Developmental diagnosis, normal and abnormal child development. Clinical methods and pediatric applications. New York: Hoeber, 1947.

Gesell A. The first five years of life. New York: Harper, 1940.

Gesell A, Thompson H. The psychology of early growth. New York: Macmillan, 1938.)

EXAMINATION SEQUENCES
0-4 Years

The basic sequence to the preschool examination is summarized below. This sequence proved to be practical and advantageous from the standpoint of producing optimal rapport with the younger children. Great pains should be taken in establishing the initial adjustment because the remaining part of the examination proceeds more naturally and smoothly from a good beginning.

1. Initial adjustment
2. Dangled bell
   (fixations)
3. Retinoscope
   Far estimate
   Intermediate estimate
   Far measure
   Near measure
   Book
4. Stereoscope
   (projection)

PROCEDURES

Adjustment

0-4 YEARS

The child is brought to the examining room by the nursery teacher. He sits on an adult chair, with a footstool for his feet. The teacher is seated beside him and is free to question him and to assist with the picture book. There is a picture on the far screen (15 feet away) when he enters the room.

Dangled Bell

The target is a metal cat bell, 1/2" in diameter, which is suspended on a heavy thread. It may be jiggled to produce sound, or twisted so that it spins. The examiner stations himself directly in front of the child, using a stool so that the eye level of child and examiner coincide.

The bell is held in median plane, at the child's eye level, within easy reaching distance (about 10 inches). It is then brought slowly toward the bridge of the child's nose. If regard is not released when the bell is near, he is asked to look at the examiner. This is repeated several times.

Instructions to the child: "See the bell?" "Watch the bell." "Look at me." "Now watch the bell and touch it."

Initially, the child's spontaneous response of eyes and hands is noted. Later, the examiner makes specific requests in order that he may observe the effect of hand participation.

Retinoscopy

Far Estimate. Pictures are serially presented on the far screen by an assistant, who operates the projector at about five feet from the screen. The examiner is at the distance of the screen and, by means of the retinoscope, observes the appearance and movement of the retinal reflex. He dictates his findings as they occur. Questioning of the child at proper intervals is done by the nearby teacher. (If the distant assistant questions the child, it often confuses children 3 years of age and younger.)

Intermediate Estimate. The same procedure as the Far Estimate is repeated, with the examiner at seven feet from the child. The child regards the pictures on the screen while the reflex is observed. A second recording is made while he is regarding the examiner.

Far Measure. While the child regards the targets before him, the examiner places lenses before the right and then the left eye to neutralize the movement and secure a measurement. The examiner now questions the child so that the attention is on the target when the measurement is made.

Near Measure. Lenses are placed before the eyes. The child is asked to regard parts of the examiner's face while the measurement is taken.

Book. The book, *Sounds the Letters Make,** was used at all ages. The introductory page of animals is presented first. The teacher holds the book and asks, "What do you see?" "Where is the cow?" Or she points and asks, "What is that?" Questioning is minimized to allow for spontaneous verbalization and pointing. Measurements are taken through lenses while the child is searching, naming and pointing.

*(Schoolfield LC, Timberlake JB. Sounds the letters make. Boston: Little Brown & Co., 1940.)

Projection

A stereoscope is mounted into a tilttop table, so that the targets rest in the center of a large undifferentiated area. The child is seated in a chair before the instrument. After he has approached the lenses, a picture is exposed before the left eye, with a blank card before the right eye. He is asked, "What do you see?" "Where is the piggy?" "Can you touch it?" After his responses have been obtained to the picture before the left eye, this is covered and the picture before the right eye is exposed. This procedure may be repeated several times. Should the child start to peer over the instrument at the picture, it is promptly covered.

(*Instrumentation:* Copeland Streak Retinoscope, Keystone Hand Stereoscope, Three Dimension Tachistoscope.)

EXAMINATION SEQUENCE**
5-10 Years

The examination for the school years from 5 to 10 was more elaborate and, typically, consisted of 17 items as follows:

1. Reaction to light
2. Acuity at far
3. Ophthalmoscopy
4. Habitual phoria at far (20 feet)
5. Habitual phoria at near (16 inches)
6. Retinoscopy at far
7. Retinoscopy at near
8. Subjective at far
9. Phoria through far subjective
10. Fusion range at far
11. Phoria through far subjective at near
12. Monocular subjective at near

12a. Phoria through monocular subjective at near

13. Binocular subjective at near

13a. Phoria through binocular subjective at near

14. Fusion range at near

15. Amplitude of accommodation
16. Stimulation and inhibition of accommodation
17. Donders push-up

**(The routine approximates that derived by A. M. Skeffington, O.D., and Associates of the Graduate Clinic Foundation in Optometry.)

PROCEDURES
5-10 Years

Reaction to Light

A light within *nearpoint* range is switched on and off and the pupillary reaction is observed.

Acuity at Far

Letters are projected on the *far* screen, starting with the 20/40 letters (or larger, when necessary). The child is asked to identify letters to the limit of his ability.

Ophthalmoscopy

With an ophthalmoscope, the media and eyegrounds are examined. This examination is usually made at the beginning, as indicated in the sequence. But at 5 and 6 years of age, it is advisable to postpone it until after the other findings have been made.

Phorias at Far

A dot target is projected on the *far* screen. A 4 diopter prism base-up is placed before the left eye, displacing the dot below the right eye target. The lateral prism before the right eye is slowly reduced from base-in (8-10 diopters) until the dots are reported to be in alignment. The prism is then moved to an extreme base-out position, and slowly reduced until the dots are in alignment. The phoria is usually taken from the two directions; but when only one direction is taken, it is from the base-in position.

Directions to the child: "Do you see one dot? Now I am going to make you see two dots. Tell me when one dot is right above the other, like the buttons on your coat." (A 5-year-old may need a concrete demonstration of "one above the other" in order to respond.)

Phorias at Near

The procedure is the same as for *Phorias at Far* except that a reduced Snellen chart is the target and the prism base-up is changed to 8 diopters. The near phorias are usually taken from one direction only (base-in toward base-out).

Retinoscopy at Far

The child looks at large letters on the *far* screen (20/200-20/70). The retinoscope is held 20" from the child and, using a +2.00 D working lens, the reflex is observed and the movement neutralized with the lenses of the phoropter. If his attention is doubtful, he may be asked to read the letters.

Retinoscopy at Near (20")

The retinoscope is held 20" from the child and his attention is maintained by asking him to count or name the examiner's fingers, which are extended as he holds the retinoscope. The movement is observed and is neutralized with the lenses of the phoropter.

Subjective at Far

The right eye is occluded. *Plus* lenses are added before the left eye until the 20/80 letters blur. Then the left eye is occluded, and *plus* lenses are added until the 20/80 letters blur. A target with radiating lines is then projected, the plus on the right is reduced and the child is asked if the lines are getting clearer and if some are clearer or blacker than the others. If there is a difference, *minus* cylinders are added at an axis opposite to that of the blackest lines until the lines appear to be equal. Then letters are shown, and the *plus* is further reduced until the 20/30 line can be read. The astigmatic correction is then checked for both axis and amount by using the flip crossed cylinder technique. The 20/20 line is then used and the *plus* is further reduced, if necessary, so that the individual is just barely able to read it.

The right eye is then occluded and the procedure is repeated. When the test is completed, the right eye and the left eye are compared and equalized as nearly as possible. The most *plus* or least *minus* through which the 20/20 (or his best acuity, if less than 20/20) line can be read binocularly is then recorded.

Subjective at Near—Monocular

The target is a five-lined grid. Illumination is lowered from the standard (about 4' candle). With the *plus* of the *far* subjective in the phoropter, a crossed cylinder with axes crossed is placed before each eye. Prisms are placed in position, with zero before the right eye and 8 diopters base-up before the left eye. Usually, the horizontal lines are reported as clearest; if so, *plus* lenses are added to the right eye until the lines are equally clear, or until the vertical lines on the top chart are darker. The same procedure is repeated with the left eye. The right and then the left eye are again checked, and the plus is reduced or added until the lines are equal or the vertical are darker in both charts. Subjective at Near—Binocular

With the results of the monocular subjective in the phoropter, the prisms are removed so that the target is no longer double. Standard illumination is reinstated. The child is asked if the vertical lines are still blacker. If so, the plus is reduced until the vertical and horizontal lines are equal or the horizontal lines are blacker. If the horizontal lines are still best, which is unusual, more plus is added.

Tolerance of Base-Out Prisms at Far

A vertical line of letters is projected on the screen, with the smallest readable type exposed. The target commonly used is of graded type with the 20/40 letters at the top. With his *far* subjective in the phoropter, prisms at zero are placed before both eyes. The prisms are simultaneously moved in base-out direction until a change in clarity or size is reported, and/or until the targets are reported to double. The prisms are then reduced until a single target is regained.

Directions to the child: He is asked to read as many letters as possible in the vertical line. A +.25 is then added, and he is asked if this blurs the letters, makes them worse. The *plus* is removed and then, as the prisms are moved, he is asked to tell when the letters change—get blurred "as I showed you"—or when he has two sets of them. On the reduction of prisms, he is asked to tell when he sees only one set of letters. It is frequently necessary to repeat questioning.

Tolerance of Base-in Prisms at Far

The procedure is the same as that for base-out tolerance, except that the prisms are moved base-in. It is not usual to experience a blur, and therefore the emphasis on instructions is for the report of doubling.

Tolerance of Base-Out Prisms at Near

The reduced Snellen chart at *nearpoint* is the target. With the *far* subjective in the phoropter, prisms at zero are placed before the eyes. The prisms are simultaneously moved in base-out direction until a change in clarity or size is reported on the smallest readable type, or until the images are reported to double. The prisms are then reduced until a single image is regained.

Tolerance of Base-In Prisms at Near

The procedure is the same as that for base-out tolerance except that the prisms are moved base-in.

Accommodation Amplitude

The target is a test card of various-sized type. When readable, the .62 M Jaeger type is used at a distance of 13". With the far subjective in the phoropter, *minus* lenses are added until the child reports the least perceptible blur. The left eye is then occluded and, if the right eye is slightly blurred, no change is made; if badly blurred, the *minus* is reduced to slight blur. If clear, *minus* is added until it blurs. The right eye is then occluded and the same procedure is again followed. Two and one-half diopters is added to the resultant findings and record is made.

Tolerance of Minus Lens

With the *far* subjective in the phoropter, the reduced Snellen chart is presented at 16". The child is requested to read the 20/20 line or the smallest readable type. *Minus* lenses are added until the letters blur (or double) and the child can no longer read the letters.

Tolerance of Plus Lens

The same procedure as that for *Minus* Lens Tolerance is followed except that plus lenses are added until the letters blur (or double).

Donders Push-up

The test card with various-sized type is presented. The child is asked to read the smallest print he can see (.37 M, if possible). The left eye is occluded, and he is asked to watch the words; then the card is gradually moved toward the eye until the type blurs and becomes unreadable. The card is moved away until the letters become clear. The left eye is then tested, and then both eyes.

The *near* findings are taken through the *far* subjective. If the child is myopic, he is examined without lenses if glasses have not been worn, or through the correction he is wearing if it is less than the present subjective.

(Instrumentation: Copeland Streak Retinoscope, American Optical Co.; Junior Phoropter, American Optical Projector Chart, Trial Case Lenses.)

PROCEDURES

Skills

Introductory Slide (Dog and Pig, DB-10)*

This slide is presented to obtain orientation to the stereoscope. It does determine whether or not the two eyes are seeing simultaneously. The slide is presented at .00 on the instrument.

The child is asked, "What can you see?" If he names only the dog or the pig, he is asked, "Can you find another picture?" "What is the dog doing?" "Are the pig and dog both there now?"

*(DB slides from Betts Ready to Read Texts, Keystone View Co.)

Visual Resolution (DB 1,2,3)

With the slideholder at .00, the binocular slide (DB1) is presented first. The child is told that this is a game to see how many dots he can find. The examiner points to the first square, saying, "There is a black dot in one of the diamonds of each square. Tell me if it is at the top, center, bottom, the left or the right." These instructions are simplified for the younger ages; the substitute instructions for these ages are given in Chapter 12.

The monocular discrimination slides are presented next—the left and then the right. When the child fails on the monocular discrimination, one eye may be occluded and, when this is done, it is indicated on the record. If the child loses his place, the pointer is placed on the side without dots.

Stereopsis (DB 6)

The slide is placed at .00. The child is asked to look at the top row of forms. The examiner points above the forms and names each one. The child is asked, "Which one stands out nearest to you?" "Which one looks as though it were standing out from the others?" Then he is asked to tell which one comes out closer to him on the next row, and so on. He may lose his place or be unable to name, for instance, the diamond. The examiner places the pointer at the right of the row and names the forms in that row for him.

Pursuit Fixation

A small flashlight containing a blue filament bulb is used. The light is held about 8" before the child, and is moved first in a clockwise and then in a counterclockwise direction. It is then moved vertically, horizontally, and obliquely. This is done first binocularly, and then monocularly.

(Instrumentation: Keystone Tel-Eye Trainer, Flashlight.)

APPENDIX B
The Ontogenetic Gradients of Visual Behavior

This section assembles visual behavior patterns in systematic ontogenetic sequence. For convenience of reference and for concreteness, the illustrative behavior patterns are listed in tabular form and are classified in 17 progressive age groups, from 4 weeks to 10 years. It should be understood that the age assignments are approximate and suggestive. They represent average trends within a relatively homogeneous population and are, of course, subject to wide individual variations.

Individual variations, however, can be more readily identified and described with the aid of a frame of reference, which the gradients aim to supply. The order of the gradient sequence is less subject to individual variation because the sequence reflects a basic ground plan of maturation. This ground plan is envisaged in terms of growth trends for five distinguishable functional fields, namely:

1. Eye-hand coordination
2. Postural orientation
3. Fixation
4. Retinal reflex
5. Projection

These gradients are designed to indicate general sequences of development. The age assignments are approximate, and should not be used as rigid norms.

1. EYE-HAND COORDINATION

4 Weeks	Stares vacantly at surroundings
	Quiets when gazes toward light of window or bright moving object.
	Fixes object brought into visual scope.
	Eye and head movements not synchronized.
	Hands predominantly fisted.
	Hand clenches rattle placed in palm, but does not retain.
8 Weeks	Eyes more mobile, but range of movement still limiited.
	Direct regard and facial response to person's face.
	Eyes follow moving person and near object beyond midplane.
	Seeks light areas.
	Coordinate compensation eye movements well-estabished.
	Retains rattle briefly.
12 Weeks	Eyes follow dangling ring 180° with blinking or jerky eye movements.
	Holds rattle actively and glances at rattle in hand when it moves.
	Regards own hand spontaneously.
	Channelizes regard for person, light, or object.

	Demands focalized light.
16 Weeks	Eyes move in active inspection: regards own hand, toy, surroundings. Gives immediate regard for a suspended toy, and can retain a toy in hand with occasional regard. In sitting, holds head steady and set forward, looks down at table top, at own hand, at an object. Releases regard out on table or to a person in immediate vicinity. Fleetingly regards 7 mm. pellet on tabletop.
20 Weeks	Sober, intensified, and focalized regard of objects on table, with corralling arm movements. Grasps cube on contact. Maintains attention within area close to body. Tries to maintain fixation of object brought to mouth, and releases regard with uncontrolled eye movements, but can refixate. In supine, pursues dangling ring with good fixation for 180 °. Grasps ring when it is held near his hand.
24 Weeks	Regards object as he is bringing to mouth, and then releases regard and looks out into space. Pursues an object but may quickly release to regard another. Looks from handle of rattle to bowl. Quickly glances at person or object and rolls eyes easily to extreme right or left. Immediately regards a presented object, and reaches and grasps it. Discriminates between strangers.
28 Weeks	Makes direct approach on pellet, but hand comes within vicinity of pellet, and rakes. This activity results in contact. Varies activity according to size and amount of material. Manipulates objects, vigorously banging, shaking, transferring, and mouthing. Regards handle of cup and may approach it but not prehend it. Releases regard to surroundings, while he bangs or mouths a toy.
32 Weeks	Aware of surroundings, and is easily distracted; watches activity around him. Impatient in familiar situations, regardful and wary in new ones. Looks for toy he has had. Confronted with mirror, regards parts of his body; moves feet and hands and tongue—and regards them; but does not touch the mirror. Turns object about in hands to explore visually. Holds one cube and manipulates another.
36 Weeks	Prehends pellet with scissor grasp. Pushes one cube with another. Feeds self a cracker. Aware of pellet in bottle. Thrusts hand part way into cup.
40 Weeks	Pulls ring by string to appropriate distance for grasp. Also dangles the ring by the string. Enjoys watching the ball rolling around on table, the ring spinning

	on the table, and the pellet as it rolls from the bottle. Drops cube with clumsy or exaggerated release. Visually alert to tabletop and surroundings, taking in whole situation.
44 Weeks	Select regard for part, and then takes in whole; round hole to formboard, ring to string, one end of crayon to other, person's face to whole body. Lifts toys high and regards; leans trunk and arms way forward in extending toy. Smooth, easy visual pursuit of object presented to him. Probes holes and grooves, and points at pellet in bottle.
48 Weeks	Picks up cube and releases in vicinity of another. Plays serially with several toys. Transposes toys from tabletop to rail or platform. When looks forward, often squints lids or blinks; or, with head center, eyes position slightly to right or left. Sweeping regard for surroundings.
52 Weeks	Extends toys to another person, enjoying give-and-take game. Releases cube adaptively. Looks selectively from round block to round hold. Spontaneously bangs one cube on another, or places one next to another and, after demonstration, attempts to build a tower.
15 Months	Manipulates book and pats pictures—especially of baby or dog. Extremes of casting and withdrawal of hands without prehending. Frequently holds objects up near eyes or out at arm's length. Hits or brushes crayon on paper. Points to objects in surroundings, using "look" or "see."
18 Months	Quite persistently regards object being manipulated and, when regard is released, overreaches. Grasp envelops object and may displace it in act, then fingers overextend in release. Points, with vocalization "uh," for objects wanted. Looks selectively at pictures in book. Aware of location of certain objects. Propensity for vertical orientation: tower of 2-3, downward stroke, toy rolling down slide.
21 Months	Clings to objects, and often brings close to face to regard. Drops object in hand when spies another. Builds a tower of 5-6 cubes. Watches movement of others, and beginning to imitate.
2 Years	Eyes and hands less closely associated. Inspects object with eyes alone. Regards own movement during scribbling. Likes to watch movement of wheels, phonograph record, eggbeater. Beginning to screw toys, and turn doorknob. Likes small objects: pebbles, tiny cars, and so on. Horizontal orientation: spontaneous horizontal strokes; places cubes

	or cars in horizontal row.
2 1/2 Years	Regard intensifies. Temporarily loses control of arms or legs (27 months). When loses regard for object at hand, may lose so completely that can't find it again. Object in another child's hand may be seen without regard for child. Overgrasps and overreleases.
3 Years	Pretends to pick up object from page of book. Matches side of blocks to hole in formboard and adapts to reversal of board. Aware of process of performance and its completion: surveys finished product. Enjoys watching the performance of another child briefly. May "read" from pictures in a book.
3 1/2 Years	Hand tremor when fine coordination required. Projects movement onto inanimate object. Watches another child's performance. Aware of the parts of a whole. While watching, apt to hold some part of own body. Brings head close to page for identification of unfamiliar picture, or holds picture away and withdraws head. May identify D for daddy, M for mommy, J for Johnnie (own name), and S for Susan (sister).
4 Years	Free and variable eye-hand relationship. Moves or rolls eyes in expressive manner. Relationship of idea and execution ambiguous. Shifts ideas in process of performance. Drawings have few details, or detail most important is enlarged. Identifies several letters.
5 Years	Coordination has reached a new maturity. He approaches an object directly, prehends it precisely, and releases it with dispatch. Likes to color within lines, to cut and paste simple things, but is not adept. Makes an outline drawing, usually one on a page, and recognizes that it is "funny." Likes to copy simple forms. Paints at an easel or on the floor with large brushes and large sheets of paper. May enjoy making letters in this manner.
6 Years	In many of his performances he makes a good start but needs some assistance and direction to complete. He is now more deliberate and sometimes clumsy. Handles and attempts to utilize tools and material. Can print capital letters which he commonly reverses. Likes to write on the blackboard, as well as to use crayons and pencils.
7 Years	Manipulation of tools is somewhat more tense, but there is more persistence.

Pencils are tightly gripped and often held close to the point. Pressure is variable, but is apt to be heavy.
Can now print several sentences, with letters getting smaller toward the end of a line. There are individual differences in size of printing; some print very small and others continue to make large letters.

8 Years — Increase in speed and smoothness of eye-hand performance, and an easy release.
Likely to be a gap between what he wants to do with his hands and what he can do.
Writes or prints all letters and numbers accurately, with only an occasional reversal. Maintains fairly uniform alignment, slant, and spacing. Likes to do this neatly, but sometimes is in too much of a hurry.

9 Years — Individual variation in skills.
Handwriting is now a tool.
Beginning to sketch in drawing. Drawings are often detailed.
Interest in watching games played by others.

2. POSTURAL ORIENTATION

4-12 Weeks — Head predominantly rotated to a preferred side.
Lies predominantly in TNR attitude.

8 Weeks — Holds head bobbingly erect.
Lying supine, looks downward and sideward but not upward to follow retreating figure.

12 Weeks — Lying supine, tilts head backward and rolls eyes upward to follow retreating figure.

16-24 Weeks — Head rotates with increasing freedom in supine position.
Symmetrical postures predominant in supine position.
Hands engage in midline.

20 Weeks — Holds head erect in sitting.

24 Weeks — Makes a bilateral prehensory approach on object on test table.
Localizes source of sound when bell is rung at side.

28 Weeks — Alternation of prehension and manipulation, which may result in transfer.

32 Weeks — Strong bilateral use of hands in approach, grasp, and manipulation, and in simultaneous holding of two objects.

36 Weeks — Trend to unilaterality shown in approach.

40 Weeks — Increased facility in head and trunk movements.

44 Weeks — Unilateral manipulation, other hand remaining passive.
Increased mobility of eyes.
Creeps to doors of room and into another room if mother is there.

48 Weeks — Unilateral manipulation with increasing use of non-dominant hand.
Pivots freely while sitting.
Tips head way back in ocular pursuit.

52 Weeks — Grasps in one hand, transfers to other and manipulates. Combining use of both hands: holds cup with one, thrusts cube in with other.

	Combination of lateral and overhand approach. (At 56 weeks, overhand approach predominates.)
	Expresses sense of "down" and "up" by wriggling and gesture.
15 Months	Walks few steps with self-starting and self-stopping.
	Increased tendency to tilt head back and to circumduct arms upward and backward.
	Beginning to use word "up."
18 Months	Strong motor drive: walks fast, runs stiffly, repetitiously seats self on low step or low chair.
	Pushes toy or walks backward to pull toy.
	Unilateral, as well as bilateral, approach and manipulation.
	Regards object at 4-5 foot distance and goes directly to it.
21 Months	Climbs onto table or high stool.
	Becomes "frozen" during activity and stares into space.
	Pulls and leads person to point out object of interest.
2 Years	Manipulates unilaterally, but occasionally makes bilateral approach.
	Reaches with exaggerated trunk-twisting and bending.
2 1/2 Years	Vacillates with bipolar orientations in free play and in manipulation: push-pull, put in-take out, and so on.
	Pushes toy with good steering.
	Walks on board slightly elevated from the ground.
3 Years	Can play in one place and watch activity across the room.
	Confines painting to own paper.
	Can stand on one foot momentarily.
3 1/2 Years	Asymmetrical lateral posturing. Withdraws one side when attacked.
	Turns sidewise to adjust to narrow opening.
	Predominant right-handed manipulation shifts to left hand (or vice versa), or to alternation.
	Stumbles over nearby objects.
	Tolerates close contact with another, but also kicks or strikes out when interfered with.
	Shows preference for indoor or outdoor play.
4 Years	Spread of general posture; less totality in bodily orientations.
	Simultaneous spontaneous gestures, as well as simultaneous movement of fingers in manipulation.
	Frequently orients from the center to sides.
	Tends to combine cube-block structures in symmetrical form.
5 Years	Greater ease and control of general bodily activity, and economy of movement. Posture is predominantly symmetrical and closely knit.
	Control over large muscles is still more advanced than control over small ones.
	Plays in one location for longer periods, but changes posture from standing, sitting, squatting.
	Likes to activate a story. Runs, climbs onto and under chairs and tables.
6 Years	Very active; in almost constant motion. Activity is sometimes clumsy as he overdoes and falls in a tumble.

Body is in active balance as he swings, plays active games with singing, or skips to music.
He is often found wrestling, tumbling, crawling on all fours, and pawing at another child, and playing tag.
Large blocks and furniture are pushed and pulled around as he makes houses, and climbs on and in them.

7 Years — Shows more caution in many gross motor activities.
Activity is variable; he is sometimes very active, and at other times very inactive.
He repeats performances persistently. Has "runs" on certain activities, such as roller skating, jumping rope, "catch."
Likes to lie prone on floor while reading, doing puzzles, and so on.

8 Years — Bodily movement is more rhythmical and graceful.
Now aware of posture in himself and others. Likes to "follow the leader."
Stance and movement are free while painting.
Very dramatic in activities, with characteristic and descriptive gestures.

9 Years — Works and plays hard. Apt to do one thing until exhausted, such as riding bicycle, running, hiking, sliding, or playing ball.
Better control of own speed, but shows some timidity of speed of an automobile, or sliding, and of fast snow when skiing.
Frequently assumes awkward postures.
Great interest in team games, and in learning to perform skillfully.

3. FIXATION (Dangled Bell)

30 Weeks — (Illustrative Case)
Both eyes turn inward, and he fixates bell, then shifts regard upward to examiner's hand, or follows with pursuit up the string.
Quick shift of regard and release. Both eyes reposture to fixate bell with equal facility.
Release is restricted to the plane of regard and is in the upward direction toward the boundary of the target.
There may be preferential regard for the hand, which precedes fixation of the smaller, suspended target.
When both hands come in and accompany the eyes in approach, the visual performance is smoother.

52 WeekS — (Illustrative Case)
Fixates bell promptly; both eyes turn in and pursue the bell as it is brought toward the nose.
Spontaneously releases regard to examiner.
(Release is made quickly, with no observable deviations or differences in the two eyes.)

21 Months — Slow to fixate; looks through the bell at examiner.
Bell is jingled by examiner to help child localize. Regards bell, but fails to converge as it is moved in.

Maintains awareness of bell, and then looks at examiner.
When the bell is again moved in, child may maintain regard without releasing to refixate. Can look up toward examiner without changing posture. (However, one eye may turn in while the other, which remains directed outward, does not come in until child brings hand in to touch the bell.)
Hand helps to locate a plane of regard, and serves to change the posture of a lagging eye, but the hand itse if does not accurately locate the target.
Overreaching is common.

24 Months Picks up target with quick glance.
Follows target in. One eye jerky.
Spontaneously releases out beyond examiner.
The eye which was jerky turning in may be slower on release.
As the target moves into near, the head may withdraw.
On occasion, one eye may turn in only slightly, or may turn in excessively.
When the hand or hands come in, the bell is scooped, pulled in, or flipped.

30 Months May make an initial left-hand approach.
Intensifies fixation on bell.
Fights to maintain fixation. Both eyes hold and converge equally.
Release with some difficulty by shifting eyes to side and then to examiner.
If blink precedes release, there is an interval between blink and release.
On repetition, one eye may be slower than the other to release, or the hand assists in release.

36 Months Fixates easily, and may also bring hand to it.
Looks from bell to examiner's hand.
When asked to watch, he may turn head very slightly to side.
Both eyes turn in, but one moves slowly and the other jerkily.
Releases, step by step, in various ways (to side, head movement, then examiner).
The eye which moved in more jerkily is the slower to release.
When bell is in close, withdraws head or brings hand to it.
Releases and refixates when in close.
On repetition, both eyes may be smoother in converging and releasing.
When fixating and asked to touch with finger, is sometimes accurate and sometimes not.
Likes to have hand in to explore, though he can also inhibit.
When hand accompanies eyes as bell moves in, convergence is smoother.

42 Months Great individual differences.
Some hold fixation and slowly come in, withdraw head a little, and spontaneously and slowly release to examiner.
Others give quick glances at bell. In release, may make a slight or

upward adjustment before regarding examiner.
Hand response is variable. Can respond to "just look" or "just point."
The hand may assist in release or help steady fixation, but it does not change the act of converging.
Many like to take hold of bell with thumb and index or with whole hand grasp, or to touch it with index, and they often smile as they do. May also hit the bell away.
A child may refuse to touch; one may refuse to regard and cover eyes; one may protest, "Don't look at me."

48 Months
Fixates bell and follows in without resistance.
Both eyes are wobbly, and one is slower and staggers more (left in all our cases).
Release is not easy. The eye slower coming in is also slower to release. May overrelease.
Takes hold or touches with hand, and eyes may or may not accompany hand.
When maintains eyes with hand on bell, the eyes are steadier.

4. RETINAL REFLEX

30 Weeks
(Illustrative Case)
Far Estimate. Dull, then slow with motion, against, meridional difference, then oscillation from slow with to against.
No difference in the two eyes.
Near Estimate. Regards examiner: definite against.
Regards toy: increased against and brightening.
Hand approaches: with.
Grasps toy: brightening and against.
Manipulates toy: wide fluctuations of with to against.

52 Weeks
(Illustrative Case)
Far Estimate. Both bright, left brighter.
Intermediate Estimate. Changes from with to against.
Right slower motion.
Near Estimate. Changes from with to rapid against.
Pellet and bottle: against, against, with, against.
Reaching: against.
Object in mouth and regard for examiner: with.
Regards examiner: with.
Walking to examiner: with.

21 Months
Far Estimate. Difficult to initiate and sustain well-defined fixation on a far target.
Attention is somewhat elicited by movement of slides.
Identification of target is registered by facial brightening, without naming; by facial brightening with a smile; and by facial brightening, with naming.
Manifestations occur in both eyes simultaneously; or in the right without left; or left without the right; or in variable alternations.

Illustrative Sequence:
(a) Indifferent or ambiguous attention to a series of slides projected on and off screen. During this preliminary warming-up period, it is difficult to get a reflex; the reflex is dull or difficult to detect.
(b) Brief brightening with recognition of target (shoes).
(c) Occasional brightening, with slight against movement or slight with movement. (This occurs during a regardful phase, during which there is not definite release or manipulation. The fixation is diffuse, but not necessarily of low intensity.) Brightening changes from binocular to monocular, briefly.
Intermediate Estimate. The motion of the reflex is somewhat more perceptible.
Slight with and slight against motions again seen.
Near Measure—Illustrative Sequence:
(a) Maintains regard for lens or even grasps it. This produces an against motion.
(b) With difficulty, attention is directed to examiner's ear or nose. This produces with motion. On improved attention, there is less with motion.
(c) While regarding the object of interest (the lens), there is an increase of against motion when regard is more strongly sustained. No release registered as he shifts regard to examiner.
(d) A definite with motion when he touches the object.

24 Months Far Estimate. Both eyes dull.
Both eyes brighten equally.
Vary from dull to bright.
Occasionally one eye is slightly brighter.
Motion is seen briefly when reflex is bright and it is against.
Brightening occurs with verbalization or smile.
Intermediate Estimate. Divides attention between screen and examiner.
Variable individual response.
Better reflex in one eye.
Illustrative Sequence: Both with, right less with than left, then right against, then left against so both against.
Now meridional difference in right only.
Far Measure. One eye, +.25 D. Other eye, -.50 D.
Lens interference.
Near Measure. +.50 D to +1.00 D, with some difference between right and left, but less than on far measure.
Slight lens interference
Book. About -1.00 D to -2.00 D.
Difference between right and left.
Slow going into minus.
No difference when points or verbalizes.

30 Months Far Estimate. One eye bright, then both eyes bright.
Fast motion: either with or against, which does not vary.

Intermediate Estimate. Regard at far screen: One against, both against.
One eye brighter and motion easier to follow.
Regard at examiner: Both against, then left momentarily brighter, the right brighter, and both with.
Far Measure. One eye, +.25 D, other eye -.25 D. (Two children, high plus; four children, slight difference in meridians in one or both eyes.)
Near Measure. About +1.00 D., with no meridional differences (one child, high plus).
Book. -.75 D (searching); -1.50 D (pinned down) (one child -3.25 D with marked self-reference).
Hand and/or verbalization associated with increase in minus.

36 Months Far Estimate. Process of brightening to fading observable, and difference in reflex of the two eyes.
Motion not consistent or easy to follow.
Scissors motion.
One eye shows with or against, while no motion is seen in the other eye; then both are with or against.
Difference in pupils or in alignment at times.
Intermediate Estimate. Similar to far, except that difference in pupils and alignment not noted.
Far Measure. -.50 D to +.50 D, with trend toward more equality (two children, meridional difference; one child, marked inequivalence).
Near Measure. About +.75 D, with more equalization than at far. Also: (1) inequivalence, (2) higher plus, which reduces when pinned down.
Book. -2.00 D (searching), -1.50 D (pinned down).
Minus is not variable; it remains -2.00 D without fluctuation when searching, and remains -1.50 D when pinned down. Also: (1) lower amounts of minus, (2) difference in right and left eyes, (3) alternation of right and left eye.

42 Months Far Estimate. Change from dull to bright, and from with to against.
In process of change occasionally see against in vertical meridian.
One eye may be brighter and have a more definite reflex, while the other is also bright.
Can note the variability of movement in one eye, with other remaining more set.
More consistent with motion is observed.
In the two oldest children in this group (44 months), there was a rapid alternation of brightness from one eye to other.
Movement can now be observed when reflex is dull.
Intermediate Estimate. Same as at far.
Far Measure (Plano to +.75 D up).
Difference in two eyes (.50 D to .75 D).
Meridional difference or an extreme difference in two eyes.
Near Measure (+.50 D to +1.00 D).
More plus than at far but about same difference, with some tendency

toward equivalence.
When extreme difference on far measure, tend to be more equal but show difference in meridians.
Book. Individual differences from -.75 D to -3.00 D.
May show inequivalence when not evident in other measures, and vice versa.
Meridional differences not consistent with other measures.

48 Months Far Estimate. Changing and variable response (bright, dull, with, against, neutral and difference in meridians).
One eye shows a brighter and more definite response.
One eye may show more variability than the other.
There is more with motion than any other type.
Intermediate Estimate. Similar to far, except that the variability is less and changes occur more slowly.
The variability is reduced when regard is at the examiner.
Far Measure. Low plus.
Difference between eyes is slight. A few show slight difference in meridians.
Near Measure. +.50 D to +1.00 D both eyes.
Difference in meridians may not occur.
Book. Good flexibility. About -1.00 D to -1.75 D.
Naming and pointing have variable effect. Two children show difference in right and left. Meridional difference reduces or disappears.

5. PROJECTION

21 Months Has difficulty in adjusting to the stereoscope. Holds hands at sides of lens well.
Looks in and regards target; may even identify picture.
When asked to touch the picture, he moves hand forward in the sagittal plane, at the side of the lens well.

24 Months Stands, peers in, and regards picture.
When asked to touch the picture, he moves arms simultaneously; then one hand goes to surface.
Right, left, or both hands go out to surface, whether picture is before right or left eye.
Slaps at picture.
Looks over top of lens well for picture.
Recognizes it is away from him—somewhere in space.

30 Months Initially responds with hand opposite to side of the picture.
Points into lens, or at side of lens well.
When hand is postured in midspace by examiner, child follows through down to surface.
Pushes at surface with full hand or manipulates target.
Retrial, again points at lens. But, with posturing clue, gets out on surface and uses index finger to point.
If differentiations of parts of picture are requested, becomes con-

fused—"Where is it?"
After initial response, uses either hand, regardless of side picture is on.

36 Months Either hand responds to the picture which is before either eye, but he is more apt to point at side where picture is.
Points at lens—"She's right there." "She's inside, over there."
When hand moves out from lens well, goes to outside of lens, then midspace, then to surface. Then backs up to outside lens, or he may withdraw head to look around outside.
If allowed to see picture, reports "two doggies" (one in lens well, one on surface).
Touching on side of picture is accurate. When projecting, places hand in vicinity in searching manner, or reaches underneath instrument, or crosses over to the picture (right to left, or left to right).

42 Months With right or left hand, persistently locates on inside or outside of lens, but usually gets to midspace and then may go to surface (an area, not good localization).
At midspace, hand goes in close to septum and may cross over to other side.
May place hand clear out to top of board, or way down under board.
Many children have a clearer response
when projecting from left to right.
Some typical remarks are:
"Can't touch, it's way over."
"In here" (lens). Examiner: "Can you touch it?" "I can't."
"Way down there—How can we get in it? We can't."
"Open up the drawer."

48 Months After identifying the picture, he locates it by pointing to center of lens well, near either right or left lens.
If he gets beyond the lens, it is to the far side of the lens or near the midseptum.
If he then gets down to surface, he locates in toward center.
When his finger is positioned in midarea, he approaches surface unsteadily, but contacts it and can point to parts of the picture.
Projection in one direction is more sure than in the other.

APPENDIX C
Selected References

Ames LB. Early individual differences in visual and motor behavior patterns: a comparative study of two normal infants by the method of cinemanalysis. J Genet Psychol, 1944; 65: 219-226.

Ames LB. The development of the sense of time in the young child. J Genet Psychol, 1946; 68: 97-125.

Ames LB. The Gesell incomplete man test as a differential indicator of average and superior behavior in preschool children. J Genet Psychol, 1943; 62: 217-274.

Ames LB, Ilg FL. Variant behavior as revealed by the Gesell developmental examination. J Genet Psychol, 1943; 63: 273-305.

Ames LB, Learned J. Imaginary companions and related phenomena. J Genet Psychol, 1946; 69: 147-167.

Ames LB, Learned J. The development of verbalized space in the young child. J Genet Psychol, 1948; 72: 63-84.

Bartley SH. Vision, a study of its basis. New York: D. Van Nostrand, 1941: xv + 350.

Bartley SH, Chute E. Fatigue and impairment in man. New York: McGraw-Hill, 1947: ix + 429.

Bender IE, Imus HA, Rothney JWM. Motivation and visual factors: individual studies of college students. Hanover, NH: Dartmouth College Publications, 1942.

Berner GE & DE. Reading difficulties in children. Arch Ophthal, Chicago, 1938: 20: 829-838.

Bielschowsky A. Lectures on motor anomalies. Hanover, NH: Dartmouth College Publications, 1940: 1-128.

Brock FW. Space perception in its normal and abnormal aspects. Optom Wkly, 1946; Aug 29 & Sept 5. 8 pp.

Carmichael L, Dearborn WF. Reading and visual fatigue. Boston: Houghton Mifflin, 1947: v + 483.

Castner BM. Handedness and eyedness of children referred to a guidance clinic. Psychol Rec, 1939; 8: 99-112.

Castner BM. Prediction of reading disability prior to first grade entrance. Am J Orthopsych, 1935; 4: 375-387.

Chavasse FB. Worth's squint or the binocular reflexes and the treatment of strabismus, 7th ed. Philadelphia: Blakiston, 1939: 1-688.

Dusser de Barenne JG. The labyrinthine and postural mechanisms. In: Murchison (ed.). Handbook of general experimental psychology. Worcester: Clark University Press, 1934: 204-246.

Ewalt HW. The Baltimore myopia control project. J Am Optom Assoc, 1946; 6: 167-185.

Franklin I. Fusion, projection and stereopsis. Am J Ophthal, 1942; 11: 1316-1336. Fulton JR. A trip to Bohol in quest of Tarsius. Yale J Biol Med, 1939; 11: 561-573.

Fulton JR. Physiology of the nervous system, 2nd ed. London: Oxford University Press, 1943: ix + 614.

Gesell A. The ontogenesis of infant behavior. In: Charmichael (Ed.) Manual of child psychology. New York: John Wiley, 1946: 295—331.

Gesell A. The tonic-neck reflex in the human infant: its morphogenetic and clinical significance. J Pediatrics, 1938; 13: 455-464.

Gesell A, et al. The first five years of life: a guide to the study of the preschool child. New York: Harper, 1940: xiii + 393.

Gesell A, Amatruda CS. Developmental diagnosis. Normal and abnormal child development. Clinical methods and pediatric applications, 2nd ed. New York: Hoeber, 1947: xvi + 496.

Gesell A, Ames LB. The development of directionality in drawing. J Genet Psychol, 1946; 68: 45-61.

Gesell A, Ames LB. The development of handedness. J Genet Psychol, 1947; 70: 141-154.

Gessel A, Ames LB. The infant's reaction to his mirror image. J Genet Psychol, 1947; 70: 141-154.

Gesell A, Blake EM. Twinning and ocular pathology. With a report of bilateral macular coloboma in monozygotic twins. Arch Ophthal, 1936; 15: 1050-1071.

Gesell A, Ilg FL (In collaboration with Ames LB, Bullis GE). The child from 5 to 10. New York: Harper, 1946: v + 465.

Gesell A, Ilg FL (In collaboration with Ames LB, Learned J). Infant and child in the culture of today. New York: Harper, 1943: v + 399.

Gesell A, Zimmerman HM. Correlations of behavior and neuropathology in a case of cerebral palsy from birth injury. Am J Psychiat, 1937; 94: 505-536.

Halstead WC. Brain and intelligence. A quantitative study of the frontal lobes. Chicago: University of Chicago Press, 1947: v + 206.

Harmon DB. How seeing involves the whole body. Architect Record, 1946; 99: 79-80.

Heuser CH. A presomite human embryo with a definite chorda canal. Contrib Embryol, 1932; 23: 134-138.

Hooker D. A preliminary atlas of early human fetal activity. Privately published, 1939: 1-95.

Hooker D. Early fetal activity in mammals. Yale J Biol Med, 1936; 8: 579-602.

Hooker D. Reflex activities in the human fetus. (In: Barker, Kounin, Wright, eds.) Child behavior and development. New York: McGraw-Hill, 1943: v + 652.

Kleitmann N. Sleep and wakefulness as alternating phases in the cycle of existence. Chicago: University of Chicago Press, 1939: xii + 638.

Kohler W, Wallach H. Figural after-effects. An investigation of visual processes. Proc Am Philos Soc, 1944-45; 88: 269-357.

Ling, BC. A genetic study of sustained visual fixation and associated behavior in the human infant, from birth to 6 months. J Genet Psychol, 1942; 61: 227-277.

Magnus R. Korperstellung. Berlin: Springer, 1924: xiii + 740. Magnus R. Animal posture. (Croonian lecture) Proc Royal Soc, 1925; 98: 339-353.

McCulloch WS. How we see shape. (Author's mimeograph.) Dept. Psychiatry, Univ of Illinois College of Medicine, Illinois Neuropsychiatric Institute, Chicago: 5 pp.

McCulloch WS. A recapitulation of the theory, with a forecast of several extensions. Annals of NY Acad Sciences Conference on Teleological Mechanisms, Vol. 50, Art 4: 259-277.

Meyer E. Comprehension of spatial relations in preschool children. J Genet Psychol, 1940; 57: 119-151.

Meyer E. Ordnene und Ordnung bei drei-bis Sechsjaehrigen Kindern.N Psychol Stud, 1934; 10: 3.

Minkowski M. Neurobiologische studien am menschlichen foetus. Abderhaldens Handbuch d. biologischen arbeitsmethoden, 1928; Lief, 253, S: 511-618.

Pitts W, McCulloch WS. How we know universals. The perception of auditory and visual forms. Bull Mathematical Biophysics, 1947; 9: 127-147.
Polyak SL. The retina. Chicago: University of Chicago Press, 1941: x + 607.
Renshaw S. Psychological optics. Optom Extension Prog, Oct 1939-Sept 1945.
Selzer CA. Lateral dominance and visual fusion. Their application to difficulties in reading, writing, spelling and speech. Harvard Monographs in Education. Cambridge: Harvard University Press, 1933: 1-119.
Thompson DW. On growth and form. Cambridge: University Press, 1942: 1116.
Walls GL. The vertebrate eye and its adaptive radiation. Michigan: Cranbook Institute of Science, 1942; 19: 111-785.
Woods AC. Report from the Wilmer Institute on the results obtained in the treatment of myopia by visual training. Trans Am Acad Ophthal, 1945: 37-65.

INDEX